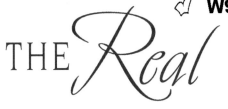

THE *Real*
SKINNY ON WEIGHT LOSS SURGERY

*An Indispensable Guide
to What You Can REALLY Expect!*

2ND EDITION

Written For Real People, By Real People!!

Julie M. Janeway, BBA, MSA, JD, ABD/PhD
Karen J. Sparks, BBA, MBEd
Randal S. Baker, MD, FACS
with
Carrie A. Liebrock, RD
Scott H. Glass, MS, MA, LLP
Nabila Ahmed-Sarwar, PharmD, BCPS, CDE

Prologue by
Cynthia K. Buffington, PhD

Foreword by
Judith Brown Clarke
Olympic Medalist, World Record Holder
Sports Illustrated® Sportswoman of the Year

Illustrations by
Liz Rehfuss

Little Victories Press™

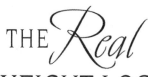

THE *Real* SKINNY ON WEIGHT LOSS SURGERY

An Indispensable Guide to What You Can REALLY Expect!

2ND EDITION

ISBN Print Ed. 978-0-9767672-2-0
Library of Congress Control Number   2005924894

Cover Design:
Robert Aulicino, Pro Art Graphics
www.aulicinodesign.com
Suzette Perry, Infinity Graphics
Okemos, Michigan
www.mycoverdesign.com

Printer:
Data Reproductions, Inc.
Auburn Hills, Michigan
www.datareproductions.com

Authors' Promotional Photos:
Tom Nakielski, Lights On Studio
Lansing, Michigan
www.lightsonstudio.com
and
Robert Neumann, Big Event Studios
Grand Rapids, Michigan
www.bigeventstudios.com

Promotional Photo Hair and
Make-up Design:
Saul Rodrigues & Danielle Ruehle
Steven L. Marvin Salon
and Wellness Spa
(An Aveda® Salon)
Holt, Michigan
www.stevenlmarvin.com

Illustrations & Graphics:
Liz Rehfuss
Lansing, Michigan

Book Layout & Interior Design:
Infinity Graphics
Okemos, Michigan
www.infinitygraphics.com

Published by:
Little Victories Press™
4371 Kinneville Road, Suite 200
Onondaga, MI 49264

— R E V I E W S —
&
R E A D E R C O M M E N T S

I just wanted to let you know that I just finished the book and loved it!! I agree with your philosophies and am thankful there are people out there like you. You had the courage not only to change your lives, but to step up to the plate and help others. Thank you.

Angie, Illinois – Registered Dietitian

If you have ever even once considered having weight loss surgery you must read this book!

Women's Lifestyle Magazine

The REAL Skinny on Weight Loss is well-written, informative, and at the same time, humorous and entertaining. The book is thorough and quite descriptive and is likely to encourage those who are ready to do whatever it takes to have a second chance at health and well-being to seek weight loss surgery, while discouraging those individuals hoping to find a "miracle procedure" that can fix their size and problems without personal effort.

Obesity Surgery
Medical Journal

I've been a bariatric nurse for five years and I've seen literally hundreds of patients go through our practice, and I learned so much from reading this book. I guess you never really know until you've walked in those shoes. All the people who work in bariatric medicine should read this book, even the surgeons!

Amy, Michigan – Bariatric Nurse

Wonderful Book!!!! I really enjoyed it and wish it had been available to me when I was thinking and then had surgery in 2004. I picked up the book because now I facilitate two bariatric support groups, and wanted to give it a read to see if it might be something I would recommend to group members. I definitely will!!

Cheryl, Indiana – Patient and Support Group Leader

I needed to learn more about possibly having weight loss surgery. I guess the best thing I learned from your book was that the place I was considering going to for my surgery was not a multi-disciplinary center. I've found a new doctor with a good team and a good program. Thanks for giving me that knowledge. You might have just saved my life.

Larry, Arizona – Prospective Patient

They relate the joys and sorrows of taking this step. They tell potential patients how to use their "tool" to make this weight-loss effort permanent. I especially liked the chapters called "Auto-Eject," which dealt with what can happen if a patient eats something that doesn't agree with the pouch, and "The Protein Safari," about how important protein is in post-op. Both were touched with a good deal of humor.

Grand Rapids Press

Hi. I just started reading your book. It is AWESOME! You guys have a great sense of humor and the book is very well written. You've done a wonderful service for us bariatric patients. Thanks!

Connie, Wisconsin – Patient and Support Group Leader

The book sets the record straight and tells the truth without all the Hollywood hype. There's no sugar-coating here, but it's funny and easy to read. It's like being with old friends.

Hillsdale News

My surgery isn't scheduled yet, but I've already read the book and I feel prepared, and I'm going back to read the book again. I already have thin hair, and the hair loss chapter (Build Your Own Cat Kit) really opened my eyes and impressed on me how important the protein is. I'd never heard of that before, but if it happens to me I'll know why, how to fix it, and be prepared to handle it. I love this book, and I've bought one for my mom and my sister so they can't say they weren't warned! I wasn't giving up my copy!

Sheryl, Michigan – Patient in Waiting

I've been working in bariatrics for a couple of years now, and this book has really helped me to understand what patients go through. I thought the book was so good, I actually purchased a copy for the surgeons in my practice out of my own money!

Lisa, Ohio – Bariatric Practice Manager

I was all set to go to a surgeon and have surgery to help me lose weight. I've struggled all my life with my weight. I thought surgery might finally be the answer. Then I read your book. I've discovered it's just too scary to me. Colour me a fraidy cat, but I just don't think I can do it! I will, however, go back to Weight Watchers® or possibly pursue something through my doctor's office and I will keep fighting to get my weight down. I'm grateful that I found out ahead of time what I would have been getting myself into. It isn't the choice for me, but I am inspired to keep fighting.

Marilynn, Ontario – Ex-Prospective Patient

As soon as I saw this book at the doctor's office I just knew it was going to really get down to brass tacks and tell me what I needed to know. I liked the witty title and it was just as witty inside. This book helped me to understand what my daughter was going to undertake when she made the decision to have surgery. It also gave me something to think about for myself. Thanks for the REAL skinny on a subject the media has seriously messed with. Now I know the truth and so does my daughter.

Al, New York – Father of Patient

Check out more reader reviews
at barnesandnoble.com and amazon.com!

⟝ DEDICATION ⟞

This book is dedicated to all those REAL people out there who are tired of dealing with their serious weight issues, and want to improve their health and quality of life. This book is for every person who has battled the scale and lost, missed far too many experiences and opportunities because of their weight, and for those whose precious lives are being shortened every minute because of health problems associated with their weight. This book is for all of you who are overweight and afraid.

For you, we offer a look at an alternative. It's not a cure, and it's not for everyone. We offer you the opportunity to investigate, to learn, and to see what real people who've had weight loss surgery go through. We offer you a choice, and maybe a chance at better health and a better life. At the very least we offer you information, and hope that there is something out there that will help you help yourself.

If you are choosing to read this book, we applaud you for your courage in continuing the fight to live life on your own terms. You deserve to get the most out of every minute life has to offer. You deserve to make the choices concerning what you do and don't experience, not have them made for you based on your size and weight. You are beautiful, you are not alone, and you are worth whatever it takes to be happy and healthy in your own body. It is for you, all our kindred spirits in the world, that we dedicate this labor of love.

— ACKNOWLEDEMENTS —

On behalf of Little Victories Press™ (LVP), Karen and I would like to extend our tremendous gratitude to the following people and businesses for their amazing support, assistance, trust, and belief in LVP and this project. Without you this book would not have come into existence, and the entire "REAL Skinny" series of books regarding weight loss surgery would not have been conceived. You are all permanently part of the Little Victories™ family, and to each of us personally, you will always be family as well: Dr. Randal Baker who made all this possible, the staff at Michigan Weight loss Specialists, who helped Dr. B., Judi Brown Clarke who is such a wonderful person and tremendous grounding force, Carrie Liebrock who reminds us to love animals and love ourselves, Scott Glass, who reminds us that with faith all things are possible, Dawn Baker for reading until she was blind, being patient, supportive and kind, and Dr. Baker's family who gave up so much time with him to allow him to be such an integral part of this endeavor, Robert Aulicino and Suzette Perry who did such a tremendous job on the cover design, and our dear friends Eugenie "Coco" Cook and Judy Burgess who never doubted for a second.

We never would have finished without the help of Kim Colton from Data Reproductions (you're a goddess), the staff at Data Reproductions (best printers on the planet), Suzette and Brian Perry at Infinity Graphics, and Liz Rehfuss (world's best "save the day" graphic artists), Dr. Nabila Ahmed-Sarwar (Pharmacy Diva and all-around loving and caring individual), Dr. Cynthia Buffington (amazingly brilliant and dedicated researcher, cherished friend, and mom to Bella and Sam), Gene Lyman, Martha Bannett, and Rod Egger (life-long friends, compatriots, and respected visionaries at Bariatrix Nutrition), Vic Giaconia (colleague, friend, and industry innovator at Building Blocks® Bariatric Vitamins), Debbie Daley, and Karl Harrison (supportive, encouraging, and amazing friends and colleagues at BariMD), and Dr. Steven Hendrick, our buddy, our colleague, and an all-around wonderful surgeon and friend. We'd also like to thank Jerry and Clarice Baker, Tom Nakielski of Lights On Studio, Robert Neumann, Steven L. Marvin, Saul Rodrigues, Danielle Ruehle, Dr. Sally Cannon, Dr. Louis Cannon, Sue and Charlie Hilton, Theresa Martone, Kimberly Stump, Gail Sobecki, Tonnie Drake, Brad Sweda, Barb Ford, Karen Kay, Dave Westcot, and all the men who participated in the research for Chapter Ten. You have all been great, and we thank you for the contributions each of you made individually to this undertaking.

We would each like to make some personal acknowledgements as well.

JULIE

Mine will be the longest as I have a tremendous number of people to thank. Without most of them I wouldn't even be alive to write this book. I love you all. First I'd like to thank my husband Matt who amazingly didn't kick me to the curb during this grueling process, or during the writing and research for the second edition.

Thanks for your support, belief in me, and for loving me fat, loving me thinner, and loving me at all. Secondly, to my mom who never waivered in her belief in me, this surgery, or this book: thanks for taking care of me, and for your proofreading and copyediting. Great job mom. To my sister Cheryl for her wise words. Thanks for the motivation. Luv ya. To my dad: thanks for really getting behind this one dad, and thanks for all those long nights in the hospital. To my niece Meggie: thanks for being such a loving kid, and for inventing funny words. To my niece Haleigh and my nephew Devin: you guys are awesome and I am so grateful for your love and belief in me. To my brother-in-law Darius: thanks for not shooting me down on this one. I appreciate that very much.

I would especially like to thank the following people because they took a mangled, barely alive woman and put her back together. You have indeed rebuilt me: better, stronger, faster. I am the 6 million dollar woman, and now I'm using my abilities to make the world a better place! Life-long gratitude goes out to: Dr. John Stubbart, Dr. John Iaccobucci, Dr. Margie White, Mickey Loomis, Dr. Edmond Ducommun, Craig Mefford, Dr. Edward Cook, Dr. Ann Hakkila, Dr. Randal Palmitier, Dr. Roy Meland, Dr. Charles Bill, Dr. Doug Leppink, Tammy Westfall, Sister Gates, the therapists and staff at Sparrow Rehabilitation, the nurses and medical staff at Spectrum Hospital, and everyone else who helped put Humpty Dumpty back together again! And last, but never least, I would like to thank the good Lord for keeping me on this planet, for giving me what I needed when I needed it, and for bringing me out of the dark to see what I was meant to do.

To Karen: Well, you know… and I know you get it. 'Nuff said. Get some sleep.

KAREN

Where to begin.…

It is difficult at best to express in words the feelings of gratitude and love to those who most influence your life. I have known since I was a very little girl that my station in this life was to assist others in their journey. Some individuals I have known for many years and others I met for only a moment in time to somehow impact their lives. Friends and family alike, to all these individuals I owe thanks as the impact they made on my life has helped to shape me into the person I am today, and provided me with what I needed to write this book.

To my parents, Everett and Barbara Sparks, who have always told me no matter what I was pursuing (and they will tell you I have pursued many things), "you can do anything you set your mind to." I love you so very much. Thank you for your love and unwavering support in my need to do the "next" thing. And despite my current successes, you know there will always still be something "new" for me to learn and do.

To my husband Bill: Thanks for "waiting" and supporting me through all those long nights. I love you.

To Julie, there are people you meet in your life who become friends and acquaintances and they enter and exit as time passes for whatever reason. Then there are those special people God puts in your life who just "know you." I believe God saved and healed you from your accident to save and heal me. Thank you for just being you. We did it my friend, we actually did it. Now...I wish you only "good" dreams...go to sleep, we have so very much more to do. God's not done with us yet.

DR. BAKER

I would first of all like to thank my wife Dawn for supporting me through the writing of this book, and life in general. A special thanks to Courtney, Arielle, Jordan, Olivia, Seth, Tessa, Caleb, Isaac, and Titus for allowing their dad to have some time to write and review chapters, even while on vacation!

I would also like to acknowledge Julie and Karen for having the vision and gumption to see this book through to completion. I have never seen any two people work so hard in such an organized way to get the facts about obesity and obesity surgery out to the lay public. Their zeal is truly motivational.

I would like to thank my partners Drs. James Foote and Paul Kemmeter for their support and esteemed character. It is a rare thing indeed to have such highly competent and truly caring surgeons as partners. Thanks also go out to our entire office staff who work tirelessly and care deeply about the welfare of the patients with whom they come in contact. Keep up the good work!

Finally, I would like to thank the Lord for His grace and for giving me such an awesome wife and family, and for allowing me to work with such wonderful people!

TABLE OF CONTENTS

ACKNOWLEDGEMENTS   vii

PROLOGUE — Obesity: A Progressive Disease   xv
By Cynthia K. Buffington, PhD

FOREWORD   xxi
By Judith Brown Clarke

INTRODUCTION   1

1   REALITY SLAP!!   5
Julie M. Janeway
Karen J. Sparks

2   EN-LIGHTENMENT   13
Julie M. Janeway
Karen J. Sparks

3   THE NEW AND IMPROVED, AMAZING,   29
ALL NATURAL LEMON DIET
Randal S. Baker MD, FACS

   Surgical Weight Loss Treatment Methods   36

   Common Potential Surgical Complications   47

   Effect of Bariatric Surgery on Co-Morbid Conditions   52

   What to Look for in a Surgical Practice   53

   Vitamin Supplementation   55

   Preventing and Dealing with Weight Regain   57

   The Effectiveness of Weight Loss Surgery   60

4   SCRAMPS, AND STRICTURE,   63
AND HICCUPS, OH MY!!
Julie M. Janeway
Karen J. Sparks

       POTENTIAL COMPLICATIONS   64

       POTENTIAL AFTER-EFFECTS   69

5   AUTO EJECT   83
Julie M. Janeway
Karen J. Sparks

6   THE "BUILD-YOUR-OWN CAT" KIT   87
Karen J. Sparks
Julie M. Janeway

7   THE SHADOWS OF MY FORMER SELF   95
Scott H. Glass, MS, MA, LLP

8   LITTLE VICTORIES   113
Karen J. Sparks
Julie M. Janeway

9   SEPARATION ANXIETY   125
Julie M. Janeway
Karen J. Sparks

PHOTO GALLERY   143

10   NO GIRLS ALLOWED!   151
Randal S. Baker MD, FACS
Julie M. Janeway
Karen J. Sparks

11   FENG SHUI FOR THE BODY AND MIND   163
Carrie A. Liebrock, RD
Scott H. Glass, MS, MA, LLP

Micronutrients   165

Macronutrients   167

    Carbohydrates   167

    Fat   169

    Water   170

    Protein   171

Functional Living Environment   175

    Movement   175

12   MEDICATION MISADVENTURES: 181
HOW TO AVOID THEM!
Nabila Ahmed-Sarwar, PharmD, BCPS, CDE

Medication Absorption Basics   182

How to Get the Right Medication for You   184

Protect Your Pouch   186

NSAID and Medication Tips Chart   188

Medication Separation Anxiety   191

How to Become Your Own Best Advocate   192

Wrap Up   193

13   THE PROTEIN SAFARI   195
         Julie M. Janeway
         Karen J. Sparks

14   THE JUNK DRAWER   203
         Julie M. Janeway
         Karen J. Sparks

         Hidden Costs Related to Weight Loss   203
         Pre-Op Emotional Issues   211
         Surgical and Physical Issues   214
         Julie and Karen's Personal Theories About Stuff   215

15   SHRINK! SHRANK! SHRUNK!   219
         Randal S. Baker MD, FACS
         Julie M. Janeway
         Karen J. Sparks

16   THE FINAL BATTLE: 227
         DEFEAT OF THE CLONES
         Randal S. Baker MD, FACS

17   ADDITIONAL RESOURCES   237

18   GLOSSARY OF TERMS   265

19   REFERENCE CITATIONS   277

⟿ PROLOGUE ⟿

Obesity: A Progressive Disease

Cynthia K. Buffington, PhD

Florida Hospital – Celebration Health Bariatric Center

How many times in your life have you gone on a diet? One?... Two?... Three?... Twenty-three times?!? My father used to tell his friends that I was his "million dollar baby" because that is the amount of money I had spent in my life on different diets and weight loss programs. In reality, the cost-to-date of my many failed attempts at long-term weight loss falls short of seven figures, but there is little doubt that I have spent a considerable amount of money on diets and weight loss programs, packaged foods, meal replacements, gymnasium memberships, anti-obesity drugs, and dozens of weight loss gimmicks, including a "torture" device that used electric shock to assist with satiety (feeling full).

In my earlier years, most of the weight management programs and devices that I used, even the electric shock, produced significant weight loss, at least temporarily. With time, however, weight regain always occurred, and with a vengeance. Not only would I recover all of my initial weight loss, but considerably more. Each time I went through one of these weight loss episodes, fewer and fewer calories were required for weight regain. Can you identify??

My frustration with long-term weight loss failure has more recently been replaced by my frustration with failed short-term weight loss attempts. It seems as though the larger and older I become, the more difficult losing weight is, and the easier it is to gain even more weight. Although I am not morbidly obese, there are still times I feel trapped in my body, not to mention frightened at the outcome all of this is having on my health. I feel as though I am rapidly approaching that dreaded number on the scales from which there may be no return. Can you relate?? So, how did we get into this situation?

Well, first of all, we have numerous so-called "survival" genes that once enabled our forefathers to store large amounts of fuel as fat when food was plentiful and to conserve calories when food was scarce. If an individual did not have these genes, they did not survive the "fast'" and their genes were not passed along to the next generation. So, we are undoubtedly the most metabolically efficient human beings that have ever been on earth, but we no longer "feast and fast." Instead, we tend to "feast and feast." Furthermore, in order to acquire food for our daily feast, we do not have to hunt or gather our food. In fact, for many of us, the only calories expended in acquiring a meal is the effort it may take to unroll the window of the car at the drive-thru of our favorite fast-food restaurant.

Additionally, technology has played a significant role in the alarming rise in obesity prevalence over the last several decades. Most of us have sedentary jobs, and then, we come home to spend the remainder of our evening in front of the television. In the U.S., children and adults spend four or more hours per day watching television and this does not include leisure time spent at the computer or playing video games, etc. All of this leads to more calories taken in than burned off through movement and activity, which contributes to fat storage and becoming overweight. If left unchecked, overweight graduates to moderate obesity, and then, on to severe and morbid obesity.

To make matters worse, the food industry has changed the types of foods that we eat, causing a substantial increase in our consumption of fat-promoting foods, *i.e.,* those high in fat, sugar, and processed grains. We have reduced our intake of the so-called "anti-obesity foods," or those foods that reduce our risk for fat accumulation. "Anti-obesity foods" include those high in fiber (beans, fruits, vegetables, nuts, whole grains), dairy foods, quality protein, and foods that provide an appropriate and adequate ratio of Omega-6 to Omega-3 essential fatty acids.

Once an individual gains weight, further weight gain becomes easier and weight loss and long-term maintenance become more and more difficult. Why is this? Science is finding that obesity is progressive, and once an individual becomes obese, fat accumulation and further weight gain is not just a matter of an imbalance between calories in and out. In fact, many obese individuals, even those with morbid obesity, are not eating all that many more calories than their leaner counterparts, yet they continue to put on weight. Actually, obesity is associated with conditions that cause more of the calories consumed from both fat and carbohydrates to be stored as fat. I used to jokingly say that everything I eat turns into fat. Actually, that statement may not be so far from the truth.

With weight gain and obesity there are a number of hormonal, metabolic, and molecular changes that increase the body's ability to accumulate fat. Such changes promote fat uptake and storage in adipose (fat) tissue and reduce the breakdown of fat even at times when the body needs fat for fuel like during exercise, in between meals, or when under stress.

Certain of the same factors that increase fat storage also increase the body's capacity to convert sugar from carbohydrate-containing foods into fat, increasing fat availability to and within adipose tissue, and contributing to fat accumulation in tissues such as muscle. An accumulation of fat in muscle occurs in association with the body's resistance to insulin uptake, and this condition reduces the utilization of sugar by muscle, making more of it available for conversion into fat.

In addition to an increased capacity for fat storage and production, obesity, and in particular, severe obesity is associated with a reduction in the body's capacity to oxidize (burn) fat, resulting primarily from a decrease in fat burning in muscle tissue. Fat is the major source of fuel used by the body for energy needs at rest or during daily activity. Most fat oxidation occurs in muscle. Therefore, any condition that reduces the oxidation of fat by muscle increases the availability of it for storage, and in this way, contributes significantly to obesity progression.

Overall then, obesity increases our body's capacity to make and store fat while reducing its ability to utilize (oxidize) fat, thus allowing for more of the calories we consume to be stored as fat. Furthermore, the changes in fat metabolism occurring with obesity not only substantially increase our risk for further weight gain, but also become more pronounced with severe obesity, creating a vicious cycle whereby obesity "begets" obesity, or "being fat makes us fatter." This is one of the reasons that it becomes more difficult to lose weight as the severity of the disease progresses.

There are a number of other conditions that occur in association with obesity that create obesity "begetting" cycles. Let's look, for instance, at emotional distress as both a cause for, and an effect of weight gain. Psychological distress, such as may occur in response to societal discrimination against obesity, activates one of the body's major stress response pathways, the *hypothalamic-pituitary-adrenal axis*. Activation of this pathway results in an increase in certain hormones, as well as changes in specific brain messengers that promote fat accumulation, stimulate appetite and food cravings, and reduce satiety or feelings of fullness. In these ways psychological distress causes weight gain and weight gain, in turn, causes psychological distress that causes even greater weight gain and psychological distress and….get the picture? Obesity "begets" obesity.

In addition to psychological stress, there are a number of obesity-induced conditions that affect appetite. There are various digestive or gut hormones and gut factors, neurochemicals (brain messengers), metabolites, hormones, and even specific products of fat tissue that regulate appetite, food selection, and satiety. Obesity causes changes in many of these appetite regulators (or their actions) in such a manner as to promote further weight gain, creating yet another obesity "begets" obesity cycle.

Are you starting to become rather overwhelmed by all of these obesity-promoting conditions that occur with weight gain? Well, there are many more, including hormone changes that lead to an increase in fat cell size and numbers, causing further weight gain which, in turn, worsens these hormone defects, etc. Adipose tissue also generates products that may have a regulatory effect on appetite, energy expenditure, and fat metabolism. Obesity causes changes in the production or actions of these adipose tissue products that result in increased fat production and storage and decreased fat utilization, causing even greater weight gain and setting in motion another obesity "begetting" cycle.

Weight gain reduces mobility, as you are likely quite aware. Joint disease, swollen legs, and sore feet are common with obesity, causing movement to be extremely painful. Obesity also reduces mobility by adversely affecting respiratory (or breathing) functions. Additionally, obesity is a contributor to a number of diseases that reduce activity or the desire to engage in such. Less activity, regardless of the cause, reduces the number of calories the body burns, increasing the risk for weight gain with further restriction of mobility, and so once again, obesity "begets" obesity.

Finally, as we are all too aware from our readings, or more likely personal experience, obesity contributes to the development of a number of diseases including diabetes, hypertension (high blood pressure), high cholesterol, heart disease, inflammatory diseases, depression, and much more. Ironically, many of these obesity-related diseases are treated with medications that cause weight gain. I remember gaining over 30 pounds of additional weight after being prescribed an antidepressant that was supposed to help the depression I had from being obese. Duh!! Does that make sense?

Obesity is also a primary cause of type 2 non-insulin dependent diabetes, yet, most diabetic medications produce weight gain. A large percentage of individuals with obesity develop osteoarthritis or other inflammatory conditions that are treated with steroids or steroid-like medications that cause weight gain. Many of the blood pressure or hypertension control medications also cause weight gain and obesity, which in turn causes hypertension. Obesity increases the risk for cancer, and certain cancer medications increase body weight. Thus, once again, obesity "begets" obesity, causing co-morbid diseases that are treated by drugs that cause weight gain and the risk for further disease.

Okay, that was a lot of information, so let's review. Obesity causes numerous changes within the body that favor fat uptake and storage, decrease fat utilization, increase appetite and food cravings, reduce feelings of fullness, cause psychological distress, reduce mobility and calories utilized by activity, and contribute to the development of diseases treated by medications that cause weight gain. Whoah! Can you see why obesity is considered a progressive disease???? Do you now have a better understanding why, as the severity of our obesity worsens, that we feel more and more trapped and hopeless? If all this is happening on its own, how can we break the obesity-promoting cycles responsible for our bondage?

With great effort individuals with obesity may be able to lose small amounts of weight with diet, exercise, behavioral changes, and in some instances, anti-obesity medication. Such weight loss, albeit small, can have a beneficial effect on overall health, but is likely to be insufficient to disrupt many of the obesity-promoting cycles. Furthermore, there is evidence that certain of the obesity "begetting" conditions, such as low fat oxidation and increased appetite, may actually be *worsened* by weight loss, increasing the risk for weight regain. These conditions, as well as the progressive nature of obesity, usually guarantee that weight loss with conventional therapy will fail to be permanent, as discussed by Dr. Baker in Chapter Three.

Although there are many valid treatments for those who are *overweight* and *obese,* experts on government panels established to provide guidelines for obesity treatment recognize bariatric surgery as the most effective treatment for *morbid obesity,* If you read the recommendations of these experts, you will notice that, in reference to obesity treatment, the word *cure* never appears. That is because, at this time, the only cure for obesity is *prevention.* Even surgery does not *cure* obesity.

Surgery is intended to produce massive weight loss that can help us break free from the bondage of obesity-promoting cycles. In addition, it provides a tool to assist in the life-long battle we must wage against the progressive nature of our disease. That's right, the battle we must wage against our disease and yes, that will involve, even after surgery, lifestyle changes such as regular exercise, healthful eating, stress-coping skills, and more. We must look at these factors as if they are the medication for our disease and know that we are required to take these medications every single day for the rest of our lives.

Surgical treatments cannot cure, but can be successful in *arresting* the progressive nature of obesity *if,* and only *if,* the bariatric patient continues to be proactive about keeping their disease state properly treated. If the patient does not provide appropriate on-going treatment in the form of proper nutrition, adequate movement and activity, nutritional supplementation, and other lifestyle changes, then the progressive nature of the disease will again take hold, and the obesity can and will come back and continue its vicious cycle.

Surgical treatment of obesity, like surgical treatment of any other progressive disease such as cancer, is a serious consideration. You should know all you can know about the treatment and what you will need to do to make sure that it is, and remains, effective for as long as possible. Just as some cancer patients may choose lesser invasive treatment methods for their cancer before resorting to surgery and other treatments that invade or seriously intrude upon the body's systems, patients with morbid obesity should also consider all of the alternatives.

You decide what is right for you at this stage in your life, under the circumstances of your life, and given your personal ability to handle and deal with your decision. Losing and maintaining the loss of any amount of weight by a medically responsible method will bring you some benefits. If nothing else, your heart, organs, and bones will be a little happier, and you may feel a little better. But, are you just looking for a short-term or partial fix? Are you looking to fight a minor battle to take a particular hill, or are you looking to win the whole world war? That's what you need to consider. If you are looking to win the whole war, then you should seriously consider one of the available surgical treatments.

Whatever you decide is right for you at this time in your life, just remember that your obesity will never get better all by itself. It will never just go away, and you will most likely never be totally "okay with it." It is a disease that is ravaging your body and shortening your life. It may not be advancing on your systems as fast as some cancers or AIDS, but it is a progressive and deadly disease. It will eventually kill you.... and me. Now is the time for us to educate ourselves, end the obesity "begetting" cycles, and make a choice to live. We hope this book helps you find what is right for you, and what will help you save your own life.

All the best of luck and health,
Cynthia K. Buffington, PhD

Dr. Buffington received her doctorate in Physiology from The University of Texas, Austin, and obtained postdoctoral fellowships in Biochemistry, Endocrinology, and Cardiology at The University of Texas and The University of Tennessee Health Science Centers. As a researcher and scientist, Dr. Buffington has earned the reputation of being one of the world's foremost authorities in the field of bariatrics. She was one of the first to recognize the low anti-oxidant potential among the morbidly obese, and she was one of the first to report vitamin D deficiencies in both post-operative and pre-operative (non-operative) Roux-en-Y gastric bypass patients.

Florida Hospital–Celebration Health Bariatric Center is where Dr. Buffington currently calls home, and serves as one of its premier research scientists and advisors. Dr. Buffington has also served as the Director of Research for U.S. Bariatric, the Director of Research for The University of Tennessee's Obesity Wellness Center, and as an Associate Professor in the University's Departments of Medicine and Preventative Medicine. She has written and published hundreds of internet columns, newspaper columns, peer-reviewed journal articles and essays, papers, case studies and abstracts on the subject of obesity, its nature as a disease, associative illnesses, the treatments and cures, and the subsequent lifetime of follow-up for even the most successful of bariatric patients. Cynthia Buffington has presented numerous reports, moderated special scientific sessions, and served on various committees for the American Society for Bariatric Surgery (now the American Society for Metabolic and Bariatric Surgery), the North American Association for the Study of Obesity, the International Federation for the Surgery of Obesity, the American Diabetes Association, and the Endocrine Society. In addition, she has authored several book chapters and numerous manuscripts and reports, along with writing a monthly research column for Beyond Change, an international bariatric newsletter.

Celebration, Florida, is proud to call Dr. Buffington a resident, and she can often be seen walking Bella and Sam, her two canine "fur-children," the lights of her life. If you visit Celebration, Florida, be sure to keep an eye out for a little electric roadster with lightning bolts on the side flying around town. That would be Dr. Buffington and the kids....

— FOREWORD —

Judith Brown Clarke

I have always believed that "everything happens for a reason." Everything happens in order to teach us some lesson, and to give us some message about what our next step in life should be. Unfortunately, it is often quite a challenge to figure out the nature of that message. I also believe there are other instances, however, when the timing of the lesson is gauged by our ability to handle, or openness to recognizing and accepting the message. This may just be one of those instances. I believe you've picked up this book, written by these particular people, at this time in your life, because you are ready for the lesson, and ready to really hear the message.

And what is the lesson? The lesson is to read this information, examine your life, ask the hard questions, and find a way to do for yourself what you need to do. And what is the message? The message is live! Live life like the gift that it is. Live it fully, completely, and happily. Live it as a competitor in the game, and not just an observer in the stands.

Getting back in the game of life is exactly what this book is designed to help you do; surgery, or no surgery. This book will hopefully cause you to think about many aspects of your life. Do you want to continue to cheer only for others, or would you really like to feel the freedom of the run and the roar of the crowd, knowing it's all for you?

It's very easy for any of us to become an observer rather than getting out there in the race and chasing the dream. Life's tough and full of many hurdles, but do you want to know you've overcome them, or would you rather watch the whole race run by you, and find yourself left sitting in the bleachers when the race is done and the people have all gone home?

It's kind of like watching a soap opera and vicariously living through the characters on the screen. What kind of life is that? (By the way, have you noticed that they never listen to you as you shout out valuable information that would save them from six weeks of bad story line?) I understand wanting to sit down and give up when the race gets hard, but the most important thing is being in the race, and not just watching it go by.

As a former Olympian (and yes, I *really* miss my former body), I understand what it means to set goals, make sacrifices, and train hard. I understand the victories and the losses. I understand the effort required to overcome the hurdles. (No, I really mean I understand it. I ran the 400-meter hurdles!) But, the most important and valuable lessons I have learned are from just being in the "game." It is not important whether you win or lose … okay sometimes it is … but in general, just being a participant has taught me more about myself than any medal or trophy I have won. Those were the lessons, and because of them I have internalized the message and truly lived.

I can hear what you're thinking now: "If you were a world-class athlete in great shape, how can you know what I feel? How can you know what it's like to be overweight and living with so many restrictions and limitations?" Well, in some ways I do, and you're right, in some ways I don't.

Many people think that athletes can't relate to people with weight problems. In fact, all my life I've carried more weight than I should. When the game you're in measures probable success or failure based on percentage of body fat compared to other competitors, and you're found to be in an "unacceptable range," you come to identify on a certain level with people who have weight issues. Your self-esteem, and self-confidence take a bit of a beating, and in that respect, it's relative.

Now, I don't profess to have experienced the prejudice, the physical pain, or even much of the emotional pain many of you have experienced. But, I can tell you that even if you are in an "unacceptable range" of body fat, you can still show the world that you can not only play the game at a world-class level, but you can win. I did, and you will too.

The reason I know you can play this game and win is because it has nothing to do with physical ability, talent, or skill. It has to do with belief in yourself, and belief in those you choose to help you. You have to work at it, believe it will happen, and make it happen. That's all it takes to reach a goal.

Athletes have to train and work at reaching their goal every day, just like weight loss patients. We're just two ends of the same spectrum – each trying to craft the body into something it's not, and yet something it needs to be. For athletes, sometimes it takes longer than expected to reach a desired level, or an injury slows them down. In either case they just have to work through the frustration, the disappointment, the waiting, and stay committed. They have to rely on the direction of their coaches, hear the cheer of their supporters, keep their eyes on the goal, and rely on their own inner strength.

When you're struggling to lose weight, it takes a long time to reach a desired level, sometimes longer than expected. Instead of injuries, you deal with related medical conditions that delay you and slow you down. But just like athletes, you have to work through the frustration, the disappointment, the waiting, and stay committed. You must rely on the direction of your multi-disciplinary medical team, hear the cheer of your supporters, and most importantly you must keep your eye on the goal, and rely on your own inner strength.

Perhaps each of the challenges or barriers we face in life is actually strength training for the soul. When you're physically strong, it's amazing how much easier external challenges can be, but the same holds true for internal strength. When you rely on your inner strength, it's amazing how much easier personal challenges can be; how much easier it can be to move beyond the lack of validation, or self-imposed barriers. We all have physical barriers of some kind that can hold us back from where we want to be, barriers to move beyond.

As far as external barriers go, it always strikes me how strongly I react to the word "no." If you tell me I can't, then it's the first thing I'll do. I'll do it just to prove to you I can, and to prove you wrong. I'll find the inner will to move that boundary you placed around me out of the way. I decide what my boundaries are, not anyone else.

Now, don't get me wrong, I have a healthy respect for boundaries. Sometimes boundaries keep us from flying off in all directions. When boundaries aren't meant for structure, however, and they're only there to inhibit, that's when the problems start. The worst of these boundaries, of course, are the ones we impose on ourselves.

We lead ourselves to believe that those boundaries cannot be moved except by a miracle. I believe, however, that you can create miracles if you really set your mind to it. Remember: when something positive happens that is not anticipated, that's a miracle. Not all miracles are of biblical proportions. Sometimes they're just little, unexpected victories that let you know you're on the right track.

When you commit yourself to achieving a goal that moves what previously seemed immovable, that is the foundation of a miracle. If you stay committed, find the right help, stay strong, and never stop believing, watch for the miracle to happen. You have everything you need to create your own miracle, and this book is hopefully going to help you start down the road toward it, in whatever direction it may lay.

The direction you'll take after reading this book will only be determined by you, but your guides along the way are some pretty incredible people who've walked a mile in your shoes, or helped others who've walked in your shoes. (You know what they say: you have to walk a mile in another man's shoes ... because then you'll be a mile away and have his shoes!) Julie Janeway and Karen Sparks have walked your path, and they know your struggles. They are your kindred souls.

I have always prided myself on my ability to identify people with true souls. This ability is not unlike the way alien abductees explain how they just "know" other alien abductees; they just feel a strange connection. Of course alien abductees then look for the "probe" mark on the back of the other person's neck to confirm their suspicions, but I haven't quite found any such external marking that confirms the true souls I meet.

When I met Julie eight years ago in the first of many laborious doctoral classes, I felt a strange connection to her. I immediately heard her soul, and our friendship was born. Now granted, I did see a probe mark on the back of her neck ... but that's another story....

Throughout my friendship with Julie, she has struggled with her weight. She has swung on the "rationale" pendulum from "God made me this way, therefore I should be grateful," all the way across to the self-loathing "I am fat, therefore I eat. I eat, therefore I am fat." But to the world, Julie was always just Julie. Her attitude was, "Here I am world, and what are you going to do about it?!" Inner turmoil safely hidden away, Julie has always compensated for lost self-esteem with her tremendous intellect, and an incredible sense of humor.

Julie's sense of humor has carried her through a lot of tough times in her life. I'm sure many of you reading this book can relate. Throughout Julie's struggle with her weight, and the life-altering journey that started with her miraculous comeback from a death-defying car accident, and took her through gastric bypass surgery, she has never lost her ability to laugh. We all need to laugh. Julie, Karen, and the others will help you laugh because life's too short not to.

I've always thought that my ability to find humor in everything was a character flaw. I've since come to discover, however, that it is the foundation of strength, and the essence of a quality life. The ability to laugh, to "let go," and to move forward is truly a gift we should cherish. The authors are sharing this gift with you in abundance in this book. Through all of the tough times I watched Julie fight through in the last six years, she's shown incredible strength, courage, and laughed her way to regaining her competitive status in the game of life.

Not only did Julie get back in the game, she dragged Karen back into the game while she was at it. When Julie introduced me to Karen, I thought: "It is true … birds of a feather do flock together." Julie and Karen are like peas in a pod. On the day I first met Karen, the introduction part was quite short, because there really was no need for small talk. We just quickly moved into the comfort of a new friendship. It was like unhooking your bra at the end of the day: a welcome relief.

This comfortable feeling of being with good friends is one of the best features of this book. Throughout it you will feel as though you are part of a personal conversation with Julie and Karen, as well as with Dr. Baker, Carrie, Scott, and Nabila. That is what I liked most about the book's tone, the ability to address a sensitive subject in a real-life, non-threatening, person-to-person manner.

The clear-cut, informative, "here-it-is, do-with-it-what-you-will" style of this book, is refreshing and honest. You'll find very funny parts mixed with very serious and engaging parts – sort of like real life. But most importantly, what you'll find is the motivation and knowledge to make a decision whether you want to work toward getting back in the game, or pack a picnic and stay in the stands.

As an athlete, and a person who has immense respect for the human body, I jumped at the chance to write the Foreword of this book because I believe in any medically sound method for becoming healthier and increasing life participation. It matters not to me whether you choose to have weight loss surgery. If you simply find the will to try and reclaim control of your health, then I applaud your strength and your Olympian efforts to save your own life.

My background has instilled in me admiration for strength, commitment, and tenacity. I've competed against the world's top track athletes, and even if I lost, I respected the work that went into their performance. For those of you who are struggling with your weight, I understand your struggle, and I admire the fortitude, commitment, and tenacity you are showing in simply reading this book. You are the real winners – the real champions. You are the everyday people who deserve the medals for perseverance and determination. When you choose not to give up, when you choose life, you are the true heroes.

If you choose to have weight loss surgery, know that the information you are receiving in this book is accurate, reliable, and necessary for the creation of your game plan. Know that it's okay if you choose surgery, and okay if you don't. Neither is a cop out. As long as you've really investigated the options, learned the facts, and discussed both with your doctor, it doesn't matter which path you choose, as long as all paths lead off the bench, and back into the game. Make a decision, commit, be strong, follow through, and keep your eye on the prize.

So, congratulations on your new journey! For some of you it will be weight loss surgery, for others it will be a new way of eating or an exercise regime, and for some it will be a combination of strategies. It really does not matter. You <u>can</u> love yourself and still have aspects of you that you want to change. That's perfectly acceptable. The most important part of this journey is to find peace, health, and life, and to learn to accept and embrace yourself for the fabulous and valuable human being you are. Demand nothing less from yourself, or others.

Always, always, always, remember to laugh … it's Botox® for the soul!

Judith Brown Clarke

Judi was born in Milwaukee, Wisconsin, moved to Kokomo, Indiana, and finished her childhood in Lansing, Michigan. She is married to husband, Hugh, and is the mother of three wonderful sons: Dorian – age 19, Mychael – age 18, and Antonio – age 8. She is also the proud owner of Chance the dog, and Sponge Bob the fish.

She holds two degrees from Michigan State University, a Bachelor of Science in Audiology & Speech Science, and a Master of Education degree. She is currently completing her doctoral dissertation for her PhD in Public Administration and Public Policy from Western Michigan University, from which she will graduate with honors. In addition to working as the Director of Minority Programs at Michigan State University, and attending to her family and dissertation, St. Paul's Episcopal Church in Lansing, Michigan, has her unconditional and total devotion.

Judi has experienced athletic success in the 400-Meter Hurdle event as a five-time National Champion, and Silver Medalist in the 1984 Olympic Games in Los Angles, California. She has held numerous National and World Records, and still owns an as yet unbroken World Record as a member of the distance medley relay team in which she ran the 400-Meter leg.

In addition, Judi was a three time Gold Medalist at the Pan-American Games, was a Silver Medalist at the World Track and Field Championships, and was a twelve time Big Ten Champion in Track and Field events. In 1986 she was inducted into the Michigan State University Hall of Fame, and in 1987 she was named as one of the "Athletes of the Year," specifically "Sportswoman of the Year" by Sports Illustrated™ magazine. Judi has also been honored by having carried the Olympic torch on its tour across America.

Judi has been a Big Ten Track and Field Coach, and a sought after, nationally recognized motivational speaker working with corporations, civic groups, and schools across the country. Her current civic responsibilities include membership on the Ingham County Women's Commission, and participating in other good works sponsored by her church.

The jump is so frightening

between where I am

and where I want to be...

because of all I may

become

I will close my eyes

and leap!

MARY ANNE RADMACHER

Welcome to the weird, wild, wonderful world of weight loss surgery! Whether you're just here for a brief visit to get the lay of the land, or you intend to make this your permanent home, we're here to answer your questions and show you around. We're the Welcome Wagon, of sorts.

In fact showing you around is exactly what this book is about. This book is for those of you who are considering having a weight loss procedure done, as well as for those of you who have already made the decision to have surgery and are at various stages in the process. We wrote this book for all the *REAL* people out there who need information on more than just the medical facts (although we provide that as well). This book is written BY REAL PEOPLE, FOR REAL PEOPLE.

We're not celebrities (except in our own minds...), and we don't have private chefs to cook our meals for us, personal trainers to help us work out, or live celebrity jet-set lifestyles. We don't have therapists on speed dial, plastic surgeons on retainer, or an endless supply of time and money to shop for clothes every time we lose weight. Not that celebrities don't have the same emotional struggles, but let's face it, the rest of the world is a whole lot easier for them. We're the working stiffs who have to do this by ourselves, and work it all in around spouses, kids, jobs, school, chores, friends, and everything else. We're the people who have real life to deal with every day, while we try to find a way to just have a "life," let alone a happy and healthy one.

The purpose of this book is to tell it like it is. In a way, it's sort of a glimpse into a "day-in-the-life" of two ordinary women from Michigan. We're not sugar-coating anything, and we leave it to you to decide whether you want to experience the same things we do or not. We're not going to tell you that with weight loss surgery you can "have it all!" Maybe you will, maybe you won't. But then maybe you'll hit the lottery tonight too.... Some people have this surgery and do end up looking like stars, models, and "celebutantes." For the other 99.9% of us, however, here's what life is like on a daily basis: sometimes funny, sometimes a little painful, but always totally real.

We're not going to tell you our life histories in this book, nor use it as a forum for working through all of our personal pain and angst from years gone by. This book isn't about how ripped off and hard-done-by we were, it's about what you can really expect if you make the decision to change your life through weight loss surgery. It's about how we came to the decision to do so, and what we've experienced since making that decision.

Our intent is to provide you with useful and practical information about the types of surgeries being done today, the risks and benefits of them, and about what you might experience as a result of having surgery to help you lose weight. If you haven't yet made the decision, then our purpose here is to give you as much useful and applicable information as we can to help you decide whether this is the right direction for you, and if it is, to give you the information necessary to help you find a surgeon who will take good and proper care of you.

To assist you with that, we've included for your consideration the good, the bad, the yukky, and the strange. We've tried not to oversimplify anything, while still making it easy to understand. Some of you have already learned a bit about weight loss surgery, while others are learning about it for the first time. If you're in the advanced group, please be patient for the sake of the beginners. Hopefully the stories will be helpful, or at least keep you amused.

You read the information and the stories, and *you* determine what weight to give them in making your decision (no pun intended). In fact, while you're reading we suggest that you make a pro/con list to help you make your decision. No one can make this decision for you, and no one knows what's scary or appealing to you, but you. So, as you read along, if something either strikes you as a very negative aspect of surgery, or a very positive aspect of surgery, write it down on your decision list for later reference.

Similarly, if you have questions that arise as you read, and you can't find the answers in the book, make a list of questions as you think of them, and tuck them in the back of the book. You can then take the book, your decision list, and your notes to a physician ('cause we will tell you how to find a good one!), and efficiently get the answers to all your questions and concerns.

Speaking of what you can't find in this book, you won't find recipes, or exercise routines, insurance information, or tax benefits. For information on those issues, we suggest (in respective order), consulting your mother or aunt, the guy in the tight t-shirt and shorts at the gym, the human resource person at your job, and an accountant that gives a free consultation to new clients. In that vein, and as we tell the college students we teach, Julie is *a* lawyer, but she's not *your* lawyer, so please don't send email with legal questions.

What you will find in this book is information on what to do if you start to lose your hair after surgery (see Chapter Six), experiences that are particular only to men (see Chapter Ten), information on medication modifications and issues (see Chapter Twelve), tips and tricks from people who've been down the path before you, a heads-up on things to avoid, and a really serious discussion about whether or not you should even read this book. We've assembled some pretty awesome people to talk to you about the technical stuff, and we made sure to pick people who have a good sense of humor so you won't be bored.

We tried to keep the book on an upbeat note, but there are certain topics or stories that just require a more serious tone. We do not intend to make light of the serious nature of having surgery, nor do we intend to treat lightly the issues with which bariatric patients must deal. What we do intend, however, is to drive home the fact that you have to keep your sense of humor, something in which we wholeheartedly believe.

As for the layout of the book, since there is more than one voice being communicated in each chapter, we had to pick a head spokesperson for each one. So, when you are reading along, the first name that appears in the list of authors for that chapter is who's doing the talking for the group — unless we explicitly tell you otherwise. (Just like a lawyer to have a loophole built in....) The other authors have contributed their thoughts, ideas, and information, but realistically, only one person can talk at a time. You'll note that a majority of the time it's Julie speaking. How fitting that we should choose a lawyer/college professor to be our mouthpiece.

Because all of us are prone to using big, obscure, or technical words, for your convenient reference we've included a glossary of terms in Chapter Eighteen. (We realize there's just never a dictionary around when you need one....) To keep the page count down, and thus the cost of the book, we only printed the most important terms in the book glossary. Also, if you'd like more information on certain topics, we've provided a list of web sites and other sources for you, again, we've included the most important ones and others can be found on the internet by way of various search engines.

Well, that's about it for all the stuff we think you might need to know before you take your wild ride through the world of weight loss surgery. We hope you find it informative, helpful, insightful, and a little fun. Keep smiling, and remember you are not alone. You have the power to change your life by whatever means necessary.

The two most important things
I did learn were that you are as powerful
and strong as you allow yourself to be,
and that the most difficult part of any endeavor
is taking the first step,
making the first decision.

ROBYN DAVIDSON

Chapter One

➤ R E A L I T Y   S L A P ! ! ➤

Julie M. Janeway
Karen J. Sparks

Well, before we start on this journey, we need to sit down and have a big emotional heart-to-heart about some things. You'll need to do a little soul searching at this point. If you're a woman reading this, you are no doubt ready for such an event. If you're a man, well as I tell my husband, just suck it up and deal with it.

First things first: do not do this for anyone else but you. If you choose to begin down this path, you must be 100% honest with yourself about why you're doing this, and for whom you are doing it. You must come to grips with who you are now, and how you got this way.

Although there are many contributing factors that help people gain weight, the reality is you got here by putting the food in your mouth all by yourself. Ultimately you are responsible for what went in, and what will go in your mouth in the future. You are in control of how you maintain your health and live your life. You have chosen the paths you've taken, and you alone, will navigate new roads in the future.

You must choose to start down this road solely to take as much control over your life, weight, and food as you had over gaining the weight and eating the food thus far. You must be doing it for your own health, and control of your own life. You must be doing it to stay alive, and to be able to directly and meaningfully participate in life. You must want to create for yourself a new healthy life and lifestyle that will allow you to do what you want, and be in control of where you want to go. You must do this to please you.

You cannot do this to please anyone else, or in hopes of changing the nature of any relationships in your life. This must be a totally selfish act. Although this act must be completely about you, it is okay for it to have derivative benefits for others. The most direct and important benefits must, however, relate solely to you.

If you are thinking of undertaking this endeavor so you can give more to your children, or your spouse, or your career, then you need to stop and re-think your motives. This endeavor must be about being in control of yourself, about feeling emotionally and physically strong, and about living to see your next birthday. These are the primary reasons and direct benefits of such an undertaking. Secondary benefits may accrue in that you will be around longer and be able to interact more with your children and spouse, but don't make them the primary purpose of the event.

Undertaking this act has to be about hitting bottom, and from the very depths of your being, truly wanting to give up this painful existence. You have to be willing to literally reinvent yourself, and you can't do that if you're not focusing on you. If you're focusing on the needs or wants of others with regard to your weight, or because you think that your weight is the only thing standing in the way of all your dreams coming true, then think again.

This process is not just about losing weight, it's about molding and re-shaping a whole new existence. It isn't just about an incision, or a medical procedure, or numbers on a scale. It's about metamorphosis. If all you're ready to do is fight your way out of the cocoon, and not undergo the long, arduous, and amazing change from being one creature to becoming another, then you need to stop and re-examine your choices. If you are willing to undergo this process of transformation, then you must now examine your expectations and anticipated outcomes, and gauge them against reality.

Reality (in case you are laboring under this massive misconception), rarely, if ever resembles anything you see on television – not even on the Discovery Channel®. The ordinary and mundane don't bring ratings and high paying sponsors. The unusual and exceptional are the mainstays of television viewership.

Many of you reading this book have watched one or more television shows documenting the life of a bariatric surgery patient. Whether it be on a talk show, or on the Discovery Health Channel®, we've all seen these amazing stories of transfiguration, white knights, true love, and dreams come true. We've all seen the people who've lost 350 or more pounds and gone from a size 38 to a 4, or from a 10x shirt to a men's large. We've heard them tell us of finding true love, of becoming championship athletes, of going from being a nobody to being a cover model for a health and fitness magazine. And those stories are for the most part true, but for every one of those people who has experienced such a one-in-ten-million experience, there's ten million who've just experienced real life.

All the people who go through this process, who just experience their daily lives (albeit in a happier and healthier way), aren't the people that talk shows and documentary producers generally care about. They're not interesting television fare because they're just you and me.

These ordinary people are the ones who lose a lot of weight, but they still wear a regular size, they still have body issues they don't like, they don't end up on a magazine cover, and they may still be looking for a decent person with whom to have a relationship and share their lives. Worse, maybe their relationship blew up because the person lost so much weight and took the time to focus on themselves. That's not good television. It hits too close to home for many viewers. People think, "I can see that in my own family room. Thanks, but no thanks."

Reality is that you might go from a size 32 to a 14, not a 4. Reality is going from a 60 in. waist to a 38, not a 28. Reality is feeling better, and stronger, and being healthier, not becoming famous. Reality is you don't get younger, although you may look younger. Reality is you'll probably have some flabby skin, and you'll still have problem areas that you hate on your body, not that you'll become a championship athlete or a cover model. Reality is that stuff starts going south about age 35. Reality is if you had a crappy marriage before you lost weight, chances are you'll still have a crappy marriage after. But reality is also that you will still be as worthy of a great life and the chance to live it as those people who experienced the unique and unusual.

The reality is this is not a magic pill, or a cure-all. Weight loss surgery doesn't guarantee a great life; it only gives you the opportunity to live a happier, healthier, and hopefully longer life. Ultimately, you still determine whether or not you have a great life. You make those choices, and you choose whether or not to fix other broken areas of your life. You choose, not anybody else.

You will still have to deal with the garbage that comes your way, and you still determine how you live your life and whether it's worth living. Everything doesn't turn to gold just because you lose the weight. What does happen is you may find you have the ability to, and the inspiration to make it better, or to make a change; to make gold out of straw if you will. Deal with that concept and you're well on your way to dealing with not being a fat person any more.

So we've got you thinking about all this painful stuff, and you think you can wrap your head around transforming your life. You believe you can do this for you, and you can have realistic expectations about the outcome. But can you deal with the fact that although you may change the weight, the appearance, and the lifestyle, you can never change the emotional memories and scars of being fat?

It's true. They never go away, but you can learn to control them and no longer let them control you. You'll always feel some pain from past rejections, missed opportunities and events, lost chances and hurtful remarks, but you don't need to live in fear of them anymore either.

You'll confront these emotional monsters, every last one of them, at least ten times throughout this process. You'll feel the pain of each one over and over again. Eventually, you'll learn to control them and realize that they're in the past, and you control the future. In contrast, you'll experience the thrills of each new victory at least ten times over as well. If you're willing to wade through this morass of emotional issues and ride the proverbial emotional roller coaster in order to get it behind you for good, then stand up and take the next step down the road to a new life.

Your new life starts with knowing yourself physically and emotionally, and being ready to make the changes needed to keep yourself alive and healthy. This self-examination will also come in handy when you hear stories about medical complications, or people who put their weight back on, or people who encountered a host of other obstacles. Remembering that you are unique physiologically, psychologically, and emotionally will help you to remember that other people's problems and issues aren't necessarily going to be your problems and issues. If you can be prepared to deal with what comes your way, or doesn't, then take another step down the road. As they say, prepare for the worst, and hope for the best.

Preparing for the worst and hoping for the best includes doing your research. In reading this book, you're doing both. It is unbelievably important for you to know what you're getting into, both medically and emotionally. You need to be fully medically informed as to your options, your limitations, the benefits, and the risks of having a bariatric procedure done. You need to fully understand all the science behind what is being undertaken, and you need to be aware of the percentage of incidence of each type of foreseeable complication.

Also, be cognizant of the fact that there can be unforeseen complications due to the unique nature of your physiology, and just because one person had thus and such, doesn't mean you'll have it too. Karen had to have her gallbladder out three months after her surgery, and I had a post-operative stricture three different times. Just because she had one type of complication didn't mean I would have it also, and vice versa. Neither instance was the fault of the surgeon, but both are known complications or after-effects of the procedure.

Complications happen. If you have one, just deal with it and move on. It doesn't mean the doctor messed up; it's just a complication derived from opening up the body and reconstructing it. It may not be a nice situation, and you may not feel like dealing with it. That's normal, but you get through it.

What is not normal is to assume the doctor made a mistake. As a lawyer myself, (and I can't believe I'm saying this...), don't run off to see an attorney if you have complications from this surgery. If you have complications not remotely associated with this type of surgery (like you're missing your left kidney afterward...), then maybe consult a lawyer. Other than that, just concentrate on getting through it with your doctor's help.

When doing your research you need to be looking at facilities and surgeons that will give you a lot of information. If you are dealing with organizations and individuals who simply want to get your insurance card and book you a surgery date, *run*, don't walk the other way. Don't play bariatric roulette with your life.

Respectable and reputable organizations should be providing a full orientation that offers detailed information on the procedure, and the risks and benefits. It should also provide substantial pre-operative medical evaluation and testing by both an internist and a surgeon to determine whether or not the patient is a medically sound candidate for surgery, and whether or not laparoscopic procedures can or should be used.

Additionally, good bariatric surgical centers require a psychological assessment of the potential patient to determine whether the patient is emotionally able to withstand the process, is going into the process with the right motivations, and whether the person has reasonable and rational expectations of the process and themselves. This is not a test, an exam, or a judgment about you as a person. You need to look at this as an assets and liabilities assessment. They will help you determine what assets you already have (including the practice team as an asset) that will help you be successful. They will also help you determine what liabilities exist so that they can help you turn them into assets and help you move toward a successful new weight loss journey. So don't be afraid, and make sure to be honest because they can't help you if they don't know what needs help.

Good treatment centers also usually require an assessment of the significant support person in the patient's life to determine whether the patient will have proper and adequate emotional support throughout the process, and to determine whether situations may exist that will sabotage or undermine the patient's success. Again, this is only to help get a good picture of the entire spectrum of the patient's assets, and potential liabilities that will require some attention to turn them into more positive factors.

Having a good support system is critical to bariatric patients. Although you must do it for yourself, you can't do it alone. There's just too much to deal with. You need people who will listen, even if they don't really understand what you're going through. They need to be people who will help you see the positive in the unknowns ahead of you, not tell you that the light at the end of the tunnel is an oncoming train. You need to have people who will love you no matter how you look, or how you change.

My husband, family, and friends were a constant source of support for me, as were Karen's family and friends. They supported us, but they didn't really understand what we were going through. Karen and I went through this process together, and without each other neither one of us would have made it because only we understood what the other was going through. Good support is the key to success, both in your personal life, and in your surgeon's office.

Persons seeking bariatric treatment should also require that their surgeon's office provide nutritional and exercise counseling, as well as be affiliated with other surgeons who are trained to handle particular bariatric related complications, or other matters if necessary. Surgeons should also provide extensive follow-up care, and patients should be ready and willing to attend all follow-up appointments, have all testing done, and follow through on the process. Surgeons should be prepared to deal with a number of issues that may follow surgery, not simply tell the patient to seek treatment from a primary care physician.

Incidentally, primary care physicians should not be solely responsible for the treatment of obesity related conditions such as high blood pressure or diabetes. These types of conditions are intricately entwined in the surgical and weight loss process, and should be monitored and attended to by the surgeon and internist in consultation with the patient's primary care or other appropriate physician. Bariatric surgery has a proven track record of effectively dealing with conditions such as high blood pressure and diabetes, and Dr. Baker will address this issue in Chapter Three.

Dr. Baker will also discuss the length of the process, and why it should not be rushed. I've personally been appalled at some of the documentaries I've seen on T.V. that showed patients having massive reconstructive plastic surgery within ten months of their bariatric surgery. At ten months your body is still losing weight and adjusting to its new form. Your skin and muscle haven't been given enough time to shrink as far as they might be able to go without surgical intervention. Perhaps the skin won't shrink back all the way, but maybe a less drastic cosmetic surgical procedure could be used if so much skin weren't being removed.

This is a process that simply can't be rushed. It operates on its own time schedule, and each patient's body responds at a different rate. But I seriously doubt that the body of anyone who loses 150+ pounds in ten months has finished adjusting in that time frame.

Because it is a lengthy process, potential surgery candidates must be prepared to be patient and compliant. We know that you might be chomping at the bit if you've already made the decision to have surgery, or you may just be wanting to jump in with both feet before you lose your nerve. Either way, don't let the *desperation factor* rush you in any stage of the process. Resist the desperation factor!!! Trust me when I say, it really works best if you listen to what they tell you and follow the instructions. They don't just tell you this stuff for the good of their health – in fact, they tell you for the good of *your* health!

Now, I admit to the fact that I am a person who needs to push and test the limits because I know that I'm a unique individual, and I don't necessarily respond physically the same way everyone else does. So when they told me not to drink orange juice, I ran right out and drank orange juice. Six hours later when I got up off the bathroom floor, I decided they were right and I shouldn't drink orange juice. It's not that you can never have orange juice again, but maybe you just shouldn't slam half a glass of pulpy orange juice three months after surgery. Just a theory....

So the point of that story (and later on you'll read so many more) is to trust in the doctors' expertise, follow their guidance and instructions, and commit yourself to the process body and soul — literally. Remind yourself that you are learning entirely new skills, and learning skills effectively means practicing them over and over. Practice your new skills of controlling your food, your health, and your lifestyle.

By the way, if you think that food controlled you before your surgery, you ain't seen nothin' yet! Once you have this surgery, food will control you like never before; but in a good way. I say that because unlike smokers or drinkers, we can't just stop eating to rid ourselves of the problem (and yes, I know quitting smoking or drinking is incredibly difficult. Don't send any hate mail !!)

We must eat to survive, and we must eat well to be healthy and thrive, but because of the nature of this surgery, you may need to eat more often each day than you did before (if you were prone to skip meals and then binge), eat less food at one sitting than you probably ever did, and eat only certain kinds of foods while staying away from others. Timing, proportions, food types, and access to acceptable foods becomes a serious challenge.

Coping with this challenge is the biggest new skill you'll master. Every single day is a new adventure. We'll talk about this later in Chapter Thirteen entitled *The Protein Safari*. Learning these new food skills is unbelievably important because if you don't, and you fall back into your old habits, you can put the weight back on. You will have gone through all of this for absolutely nothing. Don't go there.

In fact, you need to be comfortable with the fact that if you begin this journey it's a one way trip. What you'll shed along the way will be more than just pounds, and the person who concludes the journey will only resemble on the inside the person who started it.

You must be comfortable with change, and willing to conquer fear. In fact, when both Karen and I wrestled with the decision to begin down this path, we came to rely on the wise words of my sister Cheryl. She reminded us, as we've many times since reminded each other: "You can do anything afraid, that you can do unafraid."

The person who travels this road has to know they can face fear, as well as fear of the unknown. The person who starts this journey has to want to participate in life. The person who walks this path has to want to live life and take advantage of what it has to offer. The person who takes these steps has to be ready to leave a lot of pain behind and happily face the future. The person who begins this process has to want to go through the metamorphosis that will make them grateful for who they are and always have been on the inside, and finally grateful for who they have become on the outside.

Now ask yourself: "Am I that person?"

If you are that person, then you're ready to read the rest of this book. In fact, read it twice!

Welcome to the rest of your life.

*Don't be afraid
that your life will end...
be afraid that
it will never begin.*

GRACE HANSON

Chapter Two

⤖ EN-LIGHTENMENT ⤘

Julie M. Janeway
Karen J. Sparks

If you're reading this you must at least be interested in changing your life through weight loss surgery, and are ready to find out more about it in order to make a really informed decision. Congratulations on getting this far!

We've named this chapter "En-Lightenment" because that's what it is truly about: being enlightened intellectually and emotionally regarding the procedure and process of weight loss through surgery, as well as the en-"lightenment" of losing a large amount of weight, and ridding yourself of a lot of the emotional load you carry as part and parcel of being overweight. With that being said, we think it prudent to tell you a little bit about the authors of this book, as we are going to be your guides through portions of your investigation and enlightenment process. We also thought you might like to know a bit about what brought Karen and me to the decision to change our lives, and be rid of the weight forever.

JULIE

My name is Julie Janeway, and for as long as I can remember I was overweight. Not just overweight, but until high school, always the tallest kid in school too. Like you, I tried every diet under the sun, and a few of them even worked for a short while. But, the weight always came back – with a vengeance! Although I wasn't happy with the fact that I was overweight, I just always assumed that it was my lot in life, and God must have made me that way for a reason.

I spent my childhood (growing up in Canada), like most overweight kids, being teased, being picked on, always wanting to fit in, but always a little on the periphery of things socially. I missed out on a lot of things in life because of my weight, but my mother did her utmost to help me diet, teach me to like and respect myself, and make sure that I had whatever I needed to feel and look like the other kids, even if it was only a reasonable facsimile of what they had.

If a particular brand of jeans were the "in" thing, and they weren't made in my size, my mom would take me wherever I needed to go to find something close, but in a plus size. Every store on the hunt, however, was a serious and painful reminder that I couldn't just go where everybody else went to buy those jeans.

Whether or not I could wear the "in" jeans of the moment, I was an intelligent, quick-witted, extrovert in high school, and I didn't lack for friends or school activities to attend. No matter how much I tried to believe I was just like everybody else, I always knew I wasn't like everybody else because of my weight.

My intelligence and wit set me apart somewhat, but my weight was always the true dividing line between "them" and "me." I've asked a million times if I've asked once, "Why am I like this, and they're not?" Maybe I was meant to be overweight in order to force me to focus my life on other things, like education, or helping others, or advocating for others who were disenfranchised from society. Blah, blah, blah…fill in the blank with whatever reason you can think of because no doubt you've had this conversation in your head a zillion times too.

I thought getting a good education would help me feel better about myself, and it did, to a certain extent. I earned an Associate degree in Business as a paralegal, a Bachelor of Business degree, Summa Cum Laude (with four minors!), a Law degree (Magna Cum Laude), a Master degree in Business with high honors, and am now finishing my dissertation on my PhD in Public Administration and Public Policy. Although I am very proud of the fact that I put myself through school on my own dime, and pulled top grades while working a full time job, it still didn't put me right in the center of the zip code for Normal, USA In fact, if anything, it put me further away.

Do I regret getting my education? No! Knowledge is power! But, I was resigned to the fact that I was a heavy girl with a lot of education and a sharp sense of humor, and that just made me radically different from the rest of the world for many, many reasons. I figured that was how I was supposed to be, and I needed to accept it.

I was learning to accept it the best I could, but I never liked it — no, not one bit. Even after law school, I kept trying to lose weight and stay active, as owning your own law firm keeps you hopping. I was always on the hunt for another diet that might be the magic formula for me. I had never even entertained the thought of weight loss surgery, and then April 26, 2001, appeared on the calendar, and life as I knew it changed forever.

That day, I was scheduled to be in three different cities over the day. When I came back to my office after the second court appearance, I was talking to my paralegal about not wanting to drive across the state to appear at this city council hearing as I just had a bad feeling about it. I didn't really feel like it had anything to do with the hearing, I just sort of felt this impending sense of doom. My hearing was at 7:30 p.m., and by 3:30 p.m., I was actually starting to feel a little queasy about going. I even mentioned something to my paralegal, and she assured me I was just tired from driving around the state all day.

So away I went with my paralegal's voice echoing in my head that I was just tired out. As I was driving through Grand Rapids (I live in Michigan), traffic started to pick up, and I knew I'd hit rush hour. It was 5:50 p.m., and not only was it rush hour, it was happy hour too. I changed lanes from the right to the left to allow for the traffic merging onto the highway.

I noticed a brand new black Sunfire coming up the on-ramp very fast. I noticed it partly because it was moving so fast, but also because I'd been looking at buying one just days before. This particular Sunfire had completely blacked out windows, and I noticed that because completely blacked out windows are illegal in Michigan. I carried on my merry way, slowing to about 72 miles per hour in the left lane (traffic speed), and assumed all was as it should be. The black Sunfire had the entire empty right lane in which to merge, and I thought that would be that. Wrong!

The Sunfire merged into the right lane, and then decided that it had to immediately be in the left lane, and swerved directly in front of me, clipping the right front corner of my car. The hit shoved me onto the gravel shoulder of the road. I tried to correct the swerve, but the car was now sliding sideways on the gravel, and that was all she wrote folks! The car rolled twice, then went end over end, and then rolled two more times before sliding to a stop on its roof on the shoulder of the right lane of the road.

As the car began to flip over I stiffened and braced myself, and then something told me to relax or I'd end up breaking every bone in my body. So I went limp, and went for the ride of my life. After the first roll, the driver side window smashed out, and the seatbelt fixture ripped away from the wall of the car. I was no longer strapped in, so I was thrown around pretty good. At one point I was even in the back seat! As I was being tossed about, I distinctly remember thinking that this must be what running shoes feel like when they're in the dryer!

Unfortunately as the car rolled and skidded, my left leg got out the driver side smashed window, and it got pretty badly crushed. Much of my lower leg was actually missing, but I didn't know it at that time. I just remember feeling it scraping along the road, and using all my energy to lift my leg up and away from the road because I thought, "That's not good...."

The amazing thing about my accident is that not one other car hit me as I rolled in front of a pretty heavy flow of traffic on Interstate 96 at rush hour. People ran to help, and I tried to determine whether I was dead or alive. I reasoned that if I could actually have that conversation in my head, I must be alive. (I think, therefore I am....) I tried to sit up (I was now laying on the roof of the car because it was upside down), and my back was pretty sore. I remember thinking, "Oh man! I'm going to end up looking like a human question mark for at least a week over this! I've seriously pulled some muscles!"

Despite the pain in my back, I sat up anyway, and noticed all the glass around me. I didn't seem to be bleeding, so I guessed I was okay. I quickly noticed that the entire dashboard had come out of the car, and virtually nothing was where it should be. There were no windows left, the center armrest was in the back seat, and what was left of my cell phone was a tangled and melted mess.

Then I remembered my leg, and how it had been dragging on the pavement. Strangely, I couldn't feel any pain, so I thought it must just be a little cut or something. I pulled myself up far enough to look at it, and as soon as I saw it, I thought two things: "Oh crap, that's probably going to require surgery," and "Huh, fat really is yellow."

Then the pain hit me. It hit so hard that I thought the car had been hit by a semi-truck. I laid back down and just began screaming because it was the only thing I knew to do. The pain was excruciating, but somehow it confirmed for me that I was alive. People came to help, police and fire trucks eventually arrived, and I was taken to Spectrum Hospital in Grand Rapids.

Spectrum Hospital is a level one regional trauma center, and a fantastic hospital. To make a long story short (because that's another book entirely), they took phenomenal care of me for the months I spent there recovering. They saved my leg, they treated my broken back (three vertebrae and three squashed discs), and they saved my life. I'll always be eternally grateful.

So how does all this relate to this book? Well here's how it came to be. Because my leg was almost completely destroyed in the accident, they gave me little chance of keeping it. Three inches of the bone was missing for crying out loud, not to mention most of the muscles were gone. Besides all the medication and surgeries (one every second day for over a month), they said I had to be plied with as much calcium and nutrition as they could get into me to keep the bone and tissues alive.

I could have cared less about eating while I was in the hospital because I was so stoked-out on Morphine and other pain killers, plus being constantly doped up with anesthetic to go into surgery, so food was not on the priority list. They force-fed me almost, and I hated every second of it.

When I came home from the hospital, I was still completely bed-bound, and I had 'round the clock nurses and caregivers who were instructed to get as much calcium and other nutrients into me as humanly possible. By that time, I was so stinking sick of somebody trying to shove ice cream in my face, I thought I'd become homicidal! I remember pleading that I didn't want any more cheese, or milkshakes, or ice cream because I was going to put on more weight, and how would I get it off?

They told me to worry about saving my leg now, and worry about getting rid of the fat later. All fine and good if you're not on the fat end of the stick! So on the pounds went over those two and a half years of recovery. Ten, twenty, forty, eighty, a hundred pounds. Arrrgggghhhhh.....!!!!! I cringe just thinking about it! I was heavy to begin with, I didn't need any more weight. Especially when they kept telling me I would never walk again. I was determined to walk again, and I was determined to get that stupid weight off me. After all, I didn't even get to enjoy putting it on!

So I told my amazing orthopedic surgeon, Dr. John Stubbart, (the man who helped save my leg), that I was thinking about having gastric bypass surgery done, because now I was so heavy I couldn't even get out of the wheelchair by myself. I told him that I was determined to *walk* down the aisle to marry my fiance Matt, and I wasn't going to spend my married life fat, or in a wheelchair!

I also talked to him about my medical concerns, not the least of which was yet another surgery and more scars. He told me about a bariatric surgeon named Dr. Randal Baker and his two partners Dr. James Foote and Dr. Paul Kemmeter. He told me that not only were they highly qualified and experienced surgeons, but they did the gastric bypass procedure laparoscopically, so it wasn't as invasive a surgery. Less invasive means less scars, and to me that was a better option because I'd had enough invasive surgery, and the lower half of me looks like a map drawn by Rand-McNally!

So off I went to see Dr. Baker, and the rest is history. I started at 368 lbs., and was a size 28. Now I'm down 190 lbs. and am a size 12/14. I walk very well thank you very much, and my leg and back are profoundly glad I did it.

Just prior to having my surgery, however, I went back to work at a new college as a professor, and met my new boss Karen Sparks, Dean of Business Administration and Technology. We became immediate friends, almost on sight. We were kindred spirits in more ways than one.

And with that, I think now is a good time for Karen to introduce herself to you. So, here, in her own words is Karen to tell you about how she came to the decision to have weight loss surgery.

KAREN

Hello, my name is Karen Sparks. I'm going to tell you about how I came to have weight loss surgery, but to do that entails telling you a little about my life, as I didn't have any one particular defining moment or event that caused me to make the decision. Instead, it was the culmination of a lifetime of events that lead me to a surgical option. I'm not afraid to say that what you're about to read was pretty hard for me to dredge up and face again. It was very hard to write, but for better or worse, and as painful as it is, here we go....

I was heavy all of my life. Even as a very young child I knew I was different. Fat, heavy, big boned, chubby, what ever you want to call it, that was me. I've spent an incalculable amount of time in my life asking, "Why did I have to be this way?" or "Why me?" As far back as I can remember, I just wanted to be normal.

From grade school through high school, I just wanted to be like everyone else. I watched as my sister picked out cute clothes from about any store we visited. My options were limited to the "chubby girls" section at Sears or Montgomery Ward. Christmas after Christmas came and went wherein I received clothes that always had to be returned; the clothes never fit, no matter the good intentions. Christmas after Christmas came and went with me putting on a brave and happy face to cover the disappointment, embarrassment, and pain of not being normal.

Disappointment and embarrassment weren't limited to Christmas though. I never got invited to birthday parties, sleepovers, school dances, or the prom. I constantly had to hide my disappointment with a laissez-faire attitude, and half a loaf of bread and butter helped soothe the pain a bit too. Countless hours were spent crying in silence and solitude on the floor in the back of my closet.

Always an outsider, the only thing that allowed me to be a part of things was my art, a good sense of humor, and the fact that I was smart. Everyone knew that "Sparky" could draw. No one could compete with me on that, and they knew it. "Sparky" was funny, she could always take a joke, no matter how pointed or mean it might be. And "Sparky" was smart. She always had the answers, and was willing to teach others how to find them when need be. That was how I participated: on the fringe of things with a smile on my face.

I was a participant only in the background, in the shadows where I didn't have to worry about being seen, but I desperately wanted to be seen. I watched as my older brother and sister went to dances and the prom, and out on weekend dates with their boyfriends and girlfriends. I watched as they picked out the special clothes and other things that come along with the rites of passage through your teen years, and I faced the pain of knowing that somehow I would never get to share in those experiences.

Later, came my younger brother following the same path of "normal" childhood activities, special memories, and events. Instead of "normal" childhood and adolescent activities, I spent my time with my books and my drawings. I played in the school band because it was a place where I could be a part of something "normal." But still, I sat too many hours on the floor in my closet crying and asking my mom, "When will it be my turn?" "Why do I have to be this way?" "Will there ever be anyone for me?" "What did I do to deserve this?" And many, many other questions she could never answer.

I spent the greater part of my school years just wanting people to like me, and trying desperately to be like everyone else; or at least convince myself I was like everyone else. Deep in my heart I knew though, it was not going to happen for me because I wasn't "normal," and I wasn't thin.

There, too, was the pain of sitting in the kitchen with mom anxiously trying to help me in any way that she could to "diet." I distinctly remember sitting at the kitchen table at age 12 one summer day eating the tuna fish and cottage cheese mom had prepared for my lunch, as once again, we were trying to lose weight. I remember too many of those days throughout my life. I kept wishing there was a way to just lose the weight forever. Later that year, I found what I thought was my great white hope.

My first knowledge of weight loss surgery was as early as 1970, during my 7th grade year of Jr. High. At that time, I read in the local paper of a doctor who was performing stomach stapling surgery in Hudson, not too far from my hometown of Jonesville, Michigan. I knew my parents would never be able to afford it, nor would they most likely ever even consider letting me go through the surgery at such a young age. Too young to pursue the program, I pushed it to the back of my mind with all my other hopes and dreams, and suffered with my weight problems through junior high and high school.

After high school I buried myself with work, two, sometimes three jobs at a time. I spent my money in ways that I hoped would make people like me. Instead of clothes and vacations with girlfriends, I bought tens of thousands of dollars worth of ornaments and collectibles. I spent my spare time always being the one to make things better for everyone else — the fix-it person, despite my own wants and needs. There never seemed to be anyone making it better for me though. Why was I so alone, and so different?

At one time I did briefly drop 100 lbs. over a summer, but I did it in a very unhealthy way. I was taking diet pills by the handful, and the weight just dropped off. As soon as I stopped taking the drugs, however, I immediately put the weight back on plus another 150 lbs. I was terrified that my weight would never stop going up. It seemed to me that it didn't matter what I ate, it simply made me gain weight. I was losing the fight, and I couldn't get an answer to the question, "Why?"

In trying to find that answer, there comes a point where you rationalize that God made you this way for a reason. Was I destined always just to be there to help everyone else get through their lives and be happy? Was I destined to be the rock and the make-it-better person for everyone else? Maybe so. But if that was true, what did I get out of the deal? I decided that what I got must be something to make me feel better, while helping to fix everyone else's life — an education.

I decided to go to college when I was 32 years old hoping that would change things for me. Unfortunately, no matter how educated you are the "fat prejudice" still follows you around. Because of that, social situations didn't change much at college. Still, going to school became a passion, as I could be noticed for being smart there, but it held little consolation for the events to which I was not invited, was too old, or was simply forgotten about. Overall, it was no different than my previous school years. Why I thought it would be different, I don't know.

I may not have been the life of the party while at college, but I did earn a Bachelor degree in Business Administration (Summa Cum Laude), and went on for a Master degree in Business Education. I'd acquired the degrees, and I had the intelligence, yet I didn't feel a bit more normal because of my weight.

As I once again searched for a way to lose weight (and I tried them all mind you), I came to the conclusion that I was forever destined to be overweight and never to be normal. I thought I could accept that, if it weren't for the part of me that knew that with all the science and discovery in our world, someone should be able to come up with something to help me. Why weren't they finding it? Why wasn't I finding it? Then I stumbled across the concept of weight loss surgery again.

Once I began to research weight loss surgery more seriously, I came to understand that there was help out there. How to get to it became my next hurdle. After five years of research, mounds of information from the Internet, and mailings from a multitude of organizations that were willing to do the job, I was just not satisfied with any of them. Those who were good enough by my standards weren't remotely close enough geographically. I began to get really discouraged.

To be truthful, it was during the summer of 2003, that I knew I had to do something about my weight, as I was dangerously close to being in serious trouble. At that time, my weight was at its highest, 425 lbs., and I was flirting carelessly with high blood pressure. I had been researching weight loss surgery with little success in finding a program I believed to be sound, and then came the day I met Julie Janeway.

I was the Dean of Business and Technology at a small college. Julie had sent me her resume looking for work as a professor, and I just happened to need someone with her credentials and experience to head up a department. I knew we were destined to be friends from the first exchange of voicemail messages. It was Julie who shared with me her knowledge of Dr. Baker and his staff at Michigan Weight Loss Specialists in Grand Rapids, Michigan. That was a major turning point in my life. I was intrigued, if not a little wary, but I decided to find out the details.

I researched Michigan Weight Loss Specialists and Dr. Baker, went to an orientation, had all my questions answered, came home satisfied, and a little scared. What I'd waited for, a potentially permanent solution to my weight issues, was now staring me in the face. I struggled with the decision whether or not to go for it. In my head I could hear Julie's sister Cheryl telling me that I "could do anything afraid, that I could do unafraid." Believing in that, all I had to do was think about all I had missed in my life, and the decision was made.

When I had surgery I weighed 425 lbs. and was wearing a size 34 to 36. Now I have lost 245 lbs., and wear a size 14. I will never go back to where I was before. Just sitting down to write this is as much of that type of pain and heartache as I can bear, let alone actually having to relive it. I am a new person now, and I'm enjoying finding out who was hiding inside me all those years. I don't know if I could have done it alone, but Julie and I resolved to go through the process together, and together we'll help take you through it as well.

OUR SURGERIES

Karen and I went through our surgeries together…well sort of. I had my surgery done on October 29, 2003, which was the day after my birthday (Happy Birthday to me). I took a slot that was vacated by someone who had cancelled, and I only had eleven days notice. Immediately I went on the protein program that you must complete before the surgery to shrink your liver, and take some pressure off your heart, and went through a whirlwind of medical tests to make sure I was in good shape for a Roux-en-Y gastric bypass. I got through everything just Jim-Dandy-fine, and the next thing I knew I was there, and it was happening.

Karen lived through those first few weeks before and after surgery with me. She watched everything I went through during that time. She watched me trying to avoid food during that pre-op period, and she watched me get progressively more scared as the time neared. She helped me as best she could, and she made mental notes, because she was scheduled for the same surgery on December 12, 2003.

Karen had it a little tougher, pre-operatively speaking. She was on the protein program for the full two weeks prior to surgery, which covered Thanksgiving. Thanksgiving with Karen's family is one of those affairs you see on T.V. It's kind of like an Osmond family reunion: tons of relatives, lots of food, all happy happy. Karen loves these occasions, as she's such a family oriented person. It was extremely hard for her not to eat that day.

Additionally, Karen came home from the hospital the day before her birthday (which traditionally involves her family making her all her favorite foods), and she was still on the all-protein protocol through Christmas and New Years! Never a braver soul have I met. The only consolation she had during these post-surgical times was that she really didn't give a rip whether or not she ate. Surgery does that to you.

But once we were both through the surgery, we kept each other afloat. We worked at making sure the other had eaten properly, had their water allotment, and taken their vitamins. We walked together, got sick together, and encouraged each other through plateaus. Despite a few rough patches that we'll discuss in later chapters, we made it through in fine style on the buddy system, and with the careful ministerings of Dr. Baker and his staff.

Dr. Baker, Dr. Foote, Dr. Kemmeter, and the rest of the staff at Michigan Weight Loss Specialists in Grand Rapids, took extremely good care of us. In fact, every patient to whom we've spoken, has raved about the care they've received at this facility. As you search for a bariatric surgeon in your area, you should be expecting to find a surgeon who cares about you as an individual, and whose staff cares equally as much.

There are many first-rate bariatric surgeons across the country that utilize the multi-disciplinary approach to weight loss surgery. This entails the use of internal medicine specialists, behaviorists, dietitians, exercise physiologists, plastic surgeons, and of course trained bariatric (not just general) surgeons. We've included in the Additional Resources chapter a web site address for the American Society for Metabolic and Bariatric Surgery that has links to outstanding surgeons and bariatric medicine practices across the country to assist you in finding a practice that will take excellent care of you.

So you'll have an idea what to look for in a doctor, we'll kind of give you an introduction to our third co-author, Dr. Randal Baker. He's going to tell you a bit about why he became a bariatric surgeon, and then we'll sing his praises by relating to you a few of his fine qualities and credentials.

RANDAL S. BAKER, MD, FACS

So, how does one end up becoming a bariatric surgeon? I never remember waking up as a six-year-old boy declaring my intense desire to become a bariatric surgeon! In fact, after graduating from Calvin College in Grand Rapids, and Albany Medical College of New York, I never dreamed I would be involved in the battle against obesity. I had no significant exposure to bariatric surgery during medical school or residency, and planned for a quiet, hometown general surgical practice, with an emphasis in trauma and critical care.

During my Critical Care Fellowship, I did help treat several bariatric patients with significant complications who were sent to the Tertiary Care, Surgical Intensive Care Unit, but that was years before I ended up moving my practice into bariatric surgery. At the time, it didn't really pique my interest, maybe because I was only dealing with the intensive care portion of the process.

Several years later, after I became the Medical Director of the Surgical ICU and Assistant Director of the General Surgery Residency Program at Spectrum Hospital in Grand Rapids, Michigan, I was approached by one of our major HMOs to consider starting a bariatric surgical program. My practice group's physician medical practice already had a comprehensive, multi-disciplinary medical weight loss program (non-surgical). The HMO asked if we could develop a similar multi-disciplinary approach to bariatric surgery. The request grew out of the fact that many surgical programs were offering no more than surgery, providing only tidbits of information, and lacking adequate pre-operative and post-operative care.

As I was plenty busy with trauma, critical care, general surgery, and my family (wife and 7 children at this point), I was warned by other surgeons not to enter the bariatric arena, as it would completely engulf my practice, and encroach on all other elements. With the best of intentions, they also warned that morbidly obese patients were higher risk and can have significant complications, which can be taxing even for the most solid and laid back person. After much consideration and deliberation, however, and after about six months of continual prodding, the decision was made to create a surgical program. I did my didactics and medical trauma training at the University of Pittsburgh Medical Center, and I've been hooked ever since.

To this day, I do not regret this decision at all. The bariatric practice did engulf my practice such that I stopped doing trauma, and other general surgery. Our center also had the opportunity to obtain two top-notch, caring surgeons in Dr. James Foote and Dr. Paul Kemmeter, both of whom were also trained in surgery and critical care. At times the trek through establishing this program has been trying and onerous, but I have no regrets.

In fact, I'm grateful for the course my professional life has taken. I have never had the opportunity to see such great benefits accrue in people's lives as a result of surgical treatment, as I have with bariatric surgery. Words become insufficient in trying to relay the emotion I experience as patients go through a metamorphosis, and come back with tears in their eyes to describe their "new" world.

Emotion is also deep when patients experiencing complications or difficulty dealing with emotional issues go through trying times in an attempt to reach their "new" world. I can do the surgery, care for them medically, support them physically and emotionally, but I can't always make it better with a treatment or a prescription. I truly wish I could find a way to help even more.

As a result I have encouraged many of my patients to write a book about their weight loss surgery experiences, but to date, none of them had taken the challenge. Little did I know that two highly educated, motivated, and caring women would cross my path, and write what I consider to be the best-researched and written weight loss book on the market for the general public. This book is the "real deal," no sugar-coated Hollywood fairy story here.

Although greater than 90% of bariatric patients experience no significant complications, it is important that patients recognize that complications do happen and can be significant in any surgery, including weight loss surgery. It so happens, however, that most bariatric complications are over "media-ized." Over a given period of time in a large hospital several patients may have complications and even die from joint replacement, or elective, general, and plastic surgery, or complications from obesity in general, yet it's the bariatric surgical cases that draw all the media attention. So don't buy into the media hype: just do your homework, weigh the risks, and make your own decision in consultation with your doctor.

Julie and Karen have spent a lot of time and energy researching this topic and attempting to relay it in an understandable form. They also share my style of humor, so this will not be your typical, dry factoid — "here's my story" — type of publication.

As I'm truly just a humble surgeon from Grand Rapids, I'll let Julie and Karen take over now for the necessary, but boring credentials section.

Thank you Dr. Baker. Let's hear it for a truly caring guy who understands that overweight people are people too. Yeahhhh !!!!! All right, simmer down now. On to the credentials section:

As you read previously, Dr. Baker specializes in bariatric surgery and has had significant experience as a general surgeon prior to his bariatric practice. He is board certified by the American Board of Surgery and is a Fellow of the American College of Surgery. He completed a Fellowship in Critical Care and holds an additional certificate for Critical Care through the American Board of Surgery. Dr. Baker presently serves as the Medical Director of the Surgical Intensive Care Units at Spectrum Hospital, and is an Assistant Professor of Surgery at Michigan State University. He is a member of the American Society for Metabolic and Bariatric Surgery, the American Medical Association, and the Society of Critical Care Medicine.

Dr. Baker is also a 2005 award nominee for the Outstanding Achievement Award of the American Society for Metabolic and Bariatric Surgery Foundation. This award is given for significant contributions to the advancement of bariatric surgery, and representation of the highest ideals of the ASBMS. As a nominee for this award Dr. Baker stands alongside some of the greatest medical minds in the world today, and his innovative ideas and contributions are most worthy of the praise. He is also a proud past recipient of the American College of Surgeons Transplantation Award.

Dr. Baker has researched, published, and lectured extensively on the topics of morbid obesity, bariatric surgery, and surgical critical care, and is on the Editorial Board of the prestigious Obesity Surgery journal, a publication of international reputation in the medical community. He was also instrumental in the development of a bio-absorbable staple line product to decrease bleeding and leaks from staple lines.[1] This product won the 2002 American Medical Innovation of the Year award.

Following the development of that sealant, Drs. Baker, Foote, and Kemmeter presented and published a landmark study on *"The Science of Stapling and Leaks"* in the *Obesity Surgery* journal.[2] Portions of this research were presented at the International Federation for the Surgery of Obesity (IFSO) Conference in Spain in 2003. The research received the prestigious international Inamed Award, which consisted of a 60 lb. statue that had to be carted back to the USA and through customs in an unruly, coarse, wooden box.

The credentials that he considers most important though, are those of husband and father of nine (yes... **9**...) wonderful children! (No, he is not Catholic or Mormon, which are the most common questions he and his wife are asked when out in public.) He is a caring and attentive family man, and has been known to take the afternoon off work to take all of his children to see a Harry Potter movie. He's even cut meetings short with us to make sure he made it to one of his kid's basketball games (and that's one of the few good reasons to cut short a meeting with us, we'll tell you!)

In addition to all his amazing credentials, he is actually a caring doctor with a wonderful bedside manner! It helps to have a doctor with a good sense of humor, but he's also very careful not to make you laugh right after surgery. Dr. Baker is also just an all around nice person who cares deeply about his patients, attempting to help them find new, healthy, and enjoyable lives. He and his partners have surrounded themselves with staff of a similar ethic, those who have intense empathy for their patients through the "thick and thin" of the whole weight loss process.

We truly believe that there are many other "Dr. Baker" type bariatric surgeons out there that are just ready, willing, and able to help you make this important decision, and carry you through to a happy ending if you choose to proceed. We've talked to many people across the country who've had positive experiences similar to ours, and we hope you find your "Dr. Baker" soon.

Unfortunately, however, we've talked to more people who've not found a "Dr. Baker," but instead have found a "Dr. Frankenstein," or worse, a "Dr. Jekyll and Mr. Hyde." It is for them that this book came into being. We hope you'll love yourself enough to expect that your doctor will care about you the way Dr. Baker and his partners care about their patients. You deserve nothing less.

SCOTT H. GLASS, MS, MA, LLP

Scott, Scott, Scott. What to say about Scott? We just love him!! Scott is a limited licensure psychologist in Dr. Baker's practice. He holds a Master degree in Counseling Psychology from Western Michigan University, and a Master degree in Exercise Physiology from the University of Michigan. Scott received his dual Bachelor degrees from Calvin College in Grand Rapids in the areas of Physical Education, and Recreation. He has also studied Rehabilitation Psychology at Michigan State University. (Yes folks, he's yet another overachiever in the bunch. He's attended almost as many education institutions as I have!)

Scott worked as an exercise physiologist for about six years, and then moved into the counseling arena, where he has since focused the majority of his time. In working with weight loss surgery patients, he now uses both disciplines for which he was educated and trained. He is a wonderful, caring man, with a peace about him that is comforting when times are tough. Scott is able to help patients through many of their emotional, physical, behavioral, and even spiritual struggles, and we know that we couldn't have done it without him.

Scott grew up with four brothers, so we've adopted him into our families so he'd finally have some sisters. Too bad he got stuck with us!! Better luck next time, buddy!

Scott tells us that his professional goal is to improve the health, productivity, and quality of life of his patients through effective counseling and leadership. We can swear under oath (and I don't take that lightly), that he meets and exceeds his goal each and every day.

CARRIE A. LIEBROCK, RD

Carrie Liebrock needs your help! She is a registered dietitian with the most unrealistic, pathetic, plastic food models you've ever seen in your life sitting on her desk! We know they're there to give patients ideas and show portion sizes, but she really needs new plastic food that looks even remotely real! For crying out loud, little kids have more realistic plastic food than Carrie has! Send your pledges to 1-900-HELP-CARRIE-NOW (just kidding).

We tease her about her silly plastic food every time we go in her office. I even had to tease her through the tears when I had stricture difficulties and couldn't eat anything. That's how bad the plastic food is; it makes you comment even when you're being self-absorbed. Maybe that was her evil plan all along...?

Anyway, Carrie is a serious ray of sunshine at Dr. Baker's practice, goofy plastic food or not. She received her Bachelor of Science degree in Dietetics from the College of Human Ecology at Michigan State University. Two years later, Carrie completed a Dietetic Internship Certification in South Dakota, and presently serves as a registered dietitian for Drs. Baker, Foote, and Kemmeter.

Carrie has worked in several hospitals including Foote Hospital in Jackson, Michigan, Avera Sacred Heart Hospital in Yankton, South Dakota, and Covenant Health Care in Saginaw, Michigan. She's a wonderful source for nutrition information and practical weight loss strategies, and a delight to have around. We're very happy to be working with her on this project. We promise, in the interest of her patients, some of the proceeds from this book will go to buy her new plastic food.

NABILA AHMED-SARWAR, PharmD, BCPS, CDE

Hi. Karen here. I ripped the lap-top out of Julie's hands because I wanted to write the bio about Nabila. Julie needs to go feed the husband and the cats anyway.

Dr. Nabila Ahmed-Sarwar, "Nabs" to Julie and me, is the latest addition to our "Big Giant Brain" collective. Dr. Ahmed-Sarwar is a funny, kind, caring person who seeks nothing more in this world than to use her incredible heart, and her incredible intelligence to find better ways to help others. We first met her in April of 2006, when she came with a colleague from Ferris State University to assist with a presentation on drug issues and bariatric patients for our Lansing support group. We have been nothing less than ridiculously impressed since day one. Besides, she has two "fur-children" named Moto and Mao-Mao. That clinched it for us. For those of you who are the pet of a cat, you understand.

Dr. Ahmed-Sarwar is from Toronto, Canada...yes, yet another Canadian. Julie always says that the Canadians are taking over the world. She says that they are very up-front about the fact that they are taking over the world starting with the United States, it's just that nobody ever takes them seriously. She says that's why the plan will work.... I think that the reason so many of them are in the states is because secretly they disguise themselves as Canadian geese, fly across the borders into the United States and land undetected in the farmlands of rural America. Once on dry land, they venture into the cities at night, and shed their goose exteriors to shop until they drop and get big sports contracts with the NHL. Well, that's my theory and I'm sticking too it.... But, back to Dr. A.

Just recently Dr. Ahmed-Sarwar was married to Dr. Muhammad "Faisal" Sarwar, an esteemed anesthesiologist in Syracuse, New York. Julie and I had the honor of actually participating in this lavish wedding steeped in the traditions of India and Pakistan. We wore all the traditional clothes (thanks for the loan Nabs) and the jewelry too. Julie was second only to the bride in the jewelry department! Bling IS her thing!

Dr. Ahmed-Sarwar holds a bachelor of science and doctorate in Pharmacy from Midwestern University - Chicago, is a Board Certified Pharmocotherapy Specialist (BCPS), and is a Certified Diabetes Educator (CDE). Yes, you guessed it...another "Big Giant Brain!" She is currently an Assistant Professor of Pharmacy Practice at Ferris State University, and an Adjunct Assistant Professor at Michigan State University College of Human Medicine, Department of Family Practice. In addition to her teaching duties, she also runs medication therapy management and diabetes patient clinics, and until recently was a part-time community pharmacist, and has been for the last ten years so she would not forget what it was like to work every day with patients and their specific concerns and issues.

And Dr. Ahmed-Sarwar really understands people's every day concerns too. Especially when it's weight related issues, as she has fought with her weight all her life as well. Although she is not a bariatric surgery patient, she still understands the struggles, the medical issues, and the experiences of those of you reading this book. She truly works amazingly hard to help weight management patients, surgical or not, make their lives better. All you need to do is talk to her to know how sincere and committed she is to helping any person struggling with weight and weight related issues find a healthier, happier life. Plus, her infectious smile and giddy school-girl giggle just kind of make your day! So, welcome to Dr. Nabila Ahmed-Sarwar. We hope she becomes as good a friend to you as she has been to us.

Oh, I see that the husband and the cats must be under control now. Julie's back, so I guess I'll relinquish the lap-top and let her continue on with the story.

OK. Where was I... oh yes... now that we've introduced you to everyone, I bet you're wondering just how this book came to be. (Well, if you weren't we're going to tell you anyway.) It really wasn't because Dr. Baker asked us to write one. By the time he met us, he'd pretty much stopped asking patients to write a book because no one seemed to have either the time, or the inclination. Nope. This book came about in a whole different way. Here's the real skinny on the...

BIRTH OF A BOOK

The inspiration for this book came from a rather strange source: a garage sale. In the summer of 2004, Karen and I found ourselves gasping for air under a mountain of "too big" clothes. We'd already shrunk through about four sizes each when we decided to have a garage sale and let others adopt our beloved clothing. After all, many of them were never worn, and some still even had the tags attached. As each piece was lovingly hunted down in true bargain-hunter style, we simply couldn't let them rot and mold in a garage somewhere, so we put them up for sale.

As professional women, we both have to dress up for work, and the money we'd put into our clothes was significant. A garage sale was our only hope of recouping some of the cash (we needed new clothes...), and seeing our beloved treasures go to good and loving homes. Lots of people came to the sale (more for the man junk my husband had out there than for the clothes), but soon a trend began to emerge.

The majority of the women who were there to look at the clothes also had weight loss surgery. Of course, they were curious as to why two women were selling a Bloomingdale's worth of clothing, and in no time at all a bond was forming over scars, clothes, tears, and lost pounds.

What struck us though, were the stories that accompanied those scars. You see, Karen and I have virtually no scars to speak of, while *all* of the women we met had great long scars (and some of them rather vicious looking) up their torsos from their surgeries. They told stories of how they got those scars too, and all of them involved a mass of miscommunications, omissions, and outdated information.

The stories centered around women (and they told of men they knew as well), that were sick of their weight issues and sought knowledge and help from medical professionals they trusted, literally, with their lives. We heard story after story of people who went to this center, and that clinic, and received not much more service than you get from the overworked and underpaid waitress at a greasy spoon.

We heard stories like the one told to us by a young woman who went to a bariatric surgery clinic, was told briefly about the surgery, and waited while they checked to see if her insurance would pay. They sent her home to wait for an authorization, and when it was received they booked her surgery. She showed up at the hospital on surgery day, had a full open procedure done ("zippers" I call them), spent one and a half days in the hospital, and was sent home. She was told to drink Slimfast®, and come back to the office in two weeks to have her stitches out.

When she showed up two weeks later, they removed her stitches, handed her a meal plan on a single sheet of paper, and wished her well. No orientation, no pre-operative testing, no counseling, no follow-up, no nutritional counseling, no answers to her questions — nothing. Just thanks for the money and the memories lady. See ya, wouldn't want to be ya.

By the way, our young friend was experiencing horrible nausea, vomiting, and diarrhea multiple times a day. She had the shakes, and would break out in cold sweats. She said she was worried she had a heart problem because her heart would race so. When she called for help in dealing with these symptoms, her surgeon's office said it wasn't his area, and to call her primary care physician.

She was stunned when we told her that the Slimfast®, although a quality product, was not meant for bariatric surgery patients, and that the sugar content was probably causing some of her symptoms. Additionally, it has a milk base, and some patients become lactose intolerant after surgery, so that might account for some of her symptoms too. She was further dumbfounded when we told her that the large quantity of orange and apple juice she was taking in six to seven times a day was probably also making her sick; a phenomenon known as dumping syndrome (see

Chapter Five – Auto Eject). Since two weeks after her surgery, her surgeon's office misguidedly recommended she drink fruit juices all day long to curb her need to eat sweets and other foods. Apparently no one told her that too much sugar would make her sick, not to mention she was ingesting tons of calories that weren't giving her much nutrition, giving her no protein, and not helping her feel full or satisfied. We sent her to another surgeon who could properly evaluate her and help her out.

We also heard from a 5 ft. 10 in. woman who only (it's all relative...) had 90 lbs. to lose, who also had a hack-job zipper-procedure done. Although open procedures can be done well resulting in almost invisible scars, this was not one of those instances. She was in tears when she saw (or rather had to help hunt for), Karen's almost non-existent laparoscopic incision scars. We were appalled at the assembly line approach that was taken in her case as well. Again, no orientation, no counseling, no medical work-up, no follow-up. Nothing. Just here's your bill, and don't let the operating room door hit you in the butt on the way out!

When we told these people of our experiences with weight loss surgery, there were more than a few tears of envy and regret I'll tell you. We reasoned there simply had to be a place to go for people who need potentially life-saving information in order to get the real scoop and skinny from people who've been there, not just people who stand to make a profit from others' misery. Thus, this book was born.

Karen and I talked it over, and because we're two college professors whose job it is to research, write, and bring the light of knowledge to the masses (pathetic, aren't we?...), we decided that we were the perfect people to write this book; except for the medical part.

For that we needed Dr. Baker: our friend, our physician, our trusted medical savior. So we cornered him at the hospital on the way into surgery, and told him he was going to co-author a book to help people just like the patient lying there on the gurney before him. Not exactly in a position to say no, he agreed, and we had witnesses.

Actually, we did corner him at the hospital, but he was more than exhilarated to be a part of this project. He was all pumped up about it, and had thoughts and ideas just flying through his mind. He was virtually bouncing around the room with excitement as he left to go back to surgery. I often wonder about that day... and, well... I hope things went okay for that patient, and the surgery wasn't too delicate a procedure. I've never asked, but I'm sure all went just swimmingly....

So, here it is. The culmination of a lot of thinking, sharing, analysis, research, experience, and caring. We all hope that you find the answers and the information you need in this book. If nothing else, at least find the questions you need to ask to save your own life.

In the immortal (paraphrased) words
from Shakespeare's Macbeth, "Read on, MacDuff."

Chapter Three

THE NEW AND IMPROVED, AMAZING, ALL NATURAL LEMON DIET

Randal S. Baker MD, FACS

...Stay tuned for scenes from tomorrow's episode of <u>As The Stomach Turns</u>. And now a word from our sponsor:

> *(Announcer) Are you tired of struggling with your weight? Tired of all the typical diets without any success? Is the mirror considered one of your foes? Do you need more energy, and want to break free from the heavy bondage of extra weight? Does your sex life need help? Is climbing stairs a chore? Sick of the décor at Subway®? High blood pressure getting you down? Is fat around your belly, hips, and thighs a source of entertainment at family gatherings? Well the answer is finally here! Doc Baker's New and Improved, Amazing, All Natural Lemon Diet.*
>
> *Yes, you heard right. Nature has provided the necessary weight combating "delta force" in this lemon-based anti-fat, anti-oxidant, low-carb, low-sugar, anti-leptin, anti-ghrelin, appetite-suppressing, sleep-improving, non-stimulant, caffeine-free, ephedra-free, recipe-enhancing dietary supplement. One pinch of this potent concentrated lemon extract before each meal and every mouthful of food will just chase the calories away.*
>
> *Why, Hanky Snider of Hooterville, USA, lost 40 lbs. in just one month using Doc's powerful and amazing, all natural lemon-based elixir. Hanky, who once shunned being seen in public, now leads tours through extensive subterranean caves. "Many of my tour people have asked the secret of my youthful vitality, energy, and weight loss. I tell them they must check out Doc's health-inducing, all natural, cortisol-blocking, age-reversing, skin-tightening, intestinal-cleansing, fat-trapping, hair-growing supplement. It's the greatest!"*
>
> *Even model-actress Barbie Beauty lost 30 lbs. in only two weeks using the life-enhancing, strength-reviving product. "Why, I even lost weight while sleeping at night, and dropped 3 dress sizes to a 2. And I wasn't even dreaming about weight loss or exercise! Huh.... Anyway, all the studios are calling now, and I've had to hire a secretary just to answer my calls! Thanks, Doc Baker. You're my hero!"*
>
> *Sound unbelievable? Well it is!!! Doc Baker's New and Improved, Amazing, All Natural Lemon Diet is much too powerful for those of you who only have a couple of vanity pounds to lose. Noooo! You need to be seriously stretched out of shape, at least triple your high school graduation*

*weight, and dissolving from the inside out to be using Doc's Diet. And because we know you no longer want to be mistaken for a float in the Macy's Thanksgiving Day parade, we're only charging $169.99 a bottle for Doc's miracle diet compound. And, if you call now, we'll even send you a second bottle **free** because we know you really need the help. That's TWO bottles of Doc's lemon miracle for only $169.99, plus $10.00 shipping and handling.*

Just try it for yourself! Find out what millions of other grateful and satisfied customers have discovered. They're sold on Doc Baker's New and Improved, Amazing, All Natural Lemon Diet, and you will be too! There's a 100% money back guarantee if you're not totally satisfied! (Just return the bottle with original proof of purchase and the kneecaps of two West African newts and we will completely refund your money!)

What are you waiting for? Call now! 1-999-BIG-CURE. That's 1-999-BIG-CURE. Again, that's 1-999-BIG-CURE. Operators are standing by! Why be fat, ugly, and disease-ridden when you can miraculously change all that, guaranteed? Make the choice for a healthy and a leaner, more beautiful and vivacious body! Buy Doc's all natural, cortisol-binding, weight loss inducing, life-rejuvenating, lemon-based supplement! Call today!

(Results depicted are not typical. Individual results may vary.)

Does this diet diatribe sound all too familiar? A hundred years ago, "snake oil" salesmen used the same pitch to sell their tonics that were guaranteed to "cure whatever ailed ya!" Today, the weight loss "snake oil" salesmen abound, and money spent on diets and weight related products are in the billions. Just slap up some before and after pictures of non-typical customers along with some medical sounding jargon, and almost anything sells as the new version of "snake oil." An overweight, stressed-out, desperate America is looking to any and every "snake oil" salesman for help and a cure for its obesity and weight related problems.

Although we all use the terms *obese*, and *overweight* interchangeably in conversation, medical definitions of the condition exist — and yes, obesity is considered a real health "condition" and disease. The National Institutes of Health (NIH) states that a person is considered *obese* when he or she weighs 20% or more than his or her ideal body weight. At this point, the person's weight poses a real health risk. Obesity becomes *morbid* when it *significantly* increases the risk of one or more obesity related health conditions or serious diseases.

According to national and international researchers, statistics now show that 65% of the U.S. population are overweight or obese, approximately 6% of Americans are morbidly obese, 150 million Europeans are obese, and nearly 2 billion individuals worldwide are classified as overweight or obese, which is about equal to the number of those starving worldwide.[1] The United States now performs about 175,000 bariatric surgeries annually, and the world total is approximately 300,000, yet only about 1% of the eligible morbidly obese population is being offered or can receive the benefits of bariatric surgery.[2] Morbid obesity is a serious chronic disease, meaning that its symptoms build slowly over an extended period of time. The media inundates us with images of "perfect" bodies from childhood on, and yet the obesity epidemic is one of the fastest growing diseases ever! In response, people are always searching for the "easy" way out, the "magic pill," or the "silver bullet;" the instant, simple, no effort required, quick fix for being overweight.

This then, begs the question of what causes obesity. Why is obesity dramatically increasing in our society? Dr. Buffington has given you a good primer on the causes and progressive nature of obesity in the Prologue. If you skipped it, go back and read it now. It's very important stuff.

Obesity, like so many ailments such as alcoholism, is directly related to genetics and environment.[3] Many alcoholics have a genetic predisposition towards alcoholism in that drinking alcohol stimulates certain portions of their brains more so than non-alcoholics.[4]

In obesity, we see that many family relatives share the predisposition toward being overweight. In fact, identical twins separated from birth will both usually have similar weights (including obesity), despite different environmental backgrounds.[5]

Environmental concerns are also important. Overall, obesity is rising as we change our environment from that of our predecessors. We no longer have to run on foot to hunt for food, or labor physically to plant and harvest crops. We do not have to work to prepare and store food either. Food is readily available, especially in calorie dense forms, and is sold in "bigger" sizes. Portion sizes have increased dramatically over the past years as well, and our "bigger" sizes today would have been considered mega-gargantuan in the previous century.

The "typical" 20th century American arises after too little sleep, and eats a breakfast of chocolate super-frosted-sugar balls, while working hard to "hunt" for, and click on the remote to the television. They then "run" to the car, and scurry off to "work" which for many consists of an exhausting day behind a desk typing on a computer. Break time is really more of the same, including sitting and eating snack cakes, soda pop, and way too much coffee. Lunch often consists of "flying" to a fast food restaurant, and not having the gumption to refuse the obnoxious siren call to "super size" your already "bigger sized," calorie packed meal.

Today, in large part, our created environments have allowed genetic predispositions to become dominant and rampant. Poor diets and lack of exercise have even lead to obesity in people who do not have clear familial genetic predispositions.[6] According to the Surgeon General, we are as a nation, dying at varying rates from obesity, and according to a 2005 New England Journal of Medicine Study, the current generation of children will be the first generation in history to have a potentially shorter life expectancy than their parents as a result of obesity and its attendant co-morbidities.[7]

Health care professionals often fail to recognize these multifactorial genetic and environmental predispositions associated with obesity. They sometimes label patients as lazy, unmotivated, or lacking will power. Although that may occasionally be the case, these descriptors are not generally major factors in a vast majority of patient obesity conditions.[8]

As I have given lectures around the country on obesity and obesity surgery, I have confronted intense biases toward obese people. Obesity prejudice is one of the last few remaining bastions of politically correct snobbery. Studies reveal that obese people are prejudged by the general public to be lazy, stupid, unorganized, selfish, and inept.[9] When faced with two substitute teachers who did identical teaching, even school children judged the skinny sub to be the best teacher in all respects.[10] This response is simply an outcropping of a greater societal prejudice that has developed regarding overweight people – a term I call "obesism."

Obesism has infiltrated the medical community despite the intellectual knowledge that obesity is a disease. As a result, obese patients are handed prescriptions that say, "lose weight," or are given poor quality, one-sheet "diet plans," and expected to lose weight. It is like handing a long time drug addict a script that says, "Stop taking drugs." I've even heard one physician tout his well thought out, overarching, anti-obesity plan by announcing in the hospital ward "send them all to the 'fat' farm." What insight....

So, we're living in a society that is biased against overweight people, and face it, you're probably biased too. Even overweight people view other overweight people with such a bias. If we all look at overweight people with such disdain, and we can't resolve that bias even knowing it's false, then the only thing left to do is to resolve the underlying cause. Let's treat the obesity itself, without adding in any obesism biases.

In order to do that, we must base our plan on *evidence*, not just hearsay based on rumor and conjecture sprinkled liberally with personal, non-evidence-oriented gestalt (unless of course you prefer "snake oil" to scientifically based research). In this case, the evidence is overwhelming! In examining the evidence, let's start with a uniform definition and standard for the terms *overweight, obese*, and *morbidly obese.*

In order to consistently describe and properly treat obesity, a uniform medical standard is used. This is called the Body Mass Index (BMI). The BMI takes into account weight and height, but not age, gender, frame size, or muscle mass which vary significantly from patient to patient. Because these variables are so far ranging, the only way to standardize obesity is to use the two factors that can be consistently compared — height and weight. When considering a person's BMI, a 5 ft. tall, 300 lb. person is considered to be in worse medical straits than a 6 ft. 3 in. tall, 300 lb. person, no matter their age, gender, frame size, or muscle mass.

Persons considered to be *normal weight,* have a BMI under 25. Any BMI over 25 is considered to be in the *overweight* category. *Obese* refers to a BMI of 30-39. *Morbid obesity,* sometimes called *"clinically severe obesity,"* is defined as being 100 lbs. or more over ideal body weight, or having a BMI of greater than 40.

For the overweight, obese, and morbidly obese, temporary weight loss is not the solution. Temporarily losing weight, gaining it back, and then losing weight again is what we term "yo-yo" dieting. Yo-yo dieting has been shown to be detrimental to your health.[11] True weight loss success must be measured in loss of extra weight over **years** not months.

Almost every "diet miracle" in the media emphasizes the short term, initial weight loss. "I lost 10 lbs. in just seven days on the incredible green paint diet." So, maybe you lost 10 lbs. in seven days, but how did you lose it? Did you keep it off? For how long? Did you lose any more? Did you die from the stupid green paint?

The true test of a weight loss program's success is to see where participants settle in 3-5 years. Studies have shown that long-term loss of only 10-15% of excess body weight significantly improves many weight related medical problems.[12] For morbidly obese patients the data also unfortunately shows that there is a less than 2% long-term success rate for even the best medically supervised weight loss programs![13] In most studies that look at sustained weight loss for longer than 3 years, the number is closer to zero![14]

Now suppose that you were told by your physician that you had a medical condition that significantly decreased your longevity (life span), carried a significantly increased risk for multiple cancers, was associated with multiple medical problems that would require a myriad of medications, and would adversely affect virtually every organ and system in your body. Your doctor then wrote you out a prescription and said, "Here, take this. It usually works around 0% of the time long-term."

Unfortunately, most general health care professionals treat patients this way, acting as if their advice to lose weight and "diet" will have more than a modicum of a chance of success. In fact, most never track their patients' results to be able to report any reasonable or verifiable data on their treatment methods. I guess that leaves overweight patients standing out in the cold, with no way to solve their weight issues or the medically related problems. Enter: the surgical treatment option.

The NIH states that surgery for obesity is largely reserved for those approximately 100 lbs. overweight, with a BMI of 40 or greater — the morbidly obese. The NIH established recommendations regarding weight loss surgery back in 1992, and the American Society for Metabolic and Bariatric Surgery and American Society for Bariatric Physicians defer to those recommendations as well. Basically, a patient who has failed previous attempts at weight loss, with a BMI of 40 or greater is a candidate. If you have tried medically supervised programs, even if you've lost weight on those programs, it will count toward meeting the criteria if you've put the weight back on.

The NIH recommendations did not, however, define a "supervised program." As practitioners, we interpret this to mean a significant attempt at weight loss under physician supervision. The best model is a totally supervised medical program where physicians are involved and monitor all aspects of the program. Also acceptable is the situation in which a primary care doctor monitors a patient while they undergo such programs as Weight Watchers® or Jenny Craig®.

Patients who do not meet the NIH criteria because of a BMI that is too low, who are unable to stop smoking, have acute mental illness, are current substance abusers (including alcohol), have had a Myocardial Infarction (M.I.) or stroke within the previous six months, or are less than five years out from treatment for certain types of cancers, are not, in our view, candidates for weight loss surgery.

Having a BMI over 40, however, is not the only criterion for weight loss surgery. Just having a BMI over 25 can lead to multiple related medical problems, referred to as co-morbidities. Those with high-risk, co-morbid conditions, and a BMI of between 35 and 40 also meet the NIH criteria for surgery. Weight related co-morbidities include type 2 diabetes, high blood pressure (hypertension), stroke, coronary artery disease (CAD), obstructive sleep apnea (OSA), congestive heart failure (CHF), hypoventilation syndrome, gallbladder disease, hyperlipidemia (high cholesterol), headaches, gastro-esophageal acid reflux (heartburn), degenerative joint disease, polycystic ovary syndrome (PCOS), infertility, menstrual irregularities, endometrial cancer, breast cancer, prostate cancer, colon cancer, osteoarthritis (OA), cardiac and respiratory dysfunction, gout, depression, alzheimer's, premature death, deep vein thrombosis (DVT), pulmonary emboli (blood clot to lungs), stress urinary incontinence, and others.

All of these conditions can occur in the absence of obesity, but all are significantly increased when obesity is present. In time, most morbidly obese patients will develop a good number of these medical problems, often requiring multiple medications and occasionally surgery to control the maladies, and resulting in a decreased quality of life.[15]

Additionally, obesity related costs greatly affect our country's economy when you figure in the cost of medications for all of the above mentioned medical problems, and the loss of worker productivity from obesity related sickness and leave.[16] Many younger people with morbid obesity are also on disability for obesity related conditions.[17] Finally, there is the staggering amount of hard-earned, and for many, hard-come-by dollars spent on diets and weight related drugs and programs that simply have no hope of having any real effect.

So, why consider such a "radical" approach to obesity if it is basically caused by a series of unfortunate genes, and a lifetime of "poor" lifestyle choices? The simple answer: to help patients live.

The quality of life issues related to obesity are numerous and significant. Many of my morbidly obese patients often cannot sit in normal chairs or seats, perform basic hygiene, clip their own nails, work, help others in physically related tasks, or even breathe without assistance. These people may believe they have received a rotten hand in the big deal of life, and maybe they didn't play their cards well on top of it, but they deserve the same chance for a happy, healthy, productive life as anyone else. (Anyone who thinks otherwise needs a serious bias and attitude adjustment.)

Helping people find that better life is why we consider such "radical" treatments as surgical intervention. You know, that "radical-high-risk-experimental surgery that didn't work on my wife's second cousin's aunt, twice removed?" Well, this ain't your wife's second cousin's aunt, twice removed's old fashioned stomach stapling procedure anymore!

Surgical approaches to the treatment of obesity came as a result of the lack of efficacy of medical weight loss programs, and the significant adverse effects associated with morbid obesity. As I give a very basic overview of the history and status of weight loss surgery, it may help you to refer to the illustration of the gastrointestinal tract and the glossary we provided in the back of the book, if the illustrations and explanations are not sufficient.

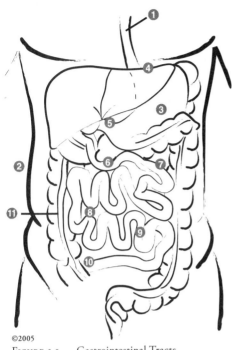

©2005

FIGURE 3.1 — Gastrointestinal Tracts

1. The esophagus is a long muscular tube, which moves food from the mouth to the stomach.

2. The abdomen contains all of the digestive organs.

3. The stomach, situated at the top of the abdomen, normally holds just over 3 pints (about 1500 ml) of food from a single meal. Here the food is mixed with an acid that is produced to assist in digestion. In the stomach, acid and other digestive juices are added to the ingested food to facilitate breakdown of complex proteins, fats, and carbohydrates into small, more absorbable units.

4. A valve at the entrance to the stomach from the esophagus allows the food to enter while keeping the acid-laden food from "refluxing" back into the esophagus, causing damage and pain.

5. The pylorus is a small round muscle located at the outlet of the stomach and the entrance to the duodenum (the first section of the small intestine). It closes the stomach outlet while food is being digested into a smaller, more easily absorbed form. When food is properly digested, the pylorus opens and allows the contents of the stomach into the duodenum.

6. The small intestine is about 15 to 20 feet long (4.5 to 6 meters) and is where the majority of the absorption of the nutrients from food takes place. The small intestine is made up of three sections: the duodenum, the jejunum, and the ileum.

7. The duodenum is the first section of the small intestine and is where the food is mixed with bile produced by the liver and with other juices from the pancreas. This is where much of the iron and calcium is absorbed.

8. The jejunum is the middle part of the small intestine extending from the duodenum to the ileum; it is responsible for digestion.

9. The last segment of the intestine, the ileum, is where the absorption of fat-soluble vitamins A, D, E and K and other nutrients are absorbed.

10. Another valve separates the small and large intestines to keep bacteria-laden colon contents from coming back into the small intestine.

11. In the large intestines, excess fluids are absorbed and a firm stool is formed. The colon may absorb protein, when necessary.

(information courtesy of Ethicon Endo-Surgery, Inc.)

Surgical Weight Loss Treatment Methods

Present surgical weight loss treatments are performed in three ways. The first is described as a *malabsorptive* technique which means that many of the calories consumed are not absorbed, and pass through the system. The second is a *restrictive* technique meaning a small pouch is created out of the stomach to give the feeling of fullness from much less food. The third option was developed combining the malabsorptive and restrictive techniques.

In the 70's the most popular surgical approach was called the *jejuno-ileal* or *intestinal bypass*, and it was purely malabsorptive. In this surgery the majority of the small intestine (where nutrients are absorbed) was bypassed by hooking up the small intestine in a different way. This procedure was easy to perform, and at first seemed to have good weight loss. The problem with this approach is that people developed severe diarrhea from the malabsorption.

In addition, many electrolytes (sodium and potassium, for example) were adversely affected and hospitalization for replacement of these electrolytes was not infrequent. Many patients developed severe protein depletion, as they could not adequately absorb protein, and this many times required an I.V. and *TPN* (liquid food via vein). Finally, the bypassed portion of small intestine grew bacteria that adversely affected the liver, sometimes leading to liver failure. As a result, this procedure was abandoned.

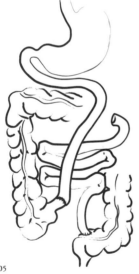
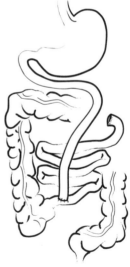

©2005

FIGURE 3.2 — Jejuno-ileal Bypass End to End

©2005

FIGURE 3.3 — Jejuno-ileal Bypass End to Side

There are three main, purely "restrictive" types of weight loss surgeries. One is called a *gastroplasty*, in which the stomach is simply stapled to form a smaller pouch, but the small intestine is left intact. The second is called a *vertical banded gastroplasty* (VBG) during which a hole is stapled in the center of the stomach, a vertical line is stapled from the top of the hole to the upper edge of the stomach, and a vertical band is attached from the side of the hole to the edge of the stomach in order to restrict food intake. The third is called an Adjustable Gastric Banding procedure, and I'll talk more about that later in the chapter.

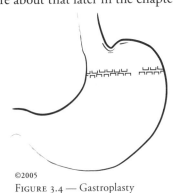

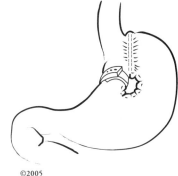

©2005
FIGURE 3.4 — Gastroplasty

©2005
FIGURE 3.5 — Vertical Banded Gastroplasty

With the development of a new technique, the *biliopancreatic diversion,* came one variant of the combination of restrictive and malabsorptive techniques. This procedure was an improvement on the jejuno-ileal bypass in that no small intestine lost function, thereby decreasing damage to the liver. Biliopancreatic diversion patients tend to suffer from protein deficiency, stomach ulcers, diarrhea, and foul smelling flatulence. A modified version of this procedure, called the *duodenal switch*, is still done today, but more so in Europe and other countries than in the U.S. It is, however, being used more in the U.S. for patients considered *super morbidly obese* or larger. In general, these procedures tend to have better overall weight loss, but at the expense of increased complications, and are not quite as popular in North America as other parts of the world.

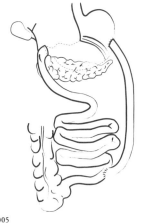

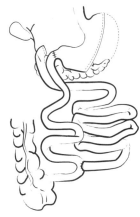

©2005
FIGURE 3.6 — Biliopancreatic Diversion

©2005
FIGURE 3.7 — Biliopancreatic Diversion with Duodenal Switch

The *Roux-en-Y gastric bypass (RYGB),* which is both malabsorptive and restrictive, was originally created in the 1960s and involves using medical staplers to create a small pouch in the top part of the stomach. To give you a good mental visual, the pouch is generally not any bigger than an egg. The rest of the stomach is not removed, but is stapled shut on top, and remains connected to the small bowel below. Bile from the gallbladder and pancreatic juices are released through the *remainder* or original portion of the stomach, and into the small intestine. The remainder portion of the stomach still creates stomach acids as well. These acids are necessary for the break-down of foods in the gastrointestinal tract.

The small intestine then carries these digestive acids downstream where they meet with the food coming in through the new small pouch, aiding in nutrient absorption. A piece of the small intestine is then brought up to the new pouch to allow empty-ing of food contents directly into the bowel (the "Roux" limb). The procedure also constructs a tiny stomach outlet, which slows the speed food leaves your new "egg" stomach. Satiety (a feeling of fullness), is created when the pouch is filled with small amounts of food that tells the brain the walls of the stomach are stretched and full.

A very small malabsorptive component is present from the bypass of some small intestine used to create the "Y" of the Roux-en-Y configuration. Several variants of the Roux-en-Y surgery exist, and if you choose to have a Roux-en-Y surgery, you should be clear which procedure your surgeon will use.

Incidentally, the name *Roux* comes from the surgeon who first divided, and re-connected the small intestine in a similar pattern, and the *Y* comes from the shape or route the intestine then takes after surgery; it looks like a capital "Y." (At least it looks like a "Y" to surgeons. Don't feel bad if you can't really see it. It's one of those "you have to be there" things.)

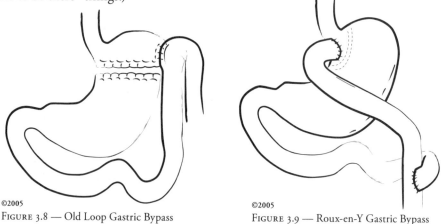

©2005
FIGURE 3.8 — Old Loop Gastric Bypass

©2005
FIGURE 3.9 — Roux-en-Y Gastric Bypass

According to many weight loss experts, the RYGB is considered to be the "gold standard" for surgical weight loss procedures as it has a good, long-term track re-cord.[18] It can be done by creating a full abdominal incision (an *open* procedure) in order to lift the liver out of the way, to access the stomach and small intestine, but the need to use this particular method has drastically decreased in recent years with the move toward laparoscopic methods.

Open procedure incisions for women tend to be about 4½-6 inches long, and about 5½-7 inches for men. The RYGB can now be done via a *laparoscope* (camera placed into the body through small incisions). Six small incisions are made in the abdomen into which instrument portals and the laparoscope are inserted. The procedure is now performed laparoscopically more often than by open incision in the U.S., although some surgeons still like to use the open procedure because they prefer to be able to feel and manipulate the tissues with their hands.

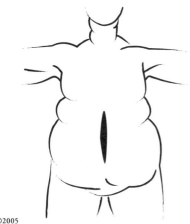
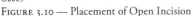
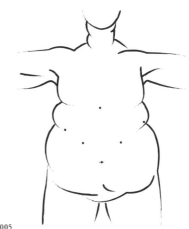

©2005

FIGURE 3.10 — Placement of Open Incision

©2005

FIGURE 3.11 — Placement of Laparoscopic Incisions

RYGB patients can plan to spend 3-4 days in the hospital if an open procedure is required. At our center, in approximately 97% of cases, my partners and I are able to perform the procedure laparoscopically, and the hospital stay is then generally 1-2 days. Patients often go back to work in 1-2 weeks following laparoscopic surgery, or 4-6 weeks after an open procedure, especially if their work involves activity such as bending or lifting.

Patients are on a liquid protein diet for approximately 2 weeks before surgery in order to shrink the liver, clear the intestinal tract of food substances. and take some weight off thereby relieving pressure on the heart. The liver must be shrunk to its smallest size possible as it sits directly in front of the stomach, and must be lifted by instruments and held out of the way. Some livers are very big and heavy, and if the liver can't be lifted out of the way with the laparoscopic instruments, the surgery may have to be converted to an open procedure involving a much bigger incision.

Shrinking the liver through use of the liquid protein diet helps the patient's chances of having a laparoscopic procedure, and with every pound gone prior to surgery, the patient's chances of cardiac and respiratory complications decrease. Patients then continue on a primarily liquid protein diet for approximately 2 weeks following surgery (protocols may vary slightly from surgeon to surgeon and patient to patient), while the stomach and small intestine heal.

Patients usually graduate to soft foods as tolerated at around 2 weeks post surgery. After 4 weeks have passed, patients may then begin eating more solid foods as tolerated. Many RYGB patients experience an intolerance of certain foods for a while, something that Julie and Karen will discuss further in the next chapter.

The advantage of the laparoscopic RYGB approach includes a decreased risk of wound infections and hernias, (which require additional surgery to repair), decreased pain, decreased length of hospital stay, and decreased post-operative restrictions. The laparoscopic approach also produces fewer adhesions (scars) on the inside of the abdomen. This means that in the future, if other unrelated surgeries are needed, there will be fewer adhesions to potentially complicate the procedure.

As with all surgeries, however, complications can develop. Leaks, strictures, bleeding, infections, pulmonary emboli, and other complications can occur. Complications from Roux-en-Y surgery will be discussed a little later in this chapter.

Overall, nationally reported mortality (death) rates from Roux-en-Y surgery are around .5% and *decreasing,* which is less than more malabsorptive procedures, but more than purely restrictive procedures.[19] At our center the mortality rate is less than .2% for RYGB. Deaths most often occur from pulmonary emboli that are blood clots that form in the legs and pass to the lung, blocking blood flow.[20] Pulmonary emboli can result from any type of surgery.

A variant of the RYGB procedure now being done is often called the *mini-Roux-en-Y.* The stomach is still stapled into a small, albeit usually longer pouch, but the small bowel is not separated to bring up a Roux limb. Instead the small bowel is connected to the pouch in a loop fashion. The procedure takes somewhat less time, but can significantly increase the risk of ulceration from bile and acid refluxing up to the pouch as the loop allows these substances easier access to the pouch. Bile and acid reflux into the pouch can be painful, and may increase the risk of cancer developing.[21] Based on this data, many bariatric surgeons do not endorse this type of bypass.

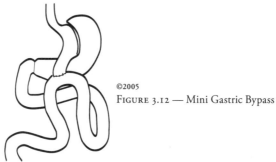

©2005
FIGURE 3.12 — Mini Gastric Bypass

Another new procedure being used is the *gastric sleeve,* also known as the *sleeve gastrectomy.* This procedure was initially employed as a first weight loss "stage" for extremely high risk patients. The thought was that performing an entire bariatric surgery would be too risky in some patients, and breaking it down into two parts might decrease those risks. In the first part of the procedure the majority of the stomach is removed to create only a sleeve of remaining stomach. After a weight loss over months to years, the surgeon could then conclude with stage two by performing an RYGB, gastric band, or duodenal switch. The sleeve gastrectomy has been found to have great early results, but additional data is needed to see how it will perform in the long-term.

Some surgeons feel that the gastric sleeve can be used for weight loss all on its own (although the medical "jury" is still out on this)[22], but it is more commonly seen as a first stop on the way to an RYGB procedure for patients who are in the *super morbidly obese* category or higher.[23] Alone it is a purely restrictive procedure. As a staged process it is restrictive and then converted to a restrictive and malabsorptive procedure.

The gastric sleeve is a procedure in which the largest side of the stomach is completely separated by a staple line and usually removed entirely, and a "sleeve" or pouch, approximately the size and shape of a small banana is created. There is no re-routing of the intestinal system, and all the rest of the anatomy is left in tact, including the natural connection of the stomach to the duodenum, normally bypassed with an RYGB.

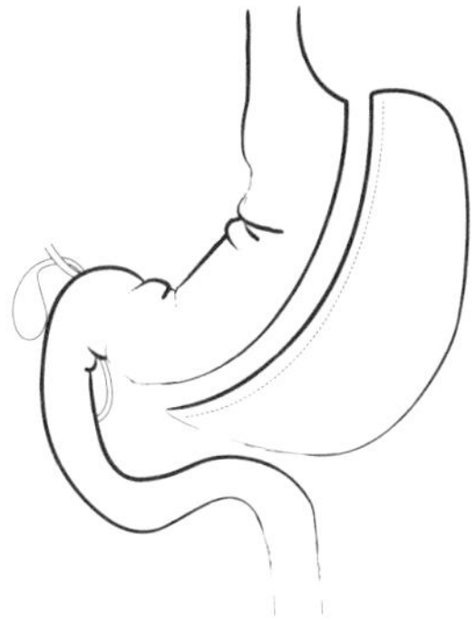

©2007
FIGURE 3.13 — Sleeve Gastrectomy

This procedure is a simpler procedure than the RYGB because of the lack of intestinal re-routing. Additionally, there is no implantation of a surgical device as in the adjustable gastric band (detailed below). There are claims that it is a safer procedure than the RYGB or the duodenal switch for those with a BMI over 60 (especially for those patients who carry a great dal of their weight in their belly), and thus, it is often used as the first stage of a two stage process to reduce the patient's BMI down to a safer level before converting it to the "gold standard" RYGB, or a duodenal switch.[24]

The gastric sleeve allows patients to lose 80 to 100 lbs. or more, shrinking the size of the liver, taking pressure off the heart and other major organs and systems in the body, and making surgical stage two of the process much safer. The sleeve can than be converted to a standard RYGB pouch, or a duodenal switch to permit additional weight loss and provide a better chance for more permanent weight loss results than with gastric sleeve alone. Both stages of the process can be performed laparoscopically allowing for better recovery times, smaller incisions, less incision related issues, and less pain.

Although the gastric sleeve may be an excellent option for those with very high BMIs, or those with very high risk factors for RYGB or duodenal switch, the sleeve is generally considered to be a temporary, not permanent, treatment for obesity. The majority of bariatric surgeons consider the gastric sleeve to be part of a staged process of obesity treatment. Some consider the staged process to be a disadvantage, and as all surgeries present risks, having multiple surgeries can be a disadvantage, despite the health benefits that can result. Additionally, many insurers still consider the gastric sleeve to be investigational and are reluctant to cover the procedure, or outright and explicitly refuse coverage. Check with your surgeon and your insurer if you believe the gastric sleeve may be an option for you.

Another recent addition to the bariatric surgery field is the laparoscopic *adjustable gastric band* (commonly referred to as a Lap-Band®). This technique involves placing an adjustable silicone band around the top of the stomach to create a small pouch. This balloon type band is connected to a port, which goes under the skin so the surgeon can inject saline solution into the band to expand it, and thus adjust the band and the size of the food "pouch" created.

Note, I said the surgeon can adjust the band, as a patient has been known to attempt to deflate the band by himself before a vacation cruise. Unfortunately, the patient kept the saline from the band in an unsterile container during the food fest, and then attempted to re-inject the now infected fluid back in the port. A nasty infection then followed, requiring removal of the band.

The band is normally described as working by creating a small pouch, thus it is a restrictive procedure. A recent landmark study revealed that the band worked best by creating satiety (fullness) not through restriction (the smallness of the pouch).[25] I believe many bands are being adjusted incorrectly as surgeons are still trying to cause weight loss solely through restriction. Adjusting the band this way leads to more problems in eating solids, and many patients then maladapt to ingesting a more liquid diet. This causes poorer weight loss and a poor overall nutritional status.

The adjustable gastric band procedure does not involve stapling the stomach or bowel, and is therefore somewhat less invasive but it does still involve surgery, anesthesia, and the laparoscopic incision sites are still necessary. The down side is that, in general, patients tend to lose weight more slowly than with the RYGB, and overall in most cases lose less weight as compared to RYGB patients.[26]

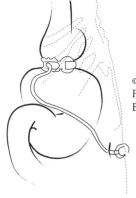

©2005
FIGURE 3.14 — Adjustable Gastric Band (Lap-Band®)

Now, please note that the band is adjustable and *reversible. Reversible* in this context means that the band can, although may never be, deflated. *Reversible* does not mean the same thing as *removable.* Although the band can technically be removed with another surgery, it is not *meant* to be removed. The band is meant to be a permanent implanted medical device that will be with you forever, not unlike a replacement joint or a pacemaker. You decide how much and how often the band works, but don't think that when you get your weight off you just run in on your lunch hour and have it removed.

Similarly, we have found a lot of patients who think that the band is meant for getting the weight off initially, but, hey, if it comes back, no big deal. I just get the doc to tighten it up again, and away the weight goes. NOT SO! This is not intended to help you continue yo-yo dieting! It is meant to be adjusted to attain a pouch of optimal size that will help you maintain your *initial* weight loss. This, like the other procedures, is meant to be a one-way, one time trip. It's not meant to be an easier way out than the other procedures.

In our experience the Lap-Band® should be considered for patients who cannot have an RYGB because they may have: crohn's disease, have had other lower abdominal surgeries that do not facilitate an RYGB procedure, have certain medical conditions such as irritable bowel syndrome (IBS) or celiac disease, are less than five years from a malignancy, or are very high risk patients that may not survive the restructuring of their stomach and gastrointestinal tract. Patients who are at the lower end of the morbid obesity scale may also be ideal patients.

It takes approximately one hour to perform this surgery, and patients are commonly in the hospital overnight. Patients usually return to work in 1-2 weeks, but must generally be evaluated on a regular basis for gradual adjustment of the band.

Patients report having good weight loss with the Lap-Band® (approximately 1-2 pounds per week). They complain of difficulty eating thick meats and breads, and like RYGB patients they must cut their food into small bites, and chew it extremely well. Also like RYGB patients, Lap-Band® patients should not drink liquids with meals, nor rely solely on calories in liquid form (juice, protein drinks, milk shakes).

The Lap-Band® patient is generally on clear liquids for the first 2 days, transitioning to soft foods for 2-4 weeks, and then to solid foods at the fourth week. Although most studies also show better weight loss with the RYGB, Lap-Band® patients who are very compliant with their weight loss program can have results that match the RYGB. (Unless one tries to self-adjust the band!)

The Lap-Band®, as well as the Midband® and the AMI Band®, commonly used in Europe and Australia respectively, (or the Swedish Adjustable Band that is currently in the FDA approval process) have their own strange little foibles and weirdo things too. The first thing is that patients need to be diligent about returning to their surgeon's office to have the band adjusted. Adjustments involve having the surgeon or a qualified allied health professional inject a needle into the port site to drain and refill the band with saline solution. The initial adjustment should occur 4-6 weeks after surgery when the patient has transitioned to solid foods. Follow-up adjustments will occur on a schedule set by the surgeon. You will have to adhere to the schedule of visits to the surgeon's office for the *rest of your life.*

Related to adjustments is the issue of proper adjustment method. Unfortunately, there are a lot of surgeons who are jumping into the adjustable gastric band arena without knowing very much about obese patients, or about how to properly use and maintain the band. Beware these clinics and centers as you will not receive the care you deserve, and you may be putting your health at seriour risk. A good surgeon has been appropriately trained on how to fill and adjust the band to help the patient achieve optimal weight loss and satiety.

If the band is *underfilled,* patients will not experience satiety, they will be able to eat big meals, and they will remain hungry and looking for food. Weight loss will not occur, or will occur slowly. If the band is *overfilled,* patients may not be able to get food down or keep it down, may experience reflux or cough after swallowing, may regurgitate food, and may develop maladaptive eating behaviors such as drinking all their calories or only eating soft foods. *Optimal* filling of the band results in patients experiencing satiety with small meals. They are not looking for food, and they do not experience the symptoms of a band that is too tight.[27]

Some surgeons feel that the band should be set as tight as possible right out of surgery to maximize weight loss. The makers of the Lap-Band® and the Center for Obesity Research and Education in Melbourne Australia where the band was developed, do not endorse this practice.[28] By overfilling the band and setting it at its tightest point right off the bat, the patient will experience tremendous difficulties as stated above. Additional difficulties may also include a narrowing of the stoma and dilation or expansion of the esophagus. Surgeons should be willing to shoot for the *optimal* setting straight away. If the optimal setting is not achieved, then adjustments should be made with an eye toward achieving the optimal band size.

Once a patient achieves goal weight or size then the patient has two options. The first, and the best is to leave the band at the point that the optimal weight loss and satiety were achieved. Why mess with success, right? The other is to loosen the band over time back to its most neutral point (as it was implanted), in order to teach the patient to eat properly without the aid of the band. Again, you'll note that I didn't mention removal of the band. The prevailing view, however, is to leave the band at the optimal fill point. If the band is in there anyway, why not let it do its job rather than sit there idle and do nothing? If you are interested in the adjustable gastric band, discuss your surgeon's philosophies on these subjects. You might just be a bit surprised at what you hear.

Another thing you might be surprised to hear is that the band has potential problems of its own. Although it is a relatively safe procedure, any implantable device can have or cause problems. No surgical procedure can claim it is completely safe. The band can cause dilation of the esophagus (the food tube from your mouth to your stomach.)[29] This can expand over time if the band is too tight and the patient keeps attempting to ingest more food in order to get adequate protein and calories. Sometimes patients just consistently overeat because they have not adjusted their behaviors and that too will cause esophageal dilation. Either way, it's not a good thing.

The band can also erode, or become infected.[30] These are known potential complications, although they occur rarely, but can require additional surgery or explantation (removal) of the band. Additionally, obstructions of the band can occur, as can tube breakages, and port displacements.[31] All of these will require additional surgery, usually on an outpatient basis to correct. Band slippage can also occur which requires a surgical intervention, although most surgeons now anchor the band to the stomach with a couple of sutures to prevent slippage.[32] I'll talk a little more about slippage in the section on complications coming up. Finally, although made of silicone, there are no reports from anywhere in the world of people being allergic to the Lap-Band®.

Issues with the band, its placement, or the adjustments are not the only things patients have to think about though. To be successful, patients must be extremely diligent about their program compliance because they do not have the malabsorptive physical component to help keep them on track with foods they eat or don't eat. Patients must be diligent about attending support groups (they're support NOT therapy!!), about learning to build a responsible relationship with food, and about getting out and moving everyday for at least 20 minutes.

Band patients have to be extremely careful about what goes in their mouths because the band doesn't really cause the dumping syndrome that can accompany other procedures when a patient eats too much sugar, too much greasy food, or too much alcohol. Band patients don't get sick, thus causing them to want to avoid foods that make them throw up and feel like they contracted Ebola Virus for three hours. Band patients can continue to put in all the foods that got them fat in the first place, just in smaller, but more frequent amounts. It is imperative that band patients be wholly committed to following their program and valuing themselves enough to do the right thing for their bodies. Support groups will help with tips and tricks, as well as getting a good pat on the back and a "good job, you look great!" once in a while.

Additionally, support groups can help patients deal with some of the weirder things that come with bands too. One of those weird things is mucous plugs. These occur when a patient has post-nasal drip, or gets a cold or the flu. Too much mucous goes down the esophagus and gets plugged at the band site. Sometimes they cause the heaves or full-on vomiting in the body's attempt to clear itself of the plug. Sometimes they just cause severe nausea. Just one of those bizarre things that's fairly low on the annoyance scale.

Another of those annoying little things is what paitnets refer to as *morning band*. Morning band seems to be a phenomenon that cause the band to be tighter in the morning making it harder to eat. The theory, and I emphase the word *theory* behind this is that during the day fluid is distributed out to all parts of the body including the extremeties. At night, when the body rests, the fluid runs back to the central part of the body and accumulates more in the organs and other areas. The stomach kind of plumps up a bit and pushes more against the band thus causing more pressure and making it harder to eat in the morning until you've been up a while and got everything moving around again. That's the theory anyway. Whatever the explanation, lots of patients report this kind of phenomenon which they tend to rate about a 1 or a 2 on the annoyance scale. It just requires a little bit of adaptation, that's all.

And speaking of adaptation, women often want to know how the Lap-Band® will affect them if they become pregnant. The band is not generally removed when a woman becomes pregnant, although it is common practice to empty the band before delivery. The band can actually help many women with their satiety and portion control during pregnancy, as the old wives' tale of "eating for two" tend to get them in hot water with weight gain. The band can be adjusted during pregnancy to accommodate any additional food intake or satiety needs that might crop up. I recommend that bariatric patients who become pregnant, with or without a Lap-Band® keep their bariatric surgeon and OB/GYN in close contact with each other.

So, as you can see, the adjustable gastric band or Lap-Band® has its own constellation of things to consider. It's not just an easier choice because people say it is safer. (By the way, it is a very safe procedure, but it is not immune to serious surgical complications). Please don't take your decision to have any surgery lightly, and do your homework. Learn all you can about any procedure you choose.

Finally, one other procedure that has some popularity in the eastern mid-west and parts of the east coast is a procedure called the *Sapala-Wood MicroPouch®*. This procedure was invented by two surgeons, Drs. Wood and Sapala, and is also referred to as *near total gastric bypass.* The procedure is essentially the same as an RYGB, but the main differences are that with an RYGB the pouch is the size of an egg versus the Sapala-Wood Micro Pouch® which is the size of a grape, and this procedure cannot be performed laparoscopically.

Micro Pouch® patients have such a small pouch that they must eat 6-8 very small meals a day. Having such a restricted food intake, patients can have a very difficult time getting enough protein and nutrients on a daily basis. As you can imagine, the biggest issue with this procedure is that it can result in severe nutrient deficiencies. Patients with this procedure MUST take appropriate vitamins and supplements to ensure against serious nutritional deficiencies and their attendant medical issues. Additionally, patients usually have to rely more heavily on protein supplements as well in order to meet the required daily protein intake, as this procedure is a variant of the RYGB and is malabsorptive as well as restrictive. Needless to say, Micro Pouch® patients must maintain a consistent and regular schedule of follow-up appointments with the surgeon, *for life,* and must becomve very accomplished at understanding the nutritional values of foods.

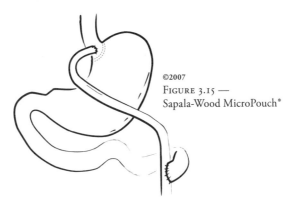

©2007
FIGURE 3.15 —
Sapala-Wood MicroPouch®

Because the procedure is not performed laparoscopically, it has an increased risk of surgical complications, especially the risk of herniation. Patients will have to be vigilant about program compliance, watching for potential complications, going to follow-up appointments, and attending support groups for guidance, tips, and help. Patients considering this procedure should evaluate why they might prefer this procedure over a standard RYGB, whether performed laparoscopically or open. Please consider carefully as you are the one who will have to do the work after the procedure.

Common Potential Surgical Complications

There are always risks with any surgery. Surgical complications can't always be prevented, but the risks can be minimized. *You and your doctor must weigh any potential complications against the risks of not having the procedure at all.* The potential complications of bariatric surgery include, but are not limited to:

Stricture: *Stenosis,* or narrowing of the connection between the stomach pouch and intestine that may require a procedure to correct the narrowing. Stricture is the most common type of complication seen with RYGB, occurring statistically in 5-15% of patients. Lap-Band® patients can experience a version of this complication if the band is too tight around the top of the stomach. Most patients notice difficulty with tolerating solids and if the opening is very tight even taking in liquids will be difficult. Nausea and vomiting can develop. Many patients describe reflux of white type "foam" and this usually indicates a tight stricture. Strictures tend to show up around three weeks after surgery although they can occur earlier or later and are treated by an endoscope placed down through the mouth into the pouch. A balloon is then used through the scope to dilate (stretch open) the tight area. Most patients only need this done one time, although occasionally strictures require several dilation sessions.

Gallstones: Historically, as many as 30% of patients were thought to develop gallstones after RYGB. This number is probably much lower and is related to the weight loss that occurs with bariatric procedures, rather than the bariatric procedure itself. Symptomatic gallstones are usually treated by removal of the gallbladder, which can most times be performed laparoscopically. The risk of gallstones can be decreased by the patient taking bile salts for 6 months after surgery, however this approach is very expensive. In the past, many surgeons advocated always taking out the gallbladder at the time of bariatric surgery. Today, however, most surgeons use a selective approach by only removing the gallbladder if the patient has gall stones and/or has symptoms from gall stones. It is a whole lot easier to take a gallbladder out laparoscopically if the patient loses significant weight as the gallbladder is directly under the liver.

Bleeding during or after surgery: This complication is seen with virtually any type of surgery, and occurs in approximately 1-2% of bariatric surgical patients. It is sometimes treated with a blood infusion, or in the case of a persistent bleed, the patient may have to return to surgery to have the source of the bleeding stopped. Bleeding can occur from the staple lines, liver, spleen, and other organs or even from an incision site. Often patients are given low doses of blood thinners (Heparin) to decrease the risk of blood clots. This can make patients more "oozy" around the time of surgery. Some bleeding though is far better than dealing with blood clots that could pass to the lungs. Use of staple buttressing material such as Seamguard®has been shown to decrease bleeding and may be helpful for decreasing this risk. Some surgeons require their patients to contineu Lovenox® or blood thinner shots for a few days to weeks after surgery to decrease the threat of a blood clot. Check with your surgeon.

Pneumonia: As with any medical procedure that involves full anesthesia, patients can develop pneumonia, or fluid in the lungs. Pneumonia occurs statistically in less than 2% of all patients. This can often be prevented by getting the patient up and about as soon as possible, as well as by having the patient breathe into a plastic device called a *spirometer* to help re-expand the lungs and prevent collapse. Patients who previously smoked or have sleep apnea and underlying lung disorders are at a higher risk for pneumonia.

Hernia: This is one of the more common complications seen in patients who have an open incision surgery. It occurs in up to 40% of non-laparoscopic RYGB surgeries. A hernia is a protrusion through an abnormal opening in the fascia layer of the abdomen that keeps the abdominal contents inside. Hernias require another operation to fix the problem, and can be complex and difficult to repair. Until much of the weight is off, the hernia can recur, as there is too much pressure on the belly, which reopens the hernia. This complication of open surgery is probably one of the most frustrating to many surgeons. It often involves reopening the edge of the hernia to find the fascia. There are usually a lot of adhesions around this area, and these must be taken down to free up the fascia all around so the hernia defect can be closed. Often some type of mesh is needed to give additional strength to the repair, although surgeons often disagree on the efficacy of mesh in this type of repair. For large hernias that develop, a company called CANICA® has created a fabulous new hernia and large wound closure system that eliminates the need for mesh implants that can become a problem later down the road. For smaller hernias, WL Gore & Associates-Medical Division, has a bio-absorbable hernia repair plug that helps repair the hernia and then harmlessly dissolves after several months. If you are a current patient who has developed a hernia, or if you develop one after surgery, then talk to your surgeon about hernia repair options other than surgical mesh. Overall this complication represents one of the major reasons to consider a laparoscopic approach.

Leaks: Leaks can occur in the staple line or at the connections of the bowel to itself, or the stomach pouch. Leaks occur in approximately 2-3% of RYGB patients. Lap-Band® patients do not usually experience this complication, although a leak originating from where the band was placed on the stomach, and the bottom of the swallowing tube has been reported. Most leaks occur within 24-36 hours and present with abnormal vital signs (temperatures, heart rates) and elevated white cell counts. A contrast swallow study is sometimes performed to help with the diagnosis of a leak. Stronger staple lines and fewer leaks are associated with the use of staple line buttressing material like Seamguard®. Leaks most often require additional surgery to attempt to close and drain the leak area in case the closure does not hold. The tissue around a leak can become weak and does not always hold sutures well so the drains assure the leak will remain "controlled" and eventually heal up over time. Ask your surgeon whether or not he/she uses staple line buttressing material. Suggest Seamguard®.

Pulmonary embolus: Commonly referred to as a blood clot in the lung, it is a risk for all persons undergoing *any* type of surgery. The clots block blood flow in part of the lung and decrease the body's ability to get enough oxygen. Statistically, the risk for this complication in all RYGB surgery is less than 1% of patients. Preventative measures for this complication are mainly in avoiding clots forming in the legs through the use of blood thinning agents and other measures.

Deep vein thrombosis (DVT): DVT means a blood clot in the large veins of the leg. While in the legs, the blood clots are painful, but they become most serious when they float up into the blood vessels of the lungs, thereby becoming pulmonary emboli. Prevention methods include wearing compression stockings, taking blood thinners, and walking as soon as possible after surgery. People at high risk for clots may need to have a filter placed in the large vein in the abdomen that drains all the leg veins. This filter can decrease the risk of clots moving to the lungs where they become a pulmonary embolism, by catching the clot before it can move that far.

Infections: Infections in the wound or abdomen can occur after any abdominal surgery. Wound infections are more common in open procedures and especially in patients who have diabetes and an open incision. Sometimes they open up the outer incision, and courses of antibiotics are needed to cure wound infections. Occasionally, a collection of infection in the abdomen (abscess) will need to be drained using CT scan directed drains.

Bowel obstruction: A partial or full blockage of the bowel can occur after abdominal surgery. Most of these blockages occur weeks to months out from surgery but can even occur *years* later. One cause for this is adhesions that can develop purely from the act of performing surgery in the abdomen. This is more common with open surgery, as the large incision causes more adhesions to form. Another type of blockage is from an internal hernia. Openings created to connect the small bowel together, or to get the small bowel up to the new pouch can open over time causing other parts of the bowel to become kinked in the openings and thus blocked. This usually requires further surgery to repair, and is often difficult to diagnose and/or locate.

Cardiac problems: The greatest risk is in patients who are the most overweight, or who have cardiac disease. Over time the heart of the obese patient enlarges and is at greater risk for problems such as heart attacks. Patients with abnormal EKGs before surgery, or patients at higher risk due to other factors may need further studies to evaluate for cardiac disease prior to surgery.

Ulcers in the pouch: Ulcers can develop in the pouch, or at the connection of the pouch to the small intestine. This can be caused by ingestion of ibuprofen (Motrin®), aspirin, NSAIDs (nonsteroidal anti inflammatories), use of steroids, smoking, or consumption of alcohol. We advise our patients to avoid all of these ulcer-promoting medications or agents. Some believe use of these drugs may increase the risk of band erosion in Lap-Band® patients but most Lap-Band® patients can take some ant-inflammatory medications. Usually, with avoidance of ulcerogenic (ulcer-causing) meds, and use of appropriate treatment medications, ulcers can be cured. Rarely, surgery is needed for nonresponsive ulcers at the connection of the stomach and small intestine (marginal ulcers). Refer to Chapter Twelve – Medication Misadventures, for more information on medications and weight loss surgery.

Cancer: There is no significant evidence that RYGB or Lap-Band® increase the risk of cancer in the stomach. In fact, stomach cancer risk may be lessened as a result of decreased acid production, and less contact between the stomach and cancer-causing edible agents like nitrosamines, which are ingested in burned meats. (Notice to my Father-in-law who likes "burned to a crisp" steak.) The "mini" RYGB procedure may increase the risk of esophageal-stomach cancer if the acid or bile reflux is significant and not well controlled. In general, any long-term weight loss actually decreases the risk of some cancers (breast, colon, uterine, prostate for example).

Erosion: The Lap-Band® can erode through the wall of the stomach to the inside of the stomach. This can be difficult to diagnose, as symptoms are vague. An infection at the skin port site may be a clue that infection has spread to the band, because if the band is now in the stomach, it may have become infected as the stomach is not entirely sterile. Sometimes patients will notice some mild abdominal pain, which may also be a subtle clue to band erosion. Band erosion is usually treated by removal of the band, and repair of the stomach were the erosion occurred. Fortunately, this now occurs infrequently.

Slippage: The band of the Lap-Band® can also "slip" so that stomach normally below the band slides up through the band. This can cause swelling and blockage of the band, and patients can develop nausea and vomiting. Difficulty with swallowing or heartburn can also develop. Some patients just don't feel as full as usual. This usually requires surgery to repair, and also occurs less frequently now as the stomach is generally sutured to itself over the top of the band.

Nausea and Vomiting: Nausea and vomiting can occur after any surgery simply in response to the anesthetics. Although rare, swelling at the surgical site from irritation or localized bleeding with a clot can also temporarily block emptying of the pouch or band. Dehydration will also exacerbate nausea and electrolyte changes, which then increase the risk of nausea and vomiting. A negative cycle may thus develop and will require I.V. fluids and electrolyte replacement. A stricture (tightening of the connection between the stomach and small intestine) can also cause nausea and vomiting and usually presents 3-4 weeks out from surgery. The small intestine and pouch can also develop what is called an *ileus,* a condition in which the intestine does not contract normally but "goes to sleep," and therefore empties poorly. This usually improves with time, but occasionally requires temporary medications for treatment.

(See note 33 — citations for statistics on complications from bariatric surgery techniques)

Although these complications occur infrequently, they do occur and it is important to have surgery at a facility that can deal appropriately with potential issues. This is not meant to be a comprehensive list, and if you are seriously considering weight loss surgery, you need to discuss with your doctor the benefits, as well as the potential complications of having surgery so that you are fully informed and comfortable with your level of knowledge. Discuss both the benefits and risks in a manner that is specific to your personal medical condition and history.

While you're reading this book, you should make notes of what *you* consider to be benefits or risks, and tuck them in the back of the book. You should also make notes of questions to ask your surgeon, and lodge them in the book as well. In fact, just take your notes, questions, and the whole book with you every time you go to your doctor's office!

Bariatric surgery offers the best-proven method of long-term weight loss for morbidly obese people. This having been said, one must note that all surgery does have risk, including the risk of death. Bariatric surgery is no different, although it does favorably compare to many "common" surgeries. For instance, the mortality rate associated with knee and hip replacement surgery can be higher than for typical bariatric cases.[34] Unfortunately, we never hear about *that* in the media.

Effect of Bariatric Surgery on Co-Morbid Conditions

The risk/benefit ratio for bariatric surgery is better than most surgery offered today. How many surgeries can decrease the risk of cancer, improve diabetes, high blood pressure, sleep apnea, arthritis, stress urinary incontinence, acid reflux, and decrease the overall risk of death? In addition, how many surgeries can dramatically improve quality of life while improving medical problems?

A recent landmark study revealed that bariatric surgery lead to an 89% reduction in the relative risk of death as opposed to those morbidly obese patients who had no surgery![35] Another meta-analysis (evaluation of multiple studies), showed that bariatric surgery not only decreases mortality rate, but also decreases the risk of developing new health related conditions and reduces healthcare utilization and direct health care costs.[36]

In fact, the following co-morbid conditions can be significantly improved and sometimes even eliminated with the utilization of weight loss surgery (excluding Lap-Band®).[37] No other therapy has produced such durable and complete control of diabetes mellitus.[38]

Hypertension (high blood pressure)	*78.5%*
Type 2 Diabetes	*86%*
Obstructive Sleep Apnea	*85.7%*
Hyperlipidemia (high cholesterol)	*70%*
Gastroesophageal Reflux Disease	*98%*
Asthma	*Not studied*

TABLE 3.1 — Co-morbidity Improvement Statistics Following Bariatric Surgery

For Lap-Band® patients, studies show the following percentages of co-morbidity improvement or resolution 36 months following surgery.[39]

Hypertension	*48%*
Type 2 Diabetes	*66%*
Obstructive Sleep Apnea	*33%*
Hyperlipidemia	*65.5%*
Gastroesophageal Reflux Disease	*87%*
Asthma	*81.8%*

TABLE 3.2 — Co-morbidity Improvement Statistics Following *Adjustable Gastric Banding* (Lap-Band®)

(Results may appear lower because weight loss is generally slower with the Lap-Band® procedure.)

What to Look for in a Surgical Practice

Surgery, however, is not a quick fix. It's not taking the "easy" way out. Patients who have surgery are given a tool — a way to lose weight like they have never before possessed, but they still have to work hard to change their habits and mindset.

As I tell my patients: it's a tool, and it's no different than a hammer or a screwdriver. You can either use the screwdriver to tighten screws, or you can intentionally poke your eye out with it playing around. You can use the hammer to drive nails, or you can whack yourself in the knee. You choose. It's no good to you if you're not using it for the purpose for which it was intended. Patients must use the tool properly to obtain optimal results.

At our center we discuss the *pouch tools*, and teach the ways to use the surgical pouch to achieve optimal weight loss. Achieving optimal weight loss means patients should avoid drinking during meals, because the food in the small pouch can be "flushed out" with liquids so the pouch can be filled again. It is important to drink fluid approximately 15-20 minutes before a meal, and then to wait until one hour afterward to drink again.

When a patient has progressed to a full compliment of foods, liquids with calories must be avoided as these will slide down through the pouch and give no sense of fullness, yet increase caloric intake. They most certainly should not be used as meal replacements. Patients need good behavioral modification support, emotional support, regular exercise, and good nutrition to achieve optimal weight loss after bariatric surgery.

Working with a comprehensive multi-disciplinary team is the best way for a patient to achieve an overall lifestyle change and maintain a healthy weight and life. A patient needs to meet with dietitians, behaviorists, exercise physiologists, and bariatric internists to truly have the best opportunity for maximal weight loss and better health.

Patients should seek surgeons with bariatric experience and proper board certification, who offer comprehensive, multi-disciplinary treatment and life-long follow-up. I believe patients are better off finding surgeons who are not "dabbling" in the bariatric area. To be properly familiar with this field of medicine, weight loss surgery should comprise at least 50% of a surgeon's practice. In addition, when evaluating a bariatric surgeon, evidence of regular continuing medical education, and active membership in outstanding bariatric medical societies (ASMBS, NAASO, IFSO) is highly recommended.

Look for a practice that is affiliated with or supports the Obesity Action Coalition as well. This is a national organization that is affiliated with the American Society for Metabolic and Bariatric Surgery (ASMBS) Foundation, and advocates on behalf of patients with weight issues everywhere. Not only do they advocate in the legal, political, and insurance arenas, but they are a leader in bringing cutting edge obesity health related information to patients, their families, and the public. I am proud to say that Julie sits on the National Board of Directors of the OAC, and

Karen, Judi, and I are members of the National Advisory Board. The OAC is served and supported by the leading physicians, researchers, educators, academics, and medical professionals in bariatrics today. People like Dr. Neil Hutcher (you've seen him many times on the Discovery Channel® bariatric programs), Dr. Robin Blackstone, Dr. Lloyd Stegemann, Dr. Christopher Still, Dr. Jacqueline Jacques, Dr. Steven Hendrick, Emily Wong-Swartz, Jeanne Blankenship, Dr. Cynthia Buffington, Dr. Scott Shikora, Dr. Harvey Sugarman, Liz Goldenberg, Dr. Walter Pories, Dr. John Baker, and many more.

Many of us write articles for the OAC newsletter and the OAC Action Alert as well, and these are wonderful benefits of membership and association with the OAC that provide patients with a wide variety of accurate and up-to-date information and resources on surgical and non-surgical weight loss and obesity issues. Be sure to redeem your free one year complimentary OAC membership courtesy of the OAC and Little Victories Press™. The information is located in the resources section. Be sure to tell your surgeon's office and support group members about the OAC too, if they don't know about it. Remember, there's strength in numbers. Look what it did for AARP! So, if you find a great practice, but they aren't involved in the OAC, introduce them, (it's free for them!), and get them on board too.

The OAC has done a lot of work in trying to bridge the gap between Medicare and access to treatment for patients. If you are a Medicare or Medicaid patient you are required to have your surgery at a Center of Excellence (COE) if you want to have Medicare/Medicaid pay for it. Centers of Excellence are surgery practices or programs that have been evaluated and accredited by the Surgical Review Corporation (SRC) or the American College of Surgeons (ACS) as having met the highest levels of efficacy, efficiency, and safety. To locate a Center of Excellence near you, check with the SRC web site at www.surgicalreview.org.

Although Medicare and Medicaid patients must have their surgeries at a Center of Excellence, COEs are not required to accept Medicare or Medicaid. Check with your surgeon's office to see if they accept this form of payment. Additionally, even COEs can institute age limits, or BMI limits for their patients as well. In fact, they can have virtually any kind of limitation they choose. So, again, check with the practice regarding their policies, procedures, insurance coverage, multi-disciplinary program, and follow-up programs before you become attached to them as your surgical practice.

A bariatric surgeon's post-operative follow-up should consist of several appointments, not just one. We like to see our patients at 2 weeks, 4 weeks, 6 weeks, 3 months, 6 months, a year after surgery, and at least annually thereafter. It's important for your doctors to periodically monitor your blood levels, nutrition, weight, and other medical issues.

You should not stop being the bariatric surgeon's patient when you come out of the operating room, and of course, you should be having this procedure done in a hospital, not in an *outpatient* surgical center. (An exception to this rule applies in cases where Lap-Band® procedures are performed by experienced surgeons on lower risk patients.)

Additionally, surgeons and internists should provide good pre-surgical care as well. Medical tests that may need to be run prior to weight loss surgery include: a sleep study, an echocardiogram or heart stress test, and gastrointestinal scope (EGD), an abdominal ultrasound, an ultrasound of the legs, blood tests, diabetes testing, a colon cancer screening if over 50 years old, a pregnancy test, or a pap smear and mammogram. If you meet with a physician who does not recommend *at least* one of these tests, no matter your age, you should probably look for another physician.

Also, female patients should be aware that pregnancy is not recommended for at least 18 months post surgery. Although that is the recommendation, we have had patients who have become pregnant as early as two weeks after surgery! (I'll give you a moment to digest that little factoid.) It should be noted that this is in direct contradiction of medical advice.

Pregnancy can be managed while the major portion of the weight loss is occurring (the first six months post-operatively), but the patient's nutrition, blood levels, and other medical issues must be very closely monitored. Often a high risk OB specialist is recommended, as well as the use of an excellent vitamin regimen.

Vitamin Supplementation

And speaking of vitamins, it is of the *utmost importance* that *all* patients having weight loss surgery *with or without* a malabsorption component understand that you will have to take vitamins every day for the *rest of your life*. We highly recommend a vitamin specifically formulated for bariatric patients. The current state of the art and science in bariatric vitamins is Building Blocks®, but there are other bariatric vitamins available.

Why a bariatric vitamin? Because they contain higher concentrations of the nutrients needed to sustain the body than regular vitamins. Weight Loss surgery patients need extra calcium, vitamin D, iron, potassium, folic acid, thiamine, zinc, and vitamin B12. All of these are critical to the good nutrition of weight loss surgery patients. Overall, these vitamins will help prevent vitamin and mineral deficiencies that can develop after surgery.

The stomach and its acids are essential in helping to absorb vitamin B12 in particular, a nutrient critical for formation of new hemoglobin, the building block for red blood cells. An RYGB changes the stomach's environment such that it is more difficult for the body to absorb vitamin B12 in food. Taking a vitamin containing B12 is essential to allow the body to avoid anemia (low hemoglobin).

Bariatric vitamins also contain appropriate amounts of vitamin B1 or thiamine. Studies are showing that not only can bariatric surgery patients suffer from thiamine deficiencies after surgery, but they often present before surgery with a thiamine deficiency as well, and that includes those patients who come in for a Lap-Band® too.[40] Thiamine and other deficiencies can cause serious medical conditions, so patients must be sure to eat good, nourishing food, attend their follow-up appointments, and continue to have lab work drawn for those appointments for the rest of their lives. Thiamine, like B12 and other nutrients is impacted by the bypass of the duodenum, so be sure to eat foods rich in these nutrients. For tips on nutrient rich foods, see the resources section.

Additionally, iron and calcium are primarily absorbed in the first part of the small intestine, which is the part that is bypassed after RYGB surgery. Patients who experience chronic blood loss during menstruation, or from bleeding hemorrhoids should stay in close contact with their doctor as they may require extra iron. Additional calcium will be necessary, and can be taken orally in vitamin supplement form, but should never be taken at the same time as iron. Low iron can cause a whole host of problems including iron deficiency anemia. Even having a cold can cause your iron levels to drop, so be sure to take appropriate iron supplements. Consult your bariatric dietitian or surgeon.

So, as you can see your vitamins and nutrition are very important. So many people think that because they feel fine (or they think they feel fine) they don't need vitamins. The reality is, you can't always feel the damage that is going on in your body from nutritional deficiencies. Once you can start to recognize symptoms, it may be too late to reverse the damage. This is one of those things you have to trust the doctors and the scientists about. We know what kind of little chemical reactions should or should not be going on in your body.

Your body has been designed over millions of years to work by processing certain nutritional inputs with other nutritional inputs. All the various types of fuel are needed to keep the engine running at peak efficiency and keep specific parts from breaking down. Your body is like your car. Your car can run on low oil, dirty transmission fluid, junky gasoline, dirty filters, grimy power steering fluid, and worn out belts, but eventually, when it starts to make noise and you notice it isn't running well anymore, you're in trouble and you may not be able to save the car that now has a cracked block. So keep an eye on your food nutrients and take your vitamins. We study this stuff so you don't have to.

Another thing you should be keeping an eye on after surgery is the development, or exacerbation of hypoglycemia or low blood sugar. You'll know if you're getting low blood sugar because you'll start to feel a little light headed, maybe get a bit shaky, or start to sweat a little. The chemical pathways in your system and the insulin response to food sometimes gets a little out of whack after surgery, so just keep an eye on these types of symptoms and be sure to report them to your surgeon or family physician. Eat well and take those vitamins!

Not only are they formulated with higher concentrations of essential nutrients, bariatric vitamins are also highly absorbable because of *chelation* (kee-lation). Many common over the counter vitamins have extremely poor absorbability. You need all the nutrients you can get out of a state-of-the-art bariatric vitamin like Building Blocks®, and quality unprocessed foods in order to maintain a healthy mind and body.

The bariatric procedures that are primarily malabsorptive in nature, caused significantly more electrolyte and vitamin deficiencies than do the procedures being used more often today. Fortunately, most of these procedures are not performed any more in the U.S. The possibility of vitamin and nutritional deficiencies, and the related effects on the body's systems emphasizes the importance of having life-long follow-up after bariatric surgery. We've included a nutrient functions and deficiency symptoms chart for you at the back of the book in the resources section. This way you'll be better informed about what to watch for, and where to find foods that contain particular nutrients to prevent deficiencies. So no excuses! Eat your fruits, vegetables, protein,and other natural goodies!

Preventing and Dealing With Weight Regain

Assuming vitamin and nutritional deficiencies are prevented, on average, RYGB patients will lose approximately 70% of their extra weight in the first year to year and a half after surgery. Lap-Band® procedure patients will lose approximately 50-60% of the total weight they have to lose over 2-3 years.[41]

After about 6 weeks to approximately 6 months, which we call the "honeymoon period" (because you can literally sleep the time away without significant hunger and the weight will come off), weight loss slows down, and you must be ready to really kick in those revised habits and lifestyle changes or the weight can eventually come back. Obesity is a progressive disease unless it is constantly attended to and treated.

There are three main reasons why patients stop losing or regain weight after RYGB surgery. The first is that the pouch can stretch. The older pouches were larger and incorporated a part of the stomach called the *fundus* which we now know stretches, causing the pouch to hold more food. Sometimes the older stretched pouches were surgically revised to remove the stretched fundus portion. As a result of the number of revisions, pouches are now made smaller, and are made to avoid the fundus as much as possible.

A second reason for weight gain can be related to stretching of the opening from the pouch. The ideal opening of the connection is between 12 and 15mm. As the opening widens, food passes through faster and easier, and does not cause as much of a feeling of fullness. Some surgeons place bands around the opening at the time of the original surgery to prevent this stretching, but these bands can erode or cause excessive tightening of the connection.

A procedure called *sclerotherapy* which involves injecting an irritant through an endoscope around the widened opening resulting in tightening of the opening is showing promise in dealing with this problem. Sclerotherapy is a good alternative to re-operation to fix a dilated or stretched anastomoses,[42] and after having performed more than 400 of them over the past few years, I can tell you that it is *not* a temporary fix as many surgeons claims. (Of course those surgeons all do re-operations and don't offer sclerotherapy as an option....) Many surgeons will either tell patients who have regained weight that they have no options other than another surgery (that will not be covered by insurance) or to continue along on the same path back to where they started.

Not many surgeons across the country actually offer sclerotherapy. It's a procedure that is done endoscopically, meaning it is done under I.V. *conscious sedation* (they put you out and you don't remember anything, but you aren't fully intubated like during surgery), and we put a long tube with a camera and tools on the end down your throat and into your gut. It only takes a few minutes and is generally covered by insurance. But it isn't just all about the procedure. It's about the re-education efforts as well.

The doc will generally ask you to come in and see the dietitian to evaluate how and what you are eating. This is not to pick on you, it is to help you. Embrace that opportunity. You will probably also be asked to see the behaviorist. Again, this is not a "them versus me" scenario. The behaviorist is not there to prevent you from getting what you want. That person is not a hurdle to be gotten past. The behaviorist is there to help you assess your assets and your liabilities in this endeavor. They are there to help you find the most successful route to weight loss, proper treatment of your disease, and happiness again.

Look at these people as part of the team, not the enemy. THEY ARE NOT THE ENEMY! The doc may also ask you to see an exercise physiologist. AGAIN, NOT THE ENEMY! This person is simply trying to help. They are all there to help educate you, or re-educate you. They are your professional support team. They will not let you go into another situation unprepared. If your first surgeon's office let you go in unprepared and set up to fail, or you let yourself forget the lessons they taught you to prepare you for a lifetime of successful weight loss, then you should not allow yourself to go into the second situation unprepared. Expect a team that will prepare you and help you succeed even it it takes a little more time than you planned.

Once you see all of these people and they feel that a sclerotherapy procedure is the right option for you, then you will see the surgeon. The surgeon will evaluate you and if he/she feels you are ready then they will book you for the procedure. Pre-procedure labs will be drawn to make sure you don't have any other problems.

On the day of the procedure, you must have someone go with you as you will have had sedation and cannot drive. You will receive other instructions as to what you can or cannot eat or drink before hand, as well as what medication you can or cannot take. When you get there they will have a nurse place an I.V. (probably the worst part of the whole thing). TIP: stay very well hydrated for several days before the procedure. It will make getting an I.V. in much, much easier. They will also take a ton of information down including a medical history.

When you are ready, they will walk you to the procedure room which looks kind of like a hospital room with equipment in it. It's not an operating room. They will ask you to lay down on the gurney. They will make sure you are comfortable (usually with warm blankets!). The doc will ask you to open your mouth and will spray some stuff in the back of your throat. It's not really that bad. Sort of like Cepacol® for a sore throat. Then they ask you to roll over on your side. The nurse arranges you a little bit, they run the sedation into your I.V., and you're out like a light.

The entire procedure takes about 15 minutes from the point the patient sits on the gurney to the point they are wheeled out on it. This procedure is not temporary.

It is meant to last your lifetime as it "scars" the smaller anastomosis in place through the process. But you are still responsible for respecting your disease of obesity and for treating it appropriately for the rest of your life. Continue to use your pouch tools responsibly, move every day, and remember that obesity never really goes away.

When you go home you will probably need to take a day or two off. No roller coaster rides, no sitting at a desk, no mowing the lawn. Take it easy. But you will have to get up and walk and move around. You will go back to eating soft foods (yogurt, scrambled eggs, soup, protein shakes) for about 2 days, and then you should be okay. Take the pain medication and keep the pain cycle broken. Don't let it get too out of hand.

Generally after 2 days, you're in pretty good shape. Now the real work begins, getting back on track with the pouch tools and the behavior modification. It's a lifestyle. There is no easy way out. This is only a tool. It's like a screwdriver. You can turn screws with it, or you can poke yourself in the eye. One is its intended purpose, the other is what you do to yourself when you're just playing around with it and don't use it properly.

Sclerotherapy is not a miracle cure. It is a wonderful option to help you get back on track and find that healtheir, happier life you were seeking and that you deserve, but it is not an easy way out. Patients are the only ones responsible for making sure that they have a successful weight loss for a lifetime. Respect yourself and respect the fact that you can undermine all of these tools and interventions, and that the obesity can get a firm grip on your life again. You make the call. It's up to you.

Anyway... back to the reasons for weight regain. The last main reason for weight gain is maladaptive eating. If one does not use the proper *pouch tools* such as avoiding fluids during meals or avoidance of liquids with calories, weight gain will usually result. The surgery tool must be used properly to achieve the best weight loss and develop a long-term healthy lifestyle.

Commitment to lifetime change is critical to maintaining the weight loss. You'll still have to work just as hard mentally and physically to get the weight off and keep it off, as you did without surgery, but with surgery you will have a far greater chance of keeping it off. The body will lose most of the weight in the beginning, but it's up to you to get it the rest of the way, and keep it healthy.

Incidentally, the body will know when to stop losing weight. It may stop for a short time several times along the way (to sort of re-set itself), but it will eventually come to a basic stop. It is the rare person who actually doesn't stop losing weight, and in those unusual cases we reverse our pouch tool techniques to encourage more caloric intake. We would encourage the increased use of liquid protein drinks that slide through the pouch, for example. The more malabsorptive procedures (the Distal RYGB, the biliopancreatic diversion, the duodenal switch, the main RYGB, and the micropouch) do have a higher incidence of malnutrition, and sometimes additional surgery is required to allow for more intestinal surface to absorb calories, especially protein.[43]

Although at first it will seem like the weight is really dropping off, it will slow down, and for that patients must be prepared. It is important to note that this is a *process*. It is a process that occurs over a fairly long time period, so don't try to rush it. Trust me, and trust Julie and Karen when we tell you that it will fly by all on its own. Let your body move on its own time schedule, and that includes plateaus, slow downs, and "shrinks" (a term they'll define for you later in the book). It took you many years to put on this weight, so it's going to take at least a year, and maybe two or three years to get it off.

And on that note, don't rush to plastic surgery. I recommend that my patients wait at least 18 months before having plastic surgery to have skin removed. The body needs time to shrink and adjust to its new size and shape. Plastic surgery for skin removal is *not* necessary in all patient cases. It should be evaluated on a case-by-case basis. We'll discuss this more in Chapter Fifteen.

The Effectiveness of Weight Loss Surgery

So, in the long run, how effective is bariatric surgery, really? Well, to quote a lawyer friend of mine (Julie!), "*it depends*." It depends on how old you are, how much you weighed before surgery, the type of procedure you had done, how motivated you were to stick to your lifestyle changes, what you eat, how much you exercise, the level of emotional support you have, your overall health, and whether or not you take your bariatric vitamins. How's that for a non-commital answer?!

Success in bariatric surgery is commonly defined as achieving loss of 50% or more of excess body weight, and maintaining that level for at least five years.[44] I would add that success could also be rated by the overall improvement in the patient's health and weight related medical conditions. Remember, for (non-surgical) medical weight loss programs, success is usually defined as loss of 10-15% of extra weight.[45] As surgeons we prefer to have at least one half or more of the extra weight dissipate and remain gone.

Patients with higher initial Body Mass Indexes (BMIs) tend to lose more total weight. Patients with lower initial BMIs tend to lose a greater percentage of their excess weight, and may be more likely to come closer to their ideal body weight.[46] Patients with type 2 diabetes tend to show less overall excess weight loss than patients without type 2 diabetes.[47] One study shows patients can maintain a 50-60% loss of excess weight 10-14 years after bariatric surgery and approximately 50% off for 20 years.[48] Patients also have significant improvement in their quality of life. Basic things like fitting into seats, walking, and general hygiene become immeasurably easier with weight loss. Weight loss surgery is effective in so many ways.

We did find one very interesting study concerning the effectiveness of weight loss surgery that we think is worth noting, however, and that concerns those patients who may be shift workers. Shift work as defined in this study is employment occurring outside the 8:00 am to 5:00 pm traditional working day. Not only would this include persons who actually work defined shifts, but it would include those persons who may be self-employed, who travel for employment, or who otherwise keep strange or erratic hours.[49] This study noted that up to 20% of workers in the United States and Europe are employed in some form of shift work.[50]

The interesting thing about this study is that it showed that shift workers lost less weight than their non-shift work counterparts when compared at 3 months, 6 months, and 12 months after surgery.[51] In fact, it was almost 1/3 less weight than their non-shift worker counterparts.[52] The study concluded that the potential for altered sleep physiology, reduced quantity of sleep, altered hormonal balance, increased tendency to disordered eating, and poorer quality of food intake were all possible reasons for the less successful weight loss. They found that nightshift workers had an increased dependence on snacks and had more frequent grazing activity. Patients' daily physical activity was also reduced due to decreased social interactions and fewer opportunities to exercise during daylight hours.[53] Finally, the researchers also found that certain hormones related to signaling hunger or satiety were dependent on established circadian (sleep) patterns, and when the normal sleep patterns are disrupted, the hormones also become imbalanced and disrupted.[54] Even though this study only addressed gastric bypass patients, it is suspected that the same results would be true for weight loss surgery patients employing any surgical method, including Lap-Band®.

Now, I mentioned this study not to dissuade, discourage, or deter anyone who does not work regular office hours. This does not mean that you will not be successful with weight loss surgery. It simply means that you will have to be a little more diligent, a little more vigilant, a little more educated, a little more compliant, and a little more communicative with your surgeon's office. Two perfect examples of "shift workers" who have been highly successful with gastric bypass are Karen and Julie. Other than surgeons, I've never met anyone else who has as goofed up and messed up work and sleep patterns as they have!! So, if you work a job that isn't 8-5, just be aware, make your surgeon and the team aware, and make sure you prove this study wrong.

Conclusion

Okay, now you know the facts about weight loss surgery, weight loss in general, and the disease of obesity. Draw your own conclusions. As for my feelings, I think that if anyone can come up with a non-surgical, medical weight loss program with significantly better long-term results than the measly 0-2% of dieters who keep their weight off long-term, they should be eligible for a Nobel Prize in medicine! Until then we need to be painfully honest about the adverse sequelae of obesity, and the poor results of our present diet, medication, and other interventions.

The risks of weight loss surgery should not be downplayed, but neither should the risks of morbid obesity. It is not intellectually honest to downplay the significant problems related to obesity and the lack of success with medication and other approaches to weight loss, while playing-up the risks of bariatric surgery. The reality now is that surgery offers the best-documented long-term way for morbidly obese patients to lose weight and become healthier. But if you prefer to ignore the facts, I have some great lemon extract on sale for only $169.99. If you act today, I might even throw in a Gin-soo knife that can cut through pennies.

Even cowards can endure hardship;

only the brave can endure suspense.

MIGNON MCLAUGHLIN

Chapter Four

SCRAMPS, AND STRICTURE, AND HICCUPS, OH MY!!

Julie M. Janeway
Karen J. Sparks

Okay. You've just read all the medical information about weight loss surgery, and you may still be finding yourself a bit curious about some of the potential complications and after-effects that can result. Well, we've decided to write a little about our experiences with complications and after-effects to help ease that curiosity.

But before we get into that, just a quick word on the topic of dealing with post-surgical complications. First, you may not have any complications, but you will have after-effects, so be prepared. You'll understand the difference between them as you read through the chapter.

Second, don't be afraid of complications because the doctors aren't afraid of them. Trust that you've chosen a physician who are more than competent and capable of handling anything that comes up, and that they are prepared and ready to appropriately deal with whatever you may experience.

Third, what other people had, you might not have; but… you might. Each person is very different, and there's no predicting what can happen. Not even your surgeon can predict what will occur or not occur. Just wait and see. We hope (knock on wood) you won't have any complications to speak of, and your after-effects will be mild, and more humorous than annoying or painful.

Fourth, be prepared to deal with whatever comes your way. It's part of the package. Remember that you've already dealt with so many more issues, so much more pain, and far worse things than whatever complications you may experience as a result of this surgery. Just grit your teeth and persevere. Chances are excellent that all will work out well in the end.

Finally, don't lose perspective, or your sense of humor. Keeping everything in perspective and relative to the entire timeline of the process is key. Your sense of humor is so important in getting you through tough times. If you start to lose your sense of humor, make sure you turn to your support network for help in fighting through the rough patches one day, or one hour, or even one minute at a time.

Now, back to complications and after-effects. We've chosen to organize this chapter by using little subheadings to keep it simple and easy to find things for later reference. We've also indicated under each subheading who had the issue, and therefore who's writing about it. If both of us had it, then it's generally me (Julie) who's writing about it. That probably means Karen's off teaching a class somewhere. But, if she alone had the issue, then she's recording her experiences for posterity all by herself. And for those of you who may be thinking that we made this stuff up, we *did* have these issues, and we did make it through. We have exciting enough lives that we don't have to make up medical issues to write about.

The following are the experiences we had with our surgeries, and you may have different experiences, or not experience these things at all. The best we can tell you is prepare for the worst, and hope for the best.

POTENTIAL COMPLICATIONS

STRICTURE
Julie

Well, we might as well start with the most common complication of weight loss surgery. Dr. Baker has explained stricture to you in the previous chapter. If you've already forgotten, go back and look it up. I'll wait........dum dee dum dum, da dee dum dee dee......... Got it? Good.

I had a stricture, which is statistically the most common complication after RYGB surgery. The stricture first occurred within a week or so following gastric bypass. I couldn't get the protein drinks down, and it eventually got to the point that I couldn't get water or any other liquid down either. The less protein and fluid I took in, the more dehydrated and starved my body got, the more tired and sick I was, and the less I cared about even trying to get anything in.

I was fairly stubborn about all this, and didn't want to bother Dr. Baker. After all, he is a very busy man, and I thought he'd think I was just a whiny, wimpy patient. So, I just sucked it up and hoped it would pass.

When I went back for my two week follow-up appointment, I broke down and told him what was going on. Of course, he couldn't believe I'd waited so long to tell anybody, but never once did he scold or berate me. He simply dove right into taking care of it, and assured me it would be okay. After examining me, listening to me cry, and asking me a number of questions, he informed me that he suspected I had a stricture and he immediately scheduled an endoscopy.

An endoscopy is a procedure that involves sending a long tube with a camera in the tip down your throat and into your stomach. The doctors can have a lovely little look around, and in the event things have constricted because of swelling or spasm, they can send a little balloon type device down there and pop it open again. All in all, it's not unlike snaking a drain. They reel it down, have a look around, push through the blockage, and reel it back up. Voila! You can dump stuff down the drain and it will run right out to the sewer system again.

So, Dr. Kemmeter, Dr. Baker's partner, was kind enough to take me in for an endoscopy. Now, for those of you who've never had an endoscopy, I will tell you that the worst part of having one is really getting the I.V. in. I was none too happy with the concept of having a complication at all, let alone having a stricture because it involved having another procedure done under sedation, which meant another I.V.

Because of my car accident, and by my personal calculations, in the previous three years I'd had about three million, four hundred sixty two thousand, seven hundred and fourteen needle and I.V. sticks, give or take a hundred or so. Also, for such a big person, I had virtually non-existent veins, and add to that the fact that I was massively dehydrated, and you can get the picture on what a pure joy it was to try and have an I.V. started.

After a few-more-than-several attempts to get the I.V. started, I not-so-calmly reminded them that I was a "hard stick," and suggested that they might find someone who was trained to start pediatric I.V.s (a little trick I learned when in the hospital with my car accident). The theory is: if you can start one on a preemie, chances are you can get one on me. I'd been a good sport to that point, but you can only play pincushion for so long. To their credit, the nurses quickly found someone who had just that sort of training, and she came down and slapped that puppy right in on the first try. I promised her a large bequest of jewelry in my will.

Following the I.V. incident, the rest was a breeze. They give you some sedation meds to start calming you down (or maybe it's just me…I don't know), and then they wheel you into the procedure room. It's not really an operating room, it's just sort of like a hospital room with more sterile medical monitors and junk in it. Anyway, they got me situated laying on my side, told me again quickly what they were going to do, then they ran some drugs in the IV, and that was it. I don't remember a thing until they were waking me up in recovery.

In recovery you're pretty groggy. You don't really know where you are or why. They seem to think that getting you to drink something is important, so I complied. Personally, in recovery, I just want to be left alone. Unfortunately they don't think that's an option. They let you lay there for around an hour or so, during which time the doctor comes and talks to you about what he or she found.

At least that's what I'm told. I don't ever remember talking to the doctor because the drugs kind of wipe out your memory for a while after the procedure. (I'm quite sure they were developed by the CIA or something.) But I know I talked to the doctor because my husband Matt swears I did (unless the CIA got to him too), and I came home with a lovely parting gift of full color before and after pictures of my insides. (I thought lovely parting gifts always included Rice-a-Roni® and Chico-San Rice Cakes®…?)

Interestingly, the color pictures are pretty drastic. It turns out that the opening from my pouch to my roux limb was mostly closed off. Overall, very little was getting through. Hey, it happens. At least they knew how to fix it. And the color photos double as pretty nifty post-modern art pieces if you frame them just right.

So that was my first experience with stricture. Unfortunately it was not my last. My little innards are pretty stubborn, and by a couple of weeks later, the opening had spasmed and strictured closed again. Back to the endoscopy suite I went.

This time I got the pediatric I.V. nurse right off the bat, so I circumvented that drama. Again, Dr. Kemmeter cranked open the stricture. Again, I went to recovery. Again, I purportedly talked to the doctor. And again, I came home with another piece for my post-modern art collection.

We were all pretty sure at this point that the opening would stay open, as most people only have to go through this once. I, of course, had to be one of the minority that has to go through it more than once. Apparently my innards are slow learners, and about a month later, I was right back in there having it done again.

Now before I go any further, I feel it necessary to stress that this is highly unusual, but not unheard of. I've already stated that I'm a person who likes to test limitations and boundaries, and apparently so does my gastrointestinal tract. I guess it just wanted to see if it could really get Dr. Kemmeter back in there a third time.

By this point, I had the process down to a science. The I.V. went right in, the procedure went without a hitch, and I got another piece of art for the collection. But before I went under, I did ask Dr. Kemmeter if there was a record for the number of times someone had to undergo this procedure. He declined to tell me in case subconsciously I'd try to break it. I also asked if there was some other measure that could be taken to hold the opening in place, and he assured me that this procedure would do the trick. Turns out he was right. I was third time lucky.

Stricture isn't fun, but it can be dealt with effectively. Many people say they have a mild sore throat for a day or so following the procedure, but I never did.… Kudos to Dr. Kemmeter. All I ever had was the need to sleep for 24 hours after each procedure. You are advised to go back to soft and liquid foods for a day or two, but past that you're up and moving around with no issues.

It's a fairly common complication of weight loss surgeries, so don't be shocked if you find yourself in an endoscopy suite afterward. I survived my strictures, and if you find yourself being visited by the stricture fairy, you will too.

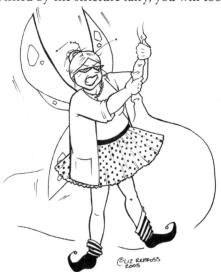

BLEEDERS AND BLOOD TRANSFUSIONS
Karen

Although I didn't have all the drama that usually accompanies anything Julie does, I, too, had a surgical complication. My complication involved a blood vessel or something that decided to leak causing a great purplish-red-black bruise on the right side of my torso. Later, we affectionately dubbed it "Lake Michigan" because that was how it was shaped.

My bruise started to form right after surgery, and as I was still enjoying the Morphine ride, I didn't notice, nor did I care. At one point, however, I tried to resituate myself in the bed, and noticed the growing discoloration. I made a mental note, and went back to dreamland.

In any hospital, trips to dreamland are only a few minutes long. It's sort of like trying to sleep on the subway, you keep waking up at every stop. In the hospital there's always a nurse or someone else there to check on something or another, or to wake you up to tell you to go to sleep. I know that's a good thing, but let's be honest; it's still annoying.

Anyway, they came in to draw blood, and when the results came back, they noticed my blood counts were low. They took my blood pressure again, and noticed that it had dropped. At that point, I was coherent just long enough to relate to the nurse my notice of "Lake Michigan" before the Morphine had me off on another adventure. (Man I love those little PCA "jeopardy" button things they give you for self-administering pain meds....)

The next thing I remember was Dr. Baker appearing in my room and telling me that he was ordering some blood because my blood level was too low. He mentioned something about a suspected bleeder, and if the infusion didn't work they'd have to go back in and find it. I mumbled through my Morphine haze that I trusted him completely, and to do whatever he thought he needed to do.

Three units of blood were hung, and my blood pressure slowly started to rise (although I don't know how, as I swear they took at least two units back out in blood samples). I was finally strong enough to have them remove the Foley catheter, and to get up to go to the bathroom.

When I went to the bathroom, I was horrified to see the toilet filled with blood, and quickly assumed I must be bleeding to death. I almost hung myself flailing about grasping for that little rope that calls for the nurse. When he came he told me everything was okay, and that it was actually a good thing because it meant that my body was expelling some of the oozing blood and my bowels were working again. My choices at that point were to believe him, or believe I would be dead in 10 minutes. I chose to believe him. Good choice.

The next problem was that my iron had dropped terribly in the process of losing and replacing my blood volume. I had to take liquid iron supplements for weeks after, which is like some sort of court-ordered punishment. I don't care what flavor they try and give it, it still tastes like you're sucking on a metal hanger. I suffered, and I mean SUFFERED through every one of those doses, but eventually that too came to an end.

Finally, my blood levels evened out, and Lake Michigan receded. Today I am just fine, and I've suffered no ill effects from my complications. I owe it all to the fact that I chose a physician who was knowledgeable, on-top of things, and was a person whom I trusted, literally with my life.

Trust is such an important thing in this situation. It wasn't the most pleasant thing I've ever gone through, but neither was it the worst. It wasn't optimal, but it was do-able. I got through it one minute at a time, and I never looked back.

THRUSH
Julie

Hi. It's me, back again. Yes, I had this one too. For those of you who don't know what thrush is, its real medical name is *candidiasis,* and it is a really nifty little infection that you generally get in your mouth. The way they diagnose it is by having you open your mouth really wide. They look at your tongue, and if it's coated with this icky white stuff that kind of looks like a thin schmeer of cream cheese, they know you have it. Babies get thrush a lot. It's not exactly lethal, but it can be life-threatening if it gets into your system and works its way to your heart or other major organs.

As I told you earlier, I was pretty sick just from dealing with the effects of my stricture, and my immune system was fairly defenseless at this point because I hadn't eaten anything in weeks. I was trying to drink skim milk because at least it had some nutrients, and it contains a high amount of protein per ounce. Never mind that I'm lactose intolerant; it was "damn the torpedoes, full steam ahead" in trying to find some form of protein that I could get in, and keep in.

The use of any antibiotics (like you get before and after surgery) can predispose toward developing thrush. Once your normal system flora (normal good bacteria) is affected, the microbe check and balance system gets out of whack. This then allows the infection to grow unchecked The problem was that I didn't know I had it, and because I was so weak and tired, it just flew down my esophagus and invaded my gastrointestinal system.

I found it ironic that nothing else could get through the stricture, but that nasty little infection just drove right through like a Mack truck. The internal thrush infection just made matters a little worse, but as soon as I went for another check-up with Dr. Baker, he found it, wrote a prescription, again listened to me cry, and again assured me I was going to be okay.

The treatment for thrush is generally a course of Nystatin®, Diflucan®, Clotrimazole®, or Fluconazole®. Ladies, if these look familiar to you, it's because you're right, they are the same drugs administered for yeast infections at the other end of the body.

Thrush is a form of yeast infection, and it is generally treated either topically or internally (orally) for a period of about 10 days or so. In my case, I was prescribed liquid Nystatin® in a pretty hefty dosage, with instructions to hold it in my mouth for about thirty seconds, swish it around, and then swallow it. I had to do this four times a day; which meant four times a day I made myself wildly sick trying to get unsick.

My thrush was particularly persistent, but as it began to beat a retreat, I got better and moved to a second course of treatment that was Diflucan® in pill form, once a day. When the stricture issue eased up and I could get some normal food in, the thrush was finally terminated. Moral of the story: You can flush the thrush!! It's not so hot to have, but in the greater scheme of things, pretty low on the "Why me, God?" list.

Neither one of us had any of the other five major types of complications. They are infection, pneumonia or lung collapse, pulmonary embolism, hernia, and bowel leakage or obstruction. Dr. Baker has talked about each of these potential complications in the previous chapter, so we believe it would be redundant to address them again; plus, we don't have any good stories to tell about them.

Suffice it to say, if you get one of these complications, you simply have to treat it like any other, and face it head on knowing you are under the care of a capable, competent, and kind surgeon who won't let you fall through the cracks. To quote a phrase, "Just pull up your big girl panties and deal with it!" (Apologies to the men reading this....)

Now on to the more fun part of this chapter: AFTER-EFFECTS!! Yeah! Everyone who has some form of weight loss surgery is going to have one or more of these weird after-effects. This is the stuff nobody tells ya, folks!!! You never hear people talk about this stuff on talk shows or the Discovery Channel®!! This is the everyday weirdness you'll deal with if you have weight loss surgery — plain and simple. It's not horrible, it's just weird. It's not deadly, it's just weird. Sometimes it's painful, but mostly....... it's just weird. It's not an all-inclusive list, just a sampling of some of the weird stuff that can happen. We've organized this section of the chapter the same way we organized the complications section, except we're going to write about them in the order in which they appeared. So without any further adieu, here they are.

POTENTIAL AFTER-EFFECTS

BLOATING AND TORSO PAIN
Julie and Karen

Ouch!! We both remember this one quite vividly. Most people experience this, and if you don't, well then they've got you on WAY too much Morphine! If you have weight loss surgery done laparoscopically the surgeon needs to fill your chest and abdominal cavity up with air so he or she can have room to maneuver things like the instruments and your liver. You know how you can spill a small glass of water, and as soon as it's out of the cup it's like a flood of biblical proportions? Well that's sort of the same principle behind how much air they put in you to do these surgeries.

The small incisions that are made in order to do the surgery are pretty well plugged up with the instruments, so not much air really escapes. When they're done the re-plumbing of your gastrointestinal tract, they take the instruments out and close the little holes. What results is basically what we like to call "the beach ball effect."

Remember as a kid (or more recently as a parent) blowing up those cheap plastic beach balls? You huff and puff, and huff and puff, and suck wind, and huff and puff, and wonder if the stupid thing will ever fill up all they way... and then you move to plug it and some of the air escapes. By this time, however, you're so tired of huffing and puffing that you don't much care as long as the darn thing floats (and if you're a parent, that the kids play with it and get lost).

The ball gets some play and is tossed around a bit, but mostly the kids just let it float around the pool. Eventually, the air just leaks out on its own, the ball goes flat, and then it goes wherever one sock always goes in the dryer. (Where is that?)

Anyway, this is pretty much what happens with the air they stuff inside you, except for the huffing and puffing part... I hope. They toss you around a bit in surgery, but then you just kind of float around while you're recovering, and eventually the air just leaks out, and you go flat. If you end up going where the one sock always goes, could you call us and let us know where that is? Thanks.

But we digress.... The point of telling you all this is that while the proverbial ball is going flat, it tends to be a little painful. You will most likely feel as though somebody broke a couple of ribs in surgery, and you'll most likely ask someone to check and see if they did. They didn't. Trust us. You'll probably feel like your rib cage is burning a little, but that's more than likely just some inflammation of the muscle tissue and the fascia. Also, it will feel as though if you roll over, all your guts will fall out. You can roll over, gently, as soon as your doctor says it's all right to do so. They won't fall out. Trust us.

So that's the bad news, but the good news is two-fold: 1) you don't have to deal with this for long; and, 2) your doctor can give you medication to help you deal with it. These sensations only last for about a week to 10 days on the whole, with each day

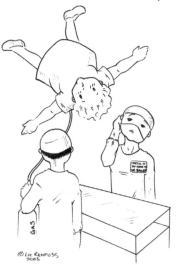

—TOO MUCH AIR—

getting a little better. Well…except the second and third days; they're pretty bad. It's kind of like working out; you're not really sore until the second day after the workout. Get it? If you have a good doctor (and you will), he or she will make sure that you have appropriate medications to help you deal with this discomfort. Julie and Karen's Prognosis: Icky, but totally survivable.

PAPER CUTS
Julie and Karen

If you've had a laparoscopic procedure, then you're going to end up with 6 little incisions about a half-inch long each. They'll most likely just put steristrips (little bandaid like things) over them to keep them closed, or they might plunk in one or two stitches under the steristrips. Either way, you're probably going to have 6 little wounds. How much do they hurt? Well, we call them paper cuts, and that's about as much as they hurt.

You know when you get a nasty paper cut, like from a file folder or cardboard? That's about what they feel like. After about 5 days, you really don't feel them anymore, assuming they don't get infected or something. But from our experience, and from the experiences of others we've talked to, you'll probably have one that will just wake up and poke you every once in a while, just to let you know it's there.

It will probably be one of the paper cuts toward the side of your torso, or the uppermost one in the front, as they seem to be the ones that rub most against clothes. For guys, the list could also include the one in your belly button if the waistband of your pants sits right there. Julie and Karen's Prognosis: Pretty low on the annoyance list. You'll recover.

ALLERGIES
Julie and Karen

There's a strange phenomenon that occurs in hospitals: the creation of allergies where none existed before. Both Karen and I developed, or maybe just discovered that we are allergic to certain types of pain medication while in hospitals. I am allergic to Dilaudid® and Demerol®, and Karen found out she is allergic to Morphine (despite the fun rides it takes her on).

It's not like you generally discover a life-threatening type allergy, although you could. You will generally discover the kind of allergy that just sort of drives you nuts by making you itch so bad you could take a steel barbeque grill brush to your hide! Karen's is technically an allergy because she itches something awful, but she doesn't break out in hives. I break out in hives and welts, so I know it's an allergy. I know that if I get hives and I don't attend to the situation promptly, my eyes and throat will begin to swell closed, and then it's not a good place to be.

Allergies are generally nothing major, just tell somebody you're uncomfortable or itchy and they'll give you some antihistamines and change your pain meds.

Note: if you begin to break out in hives, if anything begins to swell up, or you can't breathe, call for help immediately. Julie and Karen's Prognosis: Generally, no big deal. Annoying but endurable.

REVERSE HICCUPS
Julie and Karen

Now this little critter is an animal of a different sort. It's kind of unique to bariatric surgery patients, or maybe even just gastric bypass patients. All we know is that it's a very bizarre experience and condition, and it doesn't seem to go away.

As the name we've given it suggests, it feels like a form of hiccup (or hiccough for our European readers). When you have a normal hiccup, you kind of draw in air ridiculously fast. It's like there's a quick spasm, and then you're sucking in air.

But with a reverse hiccup, you still have the hiccup part, but from the point of the spasm in your gut, food and/or air also moves the opposite way through your intestines. That's the part that hurts. So it's like you're hiccupping in two directions at once. It sounds like this: HIC! OW!!

Dr. Baker tells me this is part of *peristalsis* which happens every time you eat. Peristalsis is the process of pushing food through the intestinal tract. Apparently the small intestine is always contracting, almost like a pump, but now it's hooked up high to the new pouch. The closeness of the small intestine to the upper abdomen causes more noticeable "growling" bowel sounds, and hiccups (involuntary contraction of the diaphragm) may affect the peristalsis of the pouch and small intestine such that the strange "OW" sensation occurs. Dr. Baker also noted that much more study, however, is needed to evaluate this theory.

If you have reverse hiccups too often, there's medication that can be prescribed to stop some of the spasms. Other than that, it's one of those weird things that you'll just deal with after surgery. We have no explanation for why this occurs only after surgery, but it does. And that's all we have to say about that. Julie and Karen's Prognosis: Weird, but you'll live.

AIR BUBBLES
Julie and Karen

Let us tell you right now, from the moment you come out of surgery your biggest enemy on the planet is air. To clarify: air is bad, unless you're breathing it. Air bubbles can feel like you've swallowed a VW Bug. They will cause unbelievable intestinal cramps that will have you twisting and contorting like a Cirque du Soleil performer. Air is to be avoided at all costs.

Avoiding gastrointestinal air intake involves eating slowly, chewing food very well, and avoiding all foods that cause air to enter the system. Also, not laughing while drinking something, because you tend to suck in a lot of air through your nose and then you swallow it. If you do this, you'll be experiencing the after-effect we discuss in the next chapter. (Voices of experience talking here....)

Most people swallow air while eating, especially if you are gulping. The air is generally stored in the stomach, which is usually a reservoir of sufficient size for it. After surgery, the reservoir is no longer attached to the esophagus, and only a small pouch exists to hold both air and food, thus the bloating and painful effect of gas is exponentially increased. To prevent this, you should avoid foods like broccoli, cucumbers, onions, soda pop, carbonated water, milk, peppers, bread, rice, and sometimes beans. There are others, but you'll have to make your own list of no-no's as you experience them. Air is pain. Air is your enemy.

If you are engaged by the enemy, your only survival tactic is to attempt to work it out, or wait it out. Some people say Beano® helps with the air issue, but that hasn't been our experience. If you want to try it, consult with your doctor first. Medications containing Simethicone™ such as Gas-X® strips we find helpful. Once you experience the kind of air bubble pain we're talking about, you'll learn to avoid the foods that cause the explosion or implosion of your intestines. Julie and Karen's Prognosis: Avoidable, manageable, but tolerable if necessary.

REPEATED BURPING
Karen

Related to the air bubble issue, is the issue of what we have termed Repeated Rhythmic Burping (RRB). Again, this is associated with peristalsis, but what results are repeated burps that occur in an evenly spaced rhythmic pattern. They may go on for hours. It sounds like this: Burp. Burp. Burp. Burp. Burp. (Multiply this times eighty-four more lines of text). It doesn't sound like this: Burp. Buuuurrrrrpppp!! Aaaahhhh!!

Neither one of us can figure out where all the air comes from. Julie and I can eat the same meal, eat the same amount over the same amount of time, and I'll end up with RRB, while she only gets two (and almost always two) reverse hiccups. What results is that if we're shopping when this occurs, I'm stuck in the car trying to deal with the RRB, and she's already scoped through the clearance and sale racks, and she gets all the good bargains. Meanwhile, I'm digging through my purse looking for the prescription the doctor gave me to deal with the RRB. Not fair!!

This type of thing can be headed off with a script for Cytotec®, or it's generic version Misoprostol. This medication helps to protect the lining of the stomach, but also helps to improve emptying of the pouch, which assists in moving along some of the gas. The prescription can be taken two ways. You can take it before eating, or after the burping starts. I can't really identify what's going to set it off, and I don't want to take the pills if I'm not having an issue, so I wait and take it after the RRB strikes.

I've eliminated the foods we listed previously in the "Air Bubbles" section, and many more. Sometimes I can eat a particular food and I have no problems. Other times I can eat the exact same food, and I get RRB. Go figure! But, generally about ten minutes after I take the medication, the RRB subsides. Unfortunately, that's right about the time Julie gets back in the car with the great sale shoes, and the other stuff that would have rightfully been mine were it not for the RRB ambush!! Julie and Karen's Prognosis: Annoying, strange, and totally unfair in a shopping environment.

SNEEZING WHEN YOU EAT
Julie and Karen

This has happened to both of us, but it happens to Karen far more regularly, and with far more ferocity. This one has no medical explanation we can find. It's a once-in-a-while phenomenon and is more weird than anything. Our informal survey of patients shows about 20-30% of patients experience this phenomenon.

Occasionally, you'll eat something too quickly, and the bite will have been too big. It will kind of get stuck on the way down, but it's not like you're choking or anything. While you are swallowing and trying to get it to go down, you may find that your body just creates an immediate sneeze right out of thin air.

It won't be just any old sneeze; it'll be a massive, tropical storm type sneeze, and the next thing you know the food is unstuck and moving on. Don't know what to tell you about this one folks, but we've both experienced it, as have others we've talked to, and we're just chalking this one up to the weird column. Julie and Karen's Prognosis: Whatever....

FOOD INTOLERANCES
Julie and Karen

Again, we're sure there's some long, involved medical explanation for this that includes a dissertation on enzymes, amino acids, and peptides, but all we know is that it happens to everybody who has weight loss surgery.

Every person we've ever talked to has had some sort of food intolerance issue. For some people it's immediate lactose intolerance, for others it's eggs, red meat, chicken, fish, or things that contain caffeine. It can be anything, even something you've eaten a million times — even something that's good for you like fruit, or a particular vegetable like corn or cauliflower.

We have no way of telling you what foods you'll be able to tolerate, and what ones you won't, and neither can your doctor, dietitian, or the Psychic Friends Network. This one you do on your own.

Our rule is if it makes you sick twice on two different days, separated by at least three weeks, then give it up for a while. The doctors and dietitians will tell you to wait a couple of months and try again. Some foods you'll choose to try again, like apples, or bananas, or bread. Others will have made you so sick, you turn a strange teal color just thinking about them (see our stories in the Auto Eject Chapter), and for those foods... well, maybe not so much....

We thought it important to warn you that this was coming, because it could be something as unnoticeable as black pepper, or garlic, or oregano. You'll have to experiment. Everything is an experiment!!! We should all get honorary food science degrees for dealing with this stuff!! Consider yourself warned. Now you're on your own. Julie and Karen's Prognosis: Irritating, but you'll live to tell the tale.

GALLBLADDER ISSUES
Karen

This potential after-effect of weight loss is no fun. Really, really, hope this doesn't happen, but if it does, know that it can be dealt with effectively and efficiently.

About two months after my gastric bypass surgery I began to develop a sharp stabbing pain in my side, which quickly progressed into unusual bouts of vomiting and nausea that weren't necessarily related to eating. The first time I felt the debilitating pain, I was bending down and to the right to pick something up in my kitchen, and ARRRGGHHH!, I was virtually blinded with pain, and I couldn't straighten up for about ten minutes. I thought, "That's not good...."

The second time it happened was about a week later, when I was sitting in my office. I dropped my pen, and when I leaned down and to the right to get it, I almost fell off the chair in abject agony. When I could finally straighten up, I wiped away the tears, and called Dr. Baker for help.

He scheduled an appointment for two days hence, and ordered an immediate ultrasound of my gallbladder. When I got to Dr. Baker's office, the results of the ultrasound were in, and it turned out that I had one big 2-centimeter gallstone fouling things up. Dr. Baker said it had to come out. I was profoundly glad. At that point I would have let him take an arm and a leg to get rid of that piercing pain.

Surgery was booked for about a week later. In the meantime, Dr. Baker gave me some medication to deal with the symptoms. It helped with the level of pain, but not only did the symptoms not go away, they continued to get worse.

Although the medication was dealing with the level of pain, pain became a more frequent visitor, and it brought with it its little friends "nausea" and "vomiting." At first I thought I was just eating foods that I wasn't ready for, but it turns out that most of my hurling episodes were gallbladder related. The most memorable event came one very cold night after we'd tried to eat some fajitas at a Mexican restaurant (a stupid endeavor in its own right...).

Without grossing anybody out, I spent over an hour standing in a parking lot, in the freezing cold, separating myself from what food I'd managed to consume. I was so sick I couldn't hold my head up, and it was almost three hours before I could get in the car and drive home. That night, the 45-minute ride home also included two unscheduled pit stops to separate myself from food I don't think I'd even eaten yet.

A week later I was in surgery. Interestingly, they take the gallbladder out laparoscopically when they can, and they use some of the same holes from your gastric bypass surgery. You also get two new ones about the same size. (Hey, what's a few more paper cuts between friends...?)

I was home the next day, and off work about three more only because I wanted the break. I haven't had any trouble since, and it was really no big deal to go in and have it removed. Once you've been in surgery, it takes away all the fear of the unknown. Note, gallbladder issues are the result of the weight loss, not the result of surgery *per se*. It's a potential after-effect, not a usual or direct complication of surgery.

Don't fear this potential after-effect. It happens to many people, and good surgeons will deal with it in a timely and competent manner. Julie and Karen's Prognosis: What doesn't kill you makes you stronger.

THERMOSTAT ISSUES
Julie and Karen

This one happens to almost everyone who has a drastic weight loss. When you were heavy, you probably dealt with the issue of being hot all the time (or as Karen likes to put it: "bursting into flames.") You were always complaining about being too hot, about people (read here: minions of hell) keeping the heat up too high, and you may never have understood why people whined so much about cold weather because to you it was often a welcome relief.

Remember the agony of hot, humid summer days? Remember standing in the freezer section at the grocery store for an inordinately long time? Remember wondering why skinny people never perspired, or looked like they were roasting like a Jordan almond? Well the reason is that fat is a wonderful insulator. Once you lose the fat, amazingly you're not bursting into flames anymore.

In fact, you should be prepared for just the opposite. Your poor little body is so used to being well insulated that you have to acclimatize all over again. Don't be surprised if now you're the one complaining about how cold you are, or how low people keep their thermostats (heat nazis...), or how unbelievably frigid it is outside. (There have been several occasions we've almost become convinced that a second ice age is here....)

So stock up on sweaters and sweatshirts, and get used to wearing a coat again. In fact, don't be surprised if you own more coats after surgery, than you collectively owned in all your years before surgery.

Note: issues will arise with others in your house or office as a result of your personal thermostat problem. Strangely, others will not find it humorous to discover the thermostat has gone from what appears to be 68 on the dial (ya, right!), to a comfortable and balmy 84. Ladies, your husbands may simply refuse to understand that having a space heater no more than four feet from you at all times is as necessary to life as water and air. Similarly, they're not about to understand or accept that you need more than them to keep you warm at night; at least two additional comforters will be required.

For those of you who live in warmer climates, don't think you'll escape this experience. It will probably just be less drastic. For those of you who live through cold, snowy northern winters, buckle up 'cause it's going to be one arctic-cold ride! Julie and Karen's Prognosis: S-s-s-s-survivable.

SCRAMPS!!
Julie and Karen

Scramps is a word that was invented by my niece, Meghan. Meghan suffers from a gastrointestinal disorder that has caused her terrible cramps since she was a baby.

When she was very little and learning to talk, of course she had a hard time conveying the pain she was in. As she grew and mastered language a little more, she finally learned to tell us when the *scramps* were starting so we could help her head them off, or help her through an episode.

We've adopted Meghan's term scramps because the searing, ripping pain that you can get in your legs or torso after a significant amount of weight loss is like "screaming" "cramps," or "scramps." We're not talking about your regular, every day charley horse in your calf here. We're talking about oh-my-good-golly, there must be some horrific netherworld force at work ripping my flesh from my bones, kill me now and spare me this misery — Pain!

We've found virtually no significant medical literature on this phenomenon as it relates to weight loss surgery patients, and we're in the process of convincing several medical researchers to begin a study to help explain exactly what it is, and why and when it occurs.

What goes on here feels like someone is actually ripping the muscles away from the bones in your leg! Additionally, the muscles then spasm, and each segment of your leg from joint to joint may actually twist in a different direction, making it feel as though your leg is being wrung like a dirty mop! Apparently there is a medical term for this: *tetany*. We don't care what you call it, it hurts!

Now multiply this by two if you happen to get both legs going at the same time. Somehow, one leg seems to have sympathy for the other, and says, "Hey, if you can't beat 'em, join 'em!" Sometimes the pain and spasm is so bad that you can't even get up to try and walk it out. News flash — this doesn't really work anyway....

Poor Karen gets this quite often. The first time she experienced it, we were away at an academic conference with another professor friend of ours, Judy, who is a nurse. The little college we were teaching for at the time had all of us staying in one hotel room (cheap college...). Karen began experiencing this ungodly pain in her leg. She tried to go out in the hallway and walk it off, but she was limping too badly, and it just got worse.

Judy first suggested putting ice on it, which we tried, but I knew from months of cramps similar to this (after twenty reconstructive surgeries following my car accident), that heat was probably the better way to go. Judy agreed.

I convinced Karen to get into the bathtub, pajamas and all, and I ran quite warm water in the tub as fast as I could. I had Judy massaging Karen's calf in a motion moving only toward the heart, and getting Karen to breathe deeply and stop crying.

You have to understand how much this hurts. Karen is a very strong and competent person. You don't get to be an academic Dean of over half a college campus being a whiner or a wimp. If Karen had broken down in tears, I knew we were dealing with cataclysmic pain.

After about an hour and a half, we finally got the pain under control, and got her leg to stop contorting and twisting in multiple directions at the same time. She was cold, wet, and beat up, but over all none-the-worse-for-the-wear. She could still walk, so we called it a success. We'd beaten back the leg scramps! Victory was ours!!

But what is actually worse than the leg pain, is if this occurs in your torso! PAIN! PAIN! PAIN! OW! OW! OW!

About seven months after my surgery I'd lost probably 80 lbs. or more, and I was sitting on the couch grading papers. I'd just eaten something for dinner, and about a half hour later I began to feel a little nauseous and uncomfortable, so I lay down on the couch. Immediately after changing positions I began to feel crampy discomfort, but it didn't feel like intestinal cramps. My ribs began to burn from what felt like the underside, and things in my torso just began to hurt.

I stood up and stretched my arms over my head, but that didn't work, and was making it a little worse. So I went and stretched in a doorway by hooking my hands on the upper jamb, and pulling down. That made things exponentially worse, so I lay down on the bed. I was now in a significant amount of pain, but because I'm very good in a crisis, I remained calm and rational about the situation.

Because of my analytical nature, I laid there trying to figure out what could be causing me such pain. I tried to slow my breathing down, but within about 10 minutes it became very hard to breathe, and my heart began to race. It felt as though my chest was caving in.

The pain was beginning to overwhelm me. I couldn't lie there anymore, so I got up and tried to walk around the house. I was alone, and since I live out in the country 20 minutes from a hospital, I was starting to get a little worried. I wasn't even sure if an ambulance would come all the way out there.

I was having a hard time breathing, and my heart was racing and skipping the occasional beat. I was telling myself over and over that I wasn't having a heart attack because I'm too young, I had lost a lot of weight, I have low cholesterol, and I wasn't doing anything strenuous at the time of onset. But then the doubts started to creep in: women don't experience heart attack the way men do as the pain is often atypical; maybe I'd over stressed my heart being heavy for so long, and now was the time it was going to give out; we have a history of heart problems in the family, etc.

I decided to call my mom to see if she thought I should go to a hospital, or whether I should try and wait it out. (When you're in trouble, don't you always call your mom? Or someone else's mom even...?) While I was on the phone trying to wheeze out what was happening to me, I was hit with a wave of pain that doubled me right over, and I dropped the phone. The pain caused me to let out a loud yell, and I could hear my mother on the phone hollering for me to pick it back up.

Unbeknownst to me, my husband's business partner was outside unloading equipment into the storage barn, and he heard me yell. He came running in, asking what was the matter. I could barely squeak out words at this point, and given the fact that I survived a car accident that required 6 months of hospitalization and level one trauma care, I could not believe the pain I was having.

Matt's friend grabbed the phone, and my mom told him to get me to a hospital. You have to remember that I'd had a few complications along the way, and only God knew what this was. So he threw my nightie-clad, barefoot self into the truck, and away we flew at about a million miles an hour to the closest emergency room.

The closest emergency room, by the way, is in a tiny little village in a hospital with six beds. Yup. Six beds. When I got married and moved out to the country, my husband told me that this was the closest hospital in case of an emergency. I told him in no uncertain terms that I'd literally have to be dying to go to that little tiny hospital. Be careful what you say....

We pulled up to the emergency entrance and were met by a doctor and a paramedic. They put me on a gurney and wheeled me into a curtained area that was literally three feet inside the door. No lie, the entire emergency room is smaller than my family room. They slapped oxygen and a pulse-ox monitor on me (pulse oximetry monitor — the clip thing they put on your finger), and tried to get me to tell them what was wrong.

I gasped out that I was in horrific pain, 7 months post-gastric bypass surgery, related the minimal details of my car accident 3 years before, and told them I couldn't breathe and my heart was doing funky things. They kept telling me to breathe slowly and to calm down.

I was as calm as I could get given the circumstances, because I knew that if I was having a heart attack, there was a doctor, 2 paramedics, and 3 nurses there to deal with it. I was breathing as slowly as I could, but it was hard when I couldn't expand my chest to draw in air.

They listened to my heart and lungs, they took my blood pressure, they took blood, and they took x-rays. Finally, they gave me some pain meds and some muscle relaxers. About an hour or so later it subsided. I felt like somebody had beaten the living daylights out of me with a baseball bat.

My husband showed up somewhere in the middle of all this, just about the time they were telling me that it was probably just stress, and I'd probably had a panic attack or some other psychiatric event, because they couldn't find a thing wrong with me. To me, it sounded as though they were telling me that they thought I was imagining all this, but I'm sure that's not what they meant. They simply didn't have a definitive answer, and were looking for a likely or common cause. I can assure you, however, there was something terribly, physically wrong that day.

As a person who's suffered from Post-Traumatic Stress Disorder (PTSD) as a result of my car accident, I can tell you that I am acutely familiar with panic attacks, and this was not a panic attack. This was my chest being crushed in from all sides like I was in a giant vise grip. This was almost unfathomable pain. This was purely physical in nature and had nothing to do with stress, or panic attacks, or PTSD, or anything. This was not something I wanted to experience again.

I stayed in bed the next day because I was so incredibly sore. The following day I went back to work, and told our nurse friend Judy about the ordeal. She told me that if it ever happened again to go to a bigger hospital as soon as it started, as they might be more familiar with this type of problem. She wasn't sure what it was either, but she said if it was muscle cramping, that the heart is a muscle too, and I should take it very seriously. At least she confirmed that I wasn't crazy (well, not about this anyway...).

I've had the experience several times since then, and each time I immediately headed it off with prescribed muscle relaxers and pain meds. Karen, and several others we've spoken to, have since experienced this type of scramp as well. Judy (our nurse friend), says that she has encountered patients in the ER who've lost large amounts of weight, and present with the same symptoms. Yet still, the question looms: "Why is this happening, and what causes it?" Which brings us to a conversation we had with our friend, Mark, a massage therapist.

Mark is the head of a therapeutic massage program at a local college, and he theorizes that toning exercises and massages every couple of days (even self-massages) might help prevent this experience in the legs and torso by keeping the muscles and fascia loose — a technique called *myofascial release.* Preventing dehydration also seems to help, as does keeping up your potassium (eat those bananas) and magnesium levels, and being vigilant about taking your vitamins. especially your thiamine.

What medical literature we have found refers to this pain as myofascial pain ("myo" meaning muscle, and "fascia" meaning the tissue covering the muscle). We've found documented evidence of other people presenting in an ER with exactly the same symptoms thinking they were having a heart attack. It turns out there were no heart attacks, simply the myofascial pain. No notation was made regarding whether or not any of the patients had lost large amounts of weight prior to onset.

Dr. Baker has continued to research this type of scramp, and tells us that this phenomenon is most likely from calcium or magnesium shifts associated with weight loss, or it could be related to thiamine deficiency — something many, many obese patients have although they are unaware of it. Spasms are the final result, can be significant (understatement of the century here!), and are most often noticed in the legs and at the lower end of the rib-cage. The roles calcium and magnesium play in the process of weight loss are not yet fully understood, nor are the roles played by the substances affected by calcium and magnesium well understood in situations involving losses of significant amounts of weight. At this time it is unproven as to whether it is related to too much, or not enough calcium in the body. Interestingly though, calcium is extremely important for the proper functioning of muscle, specifically for a muscle's ability to contract.

No matter the causative theory, if you experience one of these scramps, putting a heating pad on the area seems to help somewhat, also alternating ice and heat may help. It has been our experience that laying on your left side helps with your heart pounding, and giving in to the need or reaction to stretch your torso only leads to doubling the pain. We've both found that allowing your body to curl up is preferable to trying to lay out straight as far as pain levels go. Sitting up may worsen the pain as well, as your torso seems to want to try and compact together. We also suggest drinking water in small sips, and drinking as much as possible.

If you get scramps in your legs, we got a good tip from Judi Brown Clarke that really works. She told us that track athletes get a version of scramps and they deal with it by doing something they call blood washes. In essence they use the blood flow in the leg to wash through the muscle and flush out whatever is causing the cramping. If you need to give this a try, all you have to do is to raise your scramping leg as high into the air as you can until all the blood seems to have rushed out of it and your foot starts to tingle. Then swing your leg down, like off the side of the bed, and let all the blood run back into your leg. Your leg may begin to cramp up again, so if it does, just repeat the process until the scramp goes away. It may take several attempts at it, but it works pretty well overall. Judi has saved many of us from having to deal with this nasty little after-effect, so if you end up with a leg scramp, give it a try. It certainly can't hurt anymore than the scramp!

In the event of any kind of scramp, however, probably the most important thing, is to remain calm. Force yourself to calm down, relax your muscles, and breathe as slowly and deeply as possible. If you are alone when a scramp strikes, make sure you alert someone else of the situation. If others in the house are sleeping, wake someone up. Just knowing that you're not completely alone seems to help with relaxing and calming yourself. If the pain becomes too much, or you are experiencing an inability to breathe or your heart is beating erratically (not just fast), seek immediate medical attention. Better safe than sorry.

Knowing what you're going through, and not assuming that you're just stressed, or having a panic attack, will be helpful as well. If you seek medical attention, be sure to inform the doctors that you are a weight loss surgery patient, and explain in detail what you are experiencing. Make sure you have your surgeon's name and phone number with you. If you're experiencing a torso scramp, don't be at all surprised if they examine you to rule out a heart attack. Let them make sure everything is working properly, and let the safety of being with trained medical professionals who can help you in any situation assist you in trying to relax and breathe.

Just knowing that this could happen is probably one of the best pieces of information you'll get out of this book. Glad we could suffer, so you don't have to. Julie and Karen's Prognosis: This ranks ten out of ten Owies! on the Owie! Meter, but will probably not adversely affect your life expectancy.

And last, but by no means least, are our favorite after-effects of all time. Drum roll please…. (Read the next two chapters!)

They can conquer who believe they can.

VIRGIL

Chapter Five

⤛ A U T O   E J E C T ⤜

Julie M. Janeway

Karen J. Sparks

This short, but oh so very important chapter is dedicated to the phenomenon of *dumping and things that cause dumping*. For anyone who has experienced dumping syndrome, it comes as no surprise that it is being afforded its own chapter.

Dumping syndrome is something that occurs in gastric bypass patients as a result of the body's inability to absorb and process certain types of foods, or because food moves too quickly through the digestive tract. *Rapid gastric emptying* or *dumping syndrome* occurs when the small intestine fills too quickly with undigested food from the stomach.[1]

The entrance of the food material causes fluids to shift from other tissues into the intestine via osmosis. The increased fluid volume causes a rhythmic contraction that pushes food through the intestine (peristalsis), and consequently causes diarrhea. The loss of fluid from the capillaries can cause decreased blood pressure (hypotension), which may result in weakness, dizziness, and a rapid heartbeat.[2]

Early dumping begins during, or right after a meal. Symptoms of early dumping include nausea, vomiting, bloating, diarrhea, abdominal pain or cramps, feeling flushed, sweating, dizziness, weakness, rapid heartbeat, and/or shortness of breath.[3]

Late dumping happens 1-3 hours after eating. Symptoms of late dumping include weakness, sweating, dizziness, and abdominal pain or cramps.[4] Many people have one or both types, and most people have their own unique combinations of symptoms.

Make no mistake, however, if you have dumping going on, you know about it. There's no confusing it with anything else. When you're experiencing dumping, you are both afraid you're going to die, and afraid you won't.

Dumping syndrome occurs in most gastric bypass patients, although some people claim never to have experienced it (we think they are mistaken...). It's a safe bet to assume that if you have gastric bypass surgery, you will experience this thrill ride. Six Flags®, Disney World®, and the ninth ring of hell have nothing on dumping!!

If you're reading this book as a resource in helping you make a decision whether to have surgery, you also need to understand that this phenomenon doesn't happen every time you eat and doesn't happen to Lap-Band® patients. In fact, you quickly learn through the theory of negative conditioning to FOREVER avoid whatever caused it to happen in the first place!

The usual suspects include grease, sugar, rich foods like ice cream, high carbohydrate foods, eating too fast, not chewing well enough, and dehydration. Good bariatric centers will tell patients to stay away from eating sugary, greasy, rich carbohydrate filled foods. The staff members at Dr. Baker's practice in fact gave us these warnings on several occasions. As we stated earlier in this book, I tend to be a person who has to test the limits to see if they really apply to me. Yes, I was the kid who had to stick her hand on the burner to determine whether or not it was really hot.

I will now relate to you the truth about Pop-Tarts®. The truth about Pop-Tarts® is that they are in fact filled with as much sugar as the box says. I thought that maybe I could just eat half of a blueberry Pop-Tart®, and maybe if I left off the dry outer edges, it would be okay. I drastically miscalculated, and promptly spent the next six or so hours looking and feeling like a heroin addict spending her first night in detox.

To make matters worse, the phone rang while I was begging for death, and it was Karen. She could tell that I was in some sort of distress by the ghoulish way I answered the phone, and she of course immediately inquired what was wrong. When I croaked out, "I ate half a Pop-Tart®," I expected to hear some words of concern and support. Instead she quickly said she'd call me back later. Apparently, she had to get off the phone because she was spontaneously combusting with laughter on the other end of the line.

Karen did call back later (about seven hours later…) when she could finally get in enough air to form a complete sentence without busting a gut laughing. She matter-of-factly (and just a little self-righteously) told me that Dr. Baker told me not to do that. I said, "I know." She then asked me why I ate the Pop-Tart®. I said, "Well, I only ate half, and I only ate the middle." She roared laughing again, and said she'd call me back. To this day we can't walk down the Pop-Tart® aisle in the grocery store without her having a laughing fit. So, the purpose of this story is to demonstrate that the doctors and scientists have proven that sugar will cause gastric bypass patients to keel over and pray for death.

Now my stories about food limitations don't end there. I have stories about bagels, rice, birthday cake, and ice cream too. Suffice it to say, if my having to eat ice cream would create world peace, and allow me to buy and sell Bill Gates, I'd still have to think long and hard about it. By the way, because of dumping, we've conclusively proven that negative conditioning isn't just a theory. Scientists take note.

So, if panting like a dog, having your heart beat out of your chest like you're in mile 24 of a marathon, getting cramps that register on the Richter scale, having bed spins like you've been on a prom night bender, and experiencing the kind of nausea even astronauts don't get in the G-force simulator sounds like fun, then give us a call because the ice cream and Pop-Tarts® are on us.

Now I wouldn't, however, want to give you the impression that Karen is the rational compliant one in the group. In fact, I remember a little incident a couple months after her surgery in a restaurant just outside of Detroit. We were on a big shopping trip (translation: retail therapy), doing "important-woman-business," don'tcha know. We stopped to get some dinner because we needed to keep up that protein intake. I ordered some type of chicken dish because I still don't do well digesting beef. Karen decided to order a hamburger, and she ordered it with double onions, despite a warning from me not to do that.

Onions for some reason are hard to digest when you eat them in larger chunks. They seem to be okay chopped into small pieces in things like salsa, but red onions seem to be especially bad. Of course, she ordered double red onions on her burger, even though Dr. Baker told us not to eat them. To make matters worse they were cooked or carmelized which makes them very sugary. Read here: impending doom.

Karen proceeded to ditch the bun, and she cut her hamburger and onions up into very small pieces that she ate slowly and chewed very well. She stopped when she was full, and like so many other restaurant meals, put the rest in a to-go box to be later delivered to the styrofoam jungle that is her home refrigerator.

We left the restaurant and got in her car. After all, we still had so much bargain hunting to do. But alas, poor Karen succumbed to the onions. We spent the better part of an hour stuck in the freezing cold in a mall parking lot while she turned shades of green that don't even appear in nature.

But Karen is a true fighter, and as soon as she could get her head off the dashboard, she summoned up the willpower to begin the hour and a half ride home. She wouldn't even hear of letting me drive home despite the fact that she now had her head stuck out the door auto ejecting at least some of the onions. So I buckled myself in, said a prayer, and quietly emptied out one of the bags from my shopping trip in case she didn't get the window open in time as we drove. (I just thought it prudent to attempt to prevent a potentially nasty stain that the dry cleaner might not want to touch.)

Due to multiple gas station restroom stops, it took over three hours to get home that night. Now Karen has an almost freakish phobia of onions. Another aisle in the grocery store that's off limits....

The reality is, everyone who has gastric bypass surgery will eat something, advertently or inadvertently, that will cause dumping. Some people can't tolerate chicken, or beef, or fish for the longest time. Karen couldn't tolerate garlic in any form or amount for almost eight months. With other people it's potatoes, or fruit. I couldn't tolerate anything that had carbs in it like bread or pasta or potatoes for almost a year. But it can be any kind of food, even if you think you're being careful.

I ate some southern fried chicken, minus the skin, and made myself gloriously sick one day. Thank God for napkins and toilets because what is auto ejecting from you isn't too picky about the exit path.

So what can you do to limit your interactions with what can only be likened to an infantile projectile vomiting-dysentery-nervous breakdown hybrid? Drink lots of water. There are so many reasons you should be drinking lots of water (see Chapter Eleven), not the least of which is to prevent dumping. Also, chew your food well, eat slowly, and follow the instructions regarding foods to avoid.

If you end up in a dumping syndrome situation, then we advise lying on your left side (bathroom floor optional), and taking small sips of room temperature water. The rest is just waiting it out and letting it pass. It might take a half hour, and it might take six hours. We suggest stashing a pillow and a blanket behind the toilet.

Also, I think I should make a point about other things you should avoid, like drinking alcohol. Although the alcohol didn't cause dumping (but it can), I think it's important to tell you why they warn you not to drink after gastric bypass.

Once again, I decided to test my personal physical limits and test Dr. Baker's authority. I was on vacation in Florida with my husband at an outdoor restaurant on the Fort Meyers Beach boardwalk. I ordered a banana daiquiri thinking, "How much alcohol can really be in a goofy umbrella drink like that anyway?" I took three small sips of my drink over about a five-minute time span. Two hours later, when I could finally focus my eyes, my husband peeled me out of my chair, aimed me at the car, poured me in, and took my liquified body back to the hotel.

Don't drink alcohol. You might as well be main-lining it like an addict. It goes right into your blood stream in full force; and I mean *right* into your blood stream. Three sips and I was sliding under the table, screaming at a barking dog passing by, and laughing like a hyena.

Alcohol presents some serious problems for post-surgery bariatric patients. Not only does it peak in your blood stream in only 10 minutes,[5] but repeated expsoures to alcohol could cause some serious damage physically because of impaired abilities to clear the alcohol from the system and diminish toxicities related to the alcohol in the blood stream. In addition, the impaired performance of certain chemical pathways in the body as a result of morbid obesity and rapid weight loss can make the body more susceptible to the toxic and cancer-promoting effects of pollutants in the air, industrial solvents (including household cleansers), and certain drugs including acetaminophen (Tylenol®)[6]. There are a number of other physical issues that can occur with alcohol use in bariatric surgery patients, thus patients should take note and refrain from alcohol consumption other than maybe a few sips on a special occasion or something. See the information on alcohol written by Dr. Buffington in the resources section.

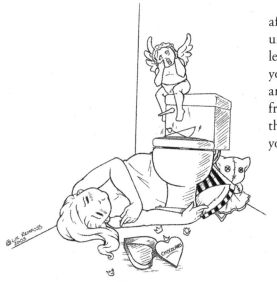

So just a word of caution here: if after gastric bypass you want to slide under the table, or dance on one, at least you'll be a cheap date. But if you would like to keep your dignity and good reputation intact, refrain from drinking alcohol. Listen when they tell you to avoid things... save yourself the trouble.

Chapter Six

THE
"BUILD-YOUR-OWN-CAT"
KIT

Karen J. Sparks
Julie M. Janeway

What did you say?... A cat with every surgery? What a deal! Or... not such a deal.... If you are a recipient of a "build-your-own-cat" kit, you can't give it back. Cat lover or not, you just have to deal with what you get. Another thing you need to understand is that your kit will arrive with little warning, and yes, unfortunately, some assembly is required.... Let me explain.

No matter what type of weight loss surgery you may undergo, they tell you there may be some hair loss due to the anesthesia, stress on the body, and actually from loss of fat in the body as well. They also warn you that if you don't take in enough protein your hair may also become dry and brittle, and begin to thin. A few lost hairs? Okay, I can deal with that.

I knew that hair loss was a possibility, and thought I was prepared. (Silly me!) I have always had a more than generous head of hair, one thing that in my mind, being overweight didn't affect (my ears are rather cute too). How was I to know that for too long I'd been taking my tresses for granted? That was all about to change.

About 4 weeks into my recovery, I noticed my hairbrush becoming fuller and fuller. I called Julie and told her I was concerned about the amount of hair being collected in my brush, and if it didn't slow down soon, I would possibly be able to use all that hair to build my own cat! So began the days of my brush containing more hair than usual, and little did I know that the first shipment of my "build-your-own-cat" kit had arrived.

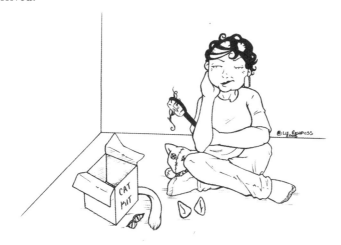

Here is where I feel I must clue you in as to my general attitude toward the feline homogeneous. As a rule, I have not always been that fond of kitties. As long as they belonged to someone else, life was good. Julie has two "cat-children," and next to God, I think they are the most important things in her life. (Husband ranks third?)

Conan O'Brien has a segment he produces on his show that pokes fun at what certain celebrities' children might look like if they should mate. Given Julie's genetically based, crazed love of cats, if Julie and Matt were to have a child, I swear it would be a cat! (I'll give you a moment to get that picture out of your head.) Needless to say, she's found more humor in the "build-your-own-cat" kit, than I have. Now that you have that background, let's move on.

At this point in my hair loss experience, I had not yet noticed any excess hair in the shower, but it has always been normal for me to see a little hair caught in the drain screen. Things were going along well — a little scrub here, a little lather there. Showers went on as usual. But then about 6 weeks post-surgery, the major shipment of my "build-your-own-cat" kit arrived. I was *SO* not prepared for that delivery.

I was getting ready for work one morning when "the kit" arrived. I had no idea that assembly of the "build-your-own-cat" kit would take place a handful at a time — or in my shower. As I ran my hands though my hair to rinse out the shampoo, I felt the loose hair caught in my fingers. Gently and fearfully pulling my hands down, I looked at them in sheer disbelief. Two tangled balls of soapy hair sat there looking back at me. Chills and nausea passed like a wave though my entire body. Looking down in the shower I realized that the fuzzy lump resembling a small, wet kitten hovering over the drain was actually a good portion of my own hair as well. I closed my eyes, and despite the water hitting me, I could feel the tears begin to slide down my face.

To tell you the truth, I was seriously scared. Scared of what was happening. Scared to look in the mirror. Scared of it getting worse. I was scared through and through. Each time I looked in the mirror in the days and weeks that followed, I began to see my brothers' receding hairlines. As I tried different ways of styling my hair to cover them up, I began to discover bald spots forming in different locations across my scalp. Would it stop? If so, when, and how?

When I took a shower I was very careful not to scrub my scalp too hard for fear of even more hair coming out. My anxiety over my hair completely disappearing doubled on a daily basis, and I began to consider what I might do. Cut my hair very, very short? Shave my head? Wear a hat? My mom suggested looking into the prospects of buying a wig. My mind worked overtime attempting to come up with a way to compensate for my hair becoming M.I.A. Dread, panic, and nausea aside, I simply wasn't going to let this beat me down.

Deciding what to do with my remaining three hairs was a dilemma. You should also know that the hair loss after-effect was not just mine. Julie experienced it as well. Julie possesses an excessively thick, full, and mostly uncontrollable, naturally curly Irish mane of dark hair — and it, too, was falling out.

Between Julie and her two cats, everywhere I sat at her house, I either had cat fur, or Julie hair on me. (I think the cats were having "sympathy" hair loss.) To a person who lived alone, and who is not used to having any pet hair on her clothes, even just a bit here and there was weird. In response to my whining about the cats shedding in sympathy with her, she told me that if I didn't want their hair (or hers) on my clothes to stay off the furniture! (She says that's why they call it "fur"niture.)

Anyway, we discussed our dilemma, considered our options, and determined we needed professional help before I went bald, the cats went bald, Julie went bald, or her husband Matt went missing under a pile of shed hair. So, I kidnapped Julie and off we went to see her hairstylist, Saul. Incidentally, you have to see a good and reputable hairstylist. Don't see the person at the $6, two-minute haircut store!! This is mega-important stuff. See someone with advanced training and education.

At the salon Saul was very kind and compassionate as Julie and I explained the dilemma with our hair. Although Julie's hair was thinning rapidly, I was in balding crisis, so we agreed on hair triage. I went first.

We began to tell Saul how this situation came about. You have to understand that at about 6 weeks post-surgery, it's still hard to tell people (strangers especially), that you've had weight loss surgery. You're still kind of sensitive about it. So, after relating that tidbit in hushed tones, we continued the story.

We told Saul how I was not exactly thrilled with the protein drink provided to me in those first few weeks, nor could I consume the required amounts. (Shortly after our surgeries they changed brands of protein drinks to SmartForme — yummy!) I simply didn't want to eat anything at all, and my initial thoughts and reactions were, "Are you kidding me here?" I forced in as much as I could, thinking it would be enough. It was to my detriment that I didn't get enough protein and nutrition in those early days following the surgery, and that compounded the hair loss.

Additionally, right after surgery you are taking in very little fat in your diet, and many researchers believe that hair loss is caused as much from low protein as it is from drastically reduced fat in the diet. We all need a certain amount of dietary fat to function properly and keep our hair in our heads, and I just hadn't been getting the requisite amount of fat, protein, vitamins, or anything else I needed! Saul listened with rapt attention.

Now, you must understand that your hair won't fall out just because you didn't eat enough protein or dietary fat the day before. This is a cumulative thing, and will take a few weeks or months to cause this kind of effect. Once you get that behind in your protein and dietary nutrients, however, you're forever playing catch-up to restore it. Don't put yourself in that situation.

I sense the panic as you read this, but not to worry. When I consulted Dr. Baker about my hair loss, he assured me my hair would restore itself. He told me just to keep up the good fight, take my vitamins, maintain the all-critical protein, use some Bariatrix' SmartForme products for additional nutrition, add some biotin if I wanted, and things would work themselves out. I had trusted this man with my life; therefore, I believed I could trust him with my hair.

Saul nodded in complete understanding of the situation. We expressed our concerns that any sort of chemical application would cause more hair loss. We related our fears of coming in with a little hair left, and going out with none. We asked for help and guidance. Saul gave me a reassuring pat, Julie a confident look, and began to explain what needed to be done.

Hairstylists are licensed professionals in most, if not all, states. If you ask for their guidance, they usually have the requisite expertise to deal with your hair-raising, hair loss predicament. Here are some of the tips our professional Aveda® hairstylist recommended.

Wash your hair every 2 or 3 days instead of every day. It doesn't need that kind of agitation. Also, coloring your hair helps to give it a fuller and thicker look because it actually expands the hair shaft. The addition of highlights and lowlights gives the illusion of fullness because it reflects more light. Add a nice cut and style (medium and shorter, but not short styles are better), and you are well on your way.

Your hair salon will probably recommend their product line as far as volumizing and thickening products. There are many excellent product lines in salons, including shampoos and conditioners, but beware the amount of styling product you use in your hair. If it weighs down the hair shaft, gravity will work against you by pulling the shaft out of the follicle, defeating your purpose. Nature based products (like those offered by Aveda®) are generally better than completely chemically contrived ones, but it becomes a personal choice.

The reality is, however, that salon products can get expensive (but if you use them correctly, they're generally comparable in the long-run). Let's face it though; unless you have an unlimited amount of disposable income, the one-stop shopping center's health and beauty aisle is looking pretty good. (But remember, although salon products may be a little pricy, like you-know-who says: "I'm worth it.")

Many products are available in your local stores that will work for adding fullness and volume at a reasonable price, including remedies like Rogaine®. For those of you who may find yourselves in situations of severe hair loss, always consult a physician before self-medicating with any of the remedies such as Rogaine®, Minoxidil®, and such. Each experience is individual, and there may be other factors contributing to your particular hair loss episode.

Besides products that simply regrow hair, there are multitudes of volumizing, thickening, and shine inducing styling products available in stores. But, be careful with getting carried away on the volumizing products; more product does not necessarily mean more volume. It just might mean more scrubbing to get it out, and more related hair loss, so cut down on the abuse you're giving your hair.

Cutting down on the abuse also means reducing the amount of blow-drying (blow dry on low, at low heat, and use fingers not brushes), and limiting the use of curling and flat irons, especially. Also, the use of hair binding items such as hair clips, ponytail bands, and the like aren't good for thinning hair, as they tend to pull on the hair shaft, and/or break it off. Our hairstylist's advice: Be kind to your hair, it's injured.

Of course, being kind to your hair necessitates following the post weight loss rules, a message we've resonated throughout this book. Drink plenty of water to keep yourself hydrated, take your Building Blocks® vitamins every day, and eat what you are supposed to in order to keep up with that all important protein quest.

Protein intake is critical not only to your overall system, but especially to your hair, which consists primarily of keratin, a type of protein. When your body is deficient in a nutrient such as protein, it begins a process of shutting down the least necessary assets, much like the electrical breakers in your house shutting down one outlet before the whole system blows out. This is why your hair falls out if your protein intake is too low for too long. Your system has shut down shipping protein to the hair, in order to continue supplying other vital systems instead. Keeping up the protein supply is the real trick.

And protein isn't the only thing. We now know that vitamin and mineral deficiencies also play a role in hair loss and hair thinning.[1] Vitamins A, C, E, B6, B12, folic acid, and biotin are all vitamins that are at risk of being deficient in a bypass patient, and coincidentally, they are also vitamins that play important roles in hair production and cell and hair health.

Minerals are also important to hair health. Calcium, copper, iron, magnesium, selenium, and zinc all contribute to keeping your hair in your head and not in your drain. Again, these are also nutrients that can become deficient in bypass patients. So, we see yet another reason for eating healthy, well balanced meals, and taking those vitamins! The people at Building Blocks® bariatric vitamins really should become some of your very best friends!

Finally, essential fatty acids are also very important to keeping your healthy hair, but we are only just beginning to understand the role they play in the average human, let alone the post-surgery bypass patient. Most people get more than enough of one of the two essential fatty acides (EFAs), that being Omega-6. We get lots of it from our foods and the oils we cook with. What we don't get much of is Omega-3, the other EFA.[2] It's found in things like salmon, mackerel, flax seed, and walnuts. Omega-3 is best obtained from food sources, but if supplementation is needed, consult your bariatric surgeon, or better yet, your bariatric dietitian for help in determining a correct dosage. They'll help you figure out how to get more Omega-3 into your daily food consumption as well. And speaking of food...

After you have had your weight loss surgery, the hardest thing is actually learning to eat again (see Chapter Thirteen). I am here to tell you that most likely you won't want to eat, but you must. It's hard, but if you like your hair just the way it is — EAT! (or drink, as the case may be...). Protein and vitamins are critical. Fact stated. Tattoo it on your forehead for future reference.

What you should also note for later reference is that if you lose your hair, you should choose to look at it as an opportunity for your first makeover (guys, this means you too). Time to update that look!

Despite the fact that I am considered a highly educated person, my sense of style and skills in promoting my own self-image were minimal at best. Being overweight for the entirety of my life, I would not engage in anything that would draw attention to myself. Hair and make-up? Why? I mean, I'm trying to hide in plain sight here!!! Why would I draw attention to myself? Geez...!!

Once you decide to have weight loss surgery, however, or if you have begun your journey already, you will start to discover another physical person emerging out of that old physical you. For me, it just so happened that she began to emerge with less hair...but emerging she was.

Because I've never been one who was concerned much with my outer presence (other than being clean and tidy), when Julie suggested we visit the stylist at her Aveda® "day-spa" to deal with the hair loss issue, I was pretty concerned that I was in a little over my head. But I trust Julie like a sister; I thought about it, and as I said, I kidnapped her from her house one day, and away we went.

When Saul suggested coloring my hair, I was a bit reticent as I've never colored my hair (gray or no gray). But since Julie has always been a hair and make-up diva, I figured I had no choice but to trust her and Saul when they told me that was what I needed. (Incidentally, Julie took away my car keys so I couldn't leave.)

Once I made that decision, I thought, "What the heck, you might as well do whatever else you think is necessary while you're at it." The two of them looked at each other with evil little grins on their faces (too evil for my liking), and they assured me that this makeover was going to help my hair loss problem, and make me feel like a whole new woman. After all, wasn't that the point of having the surgery? To become a whole new woman? They saw that my defenses were down, and they went in for the kill.

My hair loss misfortune inadvertently turned into one of the most fortunate experiences since my surgery — a serious "little victory." My hairstyle really hadn't been updated in years, and the new one brought out my features and made my face look thinner. (Yeah!) My new color and highlights worked so much better with my skin tone that it made me look younger. (Yeah!) I just couldn't believe it was me.

Saul taught me to style my hair with minimal effort, and I learned all about what was good for it, and what wasn't. Then they took me to see the make-up artist. Being an artist myself, I can appreciate the talent it takes to draw the human face, but I've never been able to draw worth anything when it came to drawing *on* my own face. I just knew that I'd end up looking like a recent graduate of clown college, but I figured I could always go and wash it off.

Julie, recognizing my trepidation (maybe the death grip on the chair gave me away?) told the make-up artist that I'd never worn make-up, and to do something extremely natural and light. She also told her to explain to me what each product was, what it was for, and to write down the order in which they were applied. I closed my eyes, and slumped back in sheer resignation to what I was sure would be my utter humiliation in looking like a carnival freak.

I was determined not to look as Danielle was applying the products, and I was only listening half-heartedly to what she was saying, but curiosity got the better of me once or twice, and I peeked. What I saw when I peeked wasn't so bad, and then I thought, "The worst is yet to come." But it never did.

When Danielle was finally finished, I took a deep breath, and squinted open one eye. I was indeed shocked at what I saw. What I saw was me — only better. She had done exactly what Julie suggested: a light and natural look that just enhanced my own features. I was amazed. I had eyelashes!! My eyebrows had shape!! I was astounded, and very, very pleased. Thinking back, I don't know why I ever thought that a trained make-up artist, or Julie, would ever let me come out looking like a Jackson Pollack painting. Must have been the fear talking.

While Julie was getting her hair repaired, I must have spent at least an hour and half sitting there looking at myself in the mirror. Was that really me? Me, who came in all frazzled at my hair loss situation? Really? Is it possible that I came in one person, and am going out another? Is it really that easy? Yup!

With the help of a good hair stylist, a little color, an appropriate hairstyle, and products to promote fullness, you can get past the hair loss issue in grand fashion. My hair has come back in good order, and the world still turns. You may think your surgeon is a miracle worker for helping you through this lifesaving surgery, but in a hair loss crisis, a good hair stylist and an accompanying friend are worth their weight in gold.

Although a full makeover is not really part of dealing with hair loss, you should do it anyway. I used to say, "Hair and make-up? Why?" Now I say, "Hair and make-up? Why? Because the new you deserves it, that's why!"

As Julie and I have stated throughout this book (and we'll say it again to anyone who'll listen), whatever comes your way, whatever the after-effect with which you must deal, do what you have to do, and move forward. Deal with it as best you can, and find the solution that works for you.

Hair loss doesn't have to happen to you, because as we've said it is almost totally preventable. Even if you don't have any hair loss issues, you should still consider going to see a good stylist anyway, just to update your look. By 6 weeks post-surgery, you'll really be starting to see the new you emerge. Give that new person a boost in the right direction, and remember: only your hairdresser really knows for sure....

Flowers grow out of dark moments.

CORITA KENT

Chapter Seven

THE SHADOWS OF
⭐ MY FORMER ⭐
SELF

Scott H. Glass, MS, MA, LLP

In this chapter we get down to serious business — no tiptoeing around. You have two main reasons not to take bariatric surgery lightly: your surgeon will be going beneath the surface of your skin to do some serious rearranging of your intestinal tract or restriction of your food intake, and you will be going beneath the surface of your psyche to operate on the shadowy memories, thoughts, and feelings that have gone unaddressed to this point. The latter deals with what's preventing you from losing the weight and keeping it off, and that is the focus of this chapter. It's not a really fun chapter, but it is an important and thought-provoking one, so hang in there with me for your own good, okay? Let's get started.

Have you ever heard the saying, "You reap what you sow?" A farmer who works hard to sow a crop will reap the reward of a good harvest. If he does not work diligently to sow and maintain a good crop, he will not get as good a harvest. The reality for you is that you, too, have reaped what you have sown. Recognizing that family history and genetics have influence as well, your obesity is a result of the choices you have made in your life. You have chosen to take in more calories than your body requires, and you have chosen to engage in more sedentary activities. These were your choices, and now you are reaping what you have sown. It's not a judgment, just a bare fact.

I have heard time and again from bariatric surgical patients that "I have had to work hard to stay this heavy." "Obesity is what I get for living foolishly." "No one forced me at gunpoint to eat that food. I chose to eat it all by myself." "At the end of the day, I chose not to go for a walk; instead I chose to watch television." Choices always have consequences. Sooner or later, everyone will reap what they have sown.

I recently met with a woman who admitted, "It was just always easier and more fun to eat." Now, well over 100 lbs. overweight, and with increasing and serious medical concerns, she experiences the cost of living in this manner. If she wishes to reap a different crop from what she has sown, she will have to change her mindset, behaviors, and really examine what she values in life.

As a culture, we value comfort. We believe we are entitled to live a comfortable life. We believe we have the right to do things that make us comfortable. After a hard day at work, we believe we deserve to take it easy. We deserve a mixed drink when we are stressed or worried. If we don't feel like cooking, we are entitled to go out to eat. As a very obese society, we have based our lifestyles and behaviors on these perceived rights and entitlements, and consequently we have reaped what we have sown.

My point is not whether you do or do not have these rights. My point is that based on these ideas, your behavior has gotten you into serious health trouble. As long as you rely on these rights and entitlements, you will not overcome your weight problem. You have other rights and entitlements to rely on, however, like the right to a healthy life and a healthy body, being entitled to engage in activities of your own choosing, to eat healthy and nutritious foods, and to make choices because they are good for you, not just popular, easy, or expected. Shift the paradigm!

Recently, the discussion in a support group centered on eating during the holidays. The attitude of the group was one of defeat. "We can't change." "Holidays only come around once in a while." "We always host the meal at our house, so I have to do the cooking." "It's tradition. People are coming in from out of town, and they will be disappointed if I don't fix their favorites. They always look forward to my cookies."

Again, I am not saying you cannot or should not do these things. What I am saying is that by continuing to hold to these preset notions and the fear of change, you lock yourself into the same behaviors that got you in trouble in the first place. Value the companionship, the family, the memories, and the experiences. Do not value the food and the obligation to maintain unhealthy behaviors. Find alternatives that can be palatable to the majority of those involved. (You can't please all of the people all of the time….) Call it progress. Call it expansion. Call it creating new traditions. Call it whatever you want, but change the reality and be prepared for somebody to be resistant to how the changes will affect their lives – after all, you were.

It is a blunt fact that people want to live their lives the way they want to live them. We do not like to be told how to live our lives. How many times over the years have your doctor or loved ones encouraged you to lose weight, to change your eating pattern, or to start exercising? Granted, these changes are difficult, but did you work at it? Were you committed to the point of doing whatever it took to meet your goal? Did you change your thinking, your viewpoints, and your outlook? Maybe, but you certainly didn't make it a pemanent change or you wouldn't be reading this book.

Take exercise for example. People will say they do not have time to exercise. Many become angry or offended when encouraged to cut back in one area of their life to make time for exercise. They maintain there just isn't time. When encouraged to get up earlier in the morning to exercise, they respond: "Oh, I am not a morning person. I could never do that." When asked, if they could go to bed a little earlier so you wouldn't be as tired in the morning, they respond, "No, I like to watch the 11:00 news and a little bit of Jay Leno," or "I just don't have time with my stressful job and busy family." People are by nature incredibly resistant to change, especially when it is perceived as "drastic" change.

Change is not easy, but the fact is that if you continue your current style of living your weight and health will get worse, and your quality of living will decrease further. Ask yourself: "Is my goal to be comfortable now, or healthy later?" Which do you value more? The answer to these questions will ultimately determine whether you should even consider weight loss surgery.

Successful weight management after bariatric surgery requires full commitment and perseverance. It is not easy. If it were, everyone would have done it and we wouldn't be writing this book! There is no cure for obesity, but, you can do it if you are serious, admit the problem, take responsibility for solving the problem, and totally commit to creating a permanent solution.

After admitting you have a problem, you must also define the problem. You might be surprised to learn that the problem is not your weight. No, really!! The excess weight is really just a symptom of a deeper problem. Turning toward food for comfort, relaxation, or just something to do is a symptom of underdeveloped, or ineffective coping skills. In today's stressful, busy lifestyles we could all use a few more coping skills!

I have said many times, one of the single best methods of managing your weight is to manage your stress and emotions effectively by developing your coping skills. Stress and emotions influence most people to overeat, and stress and emotions often keep people overeating until they are overweight or worse. So, until a person learns to manage their stress and emotion in a healthy and effective manner, that person will continue to struggle with their weight.

There is no way to just make stress and emotion completely go away. It's just life, and as we all know: life is not fair. Sorry to have to tell you this, but surgery or no surgery, you will continue to experience disappointment, failure, rejection, anger, and many other emotions. Although some of the stressors may be different, the existence of stress will remain. The trick is to learn to cope better (and don't kill the messenger!).

Coping more effectively is about breaking the less effective and often unhealthy patterns, and substituting new and healthier patterns in their place. Take, for example, a situation in which you experience frustration over something that did not work out the way you had planned. In the past, because there was nothing you could do to change the outcome, maybe you dealt with the frustration, anger, and disappointment by getting a bowl of ice cream to soothe those prickly feelings and make yourself feel better. This pattern of responding to negative emotions by using food as a salve has not really helped you feel better, and only makes you feel worse in the long-run.

A more healthy and effective method might be to first go for a walk, even a quick walk around the parking lot if you are at work, to let off the steam. Then, once you have cooled off, call a friend or co-worker and vent. Verbalizing problems and venting emotions through words really does help.

You could also just sit down, by yourself, and write out or diagram the problem from a couple of different perspectives. What are your options with that project now that the first run did not turn out as you had hoped? What are the pros and cons of each option? What did you learn from this project? How can you do it differently next time? Write down your plans for attempt number two, and know you've dealt with your emotions in a productive, positive, and non-destructive way.

When your emotions are getting the better of you, and you want to resort to your old behavior of throwing food at the problem, here is a little chart you can use to help you in coping with various emotional situations. Stick it to your refrigerator and look at it before getting a snack from now on. The following example is just to get you started. Substitute where necessary with ideas that are specific to you, such as adding to the list of emotions — sad, worried, afraid, guilty, ashamed, or hopeless.

HUNGER

When I am legitimately hungry, I will eat a small piece/portion of:

Yogurt
Cottage cheese

Cheese stick
Granola bar

Nuts
Banana
Raisins

Apple
Peanut butter and low fat crackers

Protein bar
Carrots
Melon
Sugar-free Jello® or pudding
Hard boiled egg
Bariatrix' SmartForme

OR I will drink a glass of water!

EMOTIONS

If I am experiencing an emotion, I will not get anything to eat. Instead I will do the following:

When angry I will — clean the garage or closet.

When lonely I will — call/write a friend, ask someone to meet me for a walk.

When stressed I will — write in my journal, talk to a co-worker, soak in the bathtub.

When bored I will — get out my To Do list and get on with it!

When feeling guilty over eating something I shouldn't I will — remind myself to think in the big picture, get over it, remember I am human, and move forward!

When I'm feeling defeated I will — get out my "before" picture and remember that I am in a better and healthier place than I was then.

When I am feeling _____ I will...

If, after trying some of these ideas, you realize a need for more help, do not procrastinate! Call a trusted friend or family member, or even a professional counselor or pastor. Dealing with emotions in an effective and positive way is extremely important to the success of your weight management program, whether or not you ever choose to have surgery.

If you do choose to have surgery, then developing good coping skills will help you head off problems relating emotion to food in the future. You'll have to make the drastic change of exchanging excessive eating for life participation and emotional confrontation, and all the stressors and emotions that entails. You'll have to eat right, eat less, and get moving. Well, you know what you need to do, so what keeps you from doing it? This is the $64,000 question! As you are able to identify the obstacles that interfere with what you know you should be doing, you are getting closer to the root of the problem.

Perhaps one of your obstacles to success centers on your expectations for weight loss. Think back to the expectations you had for every weight loss plan you've ever tried. Be honest with yourself. Did you have grand, high hopes of a miracle lurking in the back of your mind somewhere? Did you really hope or expect that it would somehow just melt away the fat while you slept? If you somehow harbored these kinds of expectations, then you'd better drag them out now and have a look at them before you decide on bariatric surgery.

What are your expectations for life after bariatric surgery? If you are hoping for the "extreme makeover" and "happily ever-after," you will be sorely disappointed. If you get nothing else out of this book, understand that you will probably just end up looking like an average size person. And that is okay!! You do not need to have anymore drastic changes than bariatric surgery will already bring you in your physical appearance and your inner confidence and self-esteem. You do not need to completely become something you're not, nor *should* you become something you're not! After surgery, you should essentially remain the same person on the inside that you were before surgery.

You will bring all the same attitudes, perceptions, and hurts that you have now into your life after surgery. Do not expect the surgery to change anything but decrease your weight. You can generally expect life to be pretty average, although easier and probably a little more happy. Your marital status, the quality of your close relationships, your place in life will all be quite consistent with your life before surgery. As long as you are realistic about the outcome, are accepting of yourself, are healthier than before, and are committed to not going back to your old ways, then you're on the right track.

It's not enough just to tell yourself you're being realistic, and you're okay with whatever comes your way. Don't tell your doctor or your behaviorist what you think they want to hear just so you can forge ahead in the process. Most importantly, don't tell *yourself* what you want to hear, or you won't make it through the process with any real success.

The process includes really understanding why you failed before, and correcting those behaviors and ideas now. The process includes creating a realistic and detailed image in your head of what life and the end result will be after surgery (or any weight loss plan for that matter). Creating that realistic, detailed image in your head specifically includes a realistic, detailed, long-term program for maintenance. The process doesn't come to a screeching stop the minute you drop the majority of your weight. Maintenance is incredibly important, and you can't get complacent and let your guard down.

This process you are considering requires you to be accepting of your life as it is now, willing to change for the better, and to move forward into the future and not attempt to recapture days gone by. Can you truly accept the age you are now, and live a healthy and full life from this point forward? Can you regret missed opportunities and events from your past, but move forward with expectations of creating great new life memories to replace those things that were missed in the past? Can you truly accept your body type and that you will most likely not end up with the body of a college athlete? Can you accept that life will be the same, while at the same time different once you lose the weight?

These may all be factors you've not really considered in-depth with all or many of your previous attempts at weight loss and modification of your behaviors. These may have been major reasons why you failed in the past. Others include being ready and willing to have patience with yourself, and being prepared to properly deal with setbacks, delays, and disruptions in your pre-conceived plan and timeline. Are you ready for these? Really? Are you truly prepared, and do you really understand that you will have to deal with some physical pain, some moments or periods of emotional defeat, substantial fear and anxiety, and potential feelings of regret when things don't go as you have them planned in your head? Think long and hard about these things.

You need to be comfortable with all this, and once you've really examined these issues and been honest with yourself in all the darkest corners of your mind, then, and only then, when you decide to go forward with surgery or another plan of attack, will you be truly ready to totally commit to change and a new and healthy lifestyle.

So, what does it mean to be totally committed? Total commitment is not based on emotions or feelings that change with the day. Total commitment is not based on the expectations or desires of others. If you choose surgery, it is your body that is going to be operated on. You are the one that must learn to be content with less, and with different food. Your significant other isn't the one going under the knife, facing potential surgical risks, or changing their style of living. They don't have to be totally committed.

Total commitment is not based on appearance, ability, or in any way comparing yourself with others. Total commitment is a decision to stick with something because you believe it is best, and because it is consistent with, and will enhance your personal values. Total commitment is sacrifice, going forward even though it may cost you something valuable because you believe so strongly in the end goal.

If you are of the mind that you will try the surgical route to weight loss to see if it works for you, and then, if it doesn't, simply resume life as normal, STOP! Don't proceed any further with your plan for surgery. You are setting yourself up for misery and failure. This trip cannot be purchased on a roundtrip ticket.

Hernando Cortez, a Spanish explorer, set sail for Mexico, which was at the time recently discovered. His mission was to establish a Spanish colony there. His men were grumbling and threatening to turn back because of the difficult conditions.

When they arrived on April 21, 1519, after the men had stepped on shore, Cortez set the ship on fire to prevent any thought of abandoning their new settlement. This is commitment. Despite what might lie ahead, Cortez and his men were going forward. There would be no turning back.

If anywhere in the dark shadows of your mind you are holding onto "safety" thoughts of being able to go back to your old way of doing things if you don't like doing the work necessary to get and keep the weight off, then consider Barry — learn from Barry's mistakes.

Barry was a morbidly obese man with a sedentary lifestyle, and he experienced a severe, nearly fatal heart attack at age 40. His doctor told him that he needed to make significant changes in his lifestyle to improve his health. He took his doctor's recommendations seriously. He stopped drinking alcohol, stopped smoking, started exercising, and even discontinued some of his friendships because of their unhealthy influence on him. He began working fewer hours to decrease his stress, and learned to relax. He maintained these changes for about two years.

But then when the coast seemed clear, and it was smooth sailing ahead, he gradually returned to his former lifestyle. In his mid-forties Barry developed a severe panic disorder and, for a time, was unable to come out of his bedroom. With intense counseling, he re-entered society again, gradually increased his activity, and rekindled relationships with family and friends.

His counselor and family worked with him to make drastic lifestyle changes. He enjoyed improved health and increased quality of life, but, again, he maintained these healthy lifestyle changes for only about two years. Why? He admitted that although he enjoyed the improved health, he did not enjoy the behaviors, or the style of living necessary to maintain his improved health. In both situations he became complacent and gradually returned to his former lifestyle patterns, thereby increasing his risk to repeat the cycle all over again.

Eventually, Barry again put on a significant amount of weight as a result of returning to these old behaviors. He was once again advised by his doctor to get his life and his health under control or he wouldn't make it out of his forties. Barry took the doctor very seriously, and sought yet another way to modify his lifestyle to do what he could to ensure a longer, healthier life. Barry decided to have weight loss surgery.

During Barry's behavioral assessment, it was observed and explained to him that even his near-death experience did not keep his attention very long. Barry finally admitted to himself that he would rather live his life in a manner that was easy and enjoyable, than to adhere to the less comfortable lifestyle recommendations that would result in health and longevity. He was referred to counseling to help him explore his thinking and expectations if he wanted to go forward with bariatric surgery.

Barry went to counseling, and fudged his way through by telling the counselor all he thought she wanted to hear. Her report was positive and declared Barry a good candidate for surgery from an emotional standpoint. He had the surgery, still thinking it would be the magic pill to end his obesity and related health torments. He made it through the surgery without complication, and began to see the weight drop off.

While he was losing the weight in the honeymoon period, it did in fact seem to be the magic pill. Barry never changed a single habit, however, and to this day, four years later, Barry has gained back all the weight, and then some, and his co-morbidities have all returned. Barry has made his decisions about what he values in life. How sad that his life will be so short.

So, what about you? What do you value? A healthy vital life in the long run with a few concessions and fewer beers and burgers, or all you can eat at the big food buffet of life? Remember: the buffet closes. It's not open forever, and you can only eat just so much before you die in the attempt.

Every bariatric patient desires to lose weight, but only committed persons are willing to make the difficult decisions. It takes hitting bottom and deciding to climb back up a different way than you came down to be successful. Successful weight loss requires more than desire. Desire alone produces nothing but frustration. Desire produces action only when combined with commitment.

So, are you ready to give up some things in order to gain others? Are you ready, willing, and able to accept help? Are you ready, willing, and able to follow directions from trained professionals prepared to guide you and care about your success? Are you ready to get rid of old habits forever? Are you ready to leave your uncomfortable "comfort zone?" Be honest, and when you come to an answer, then decide on your next course of action.

If your next course of action is bariatric surgery, then you will enjoy remarkable change with your weight and appearance, however, these external changes will not compare with the degree of change you will experience on the inside. It is in the shadows of our inner thoughts, feelings, and memories where fear, anger, and self-defeating thoughts hide.

The emotional world can be shadowy. Looking into the shadows can be intimidating, frightening, and overwhelming. It's hard to see anything clearly. Fear hides in the shadows. Pain hides in the shadows. This is the domain of unresolved feelings and emotions. All that hides in the shadows can rise up against you when least expected. Knowing this engenders fear and reticence. Part of your journey to weight loss success is about getting rid of the fear.

Now, before we delve into this, it is important to clarify that obesity is not caused solely from painful, unresolved emotions. Obesity is a complex disease with numerous factors contributing to it. Some are within your control, and others are not. So, given these parameters, it is important for you to accept and enjoy who you are, control what you can, and deal with anything else without food as a crutch.

It is also important, however, to be truthful with yourself. Self-righteousness, entitlement, justification, and denial, are at the opposite ends of the spectrum from truth. To the degree we make excuses, or justify, or minimize why we continue our unhealthy patterns, we are in denial, and denial is the opposite of truth. But, just because we deny a problem, or deny the importance or significance of the problem, does not mean there is no problem on which to work.

We all have tendencies toward denial. We all want to think well of ourselves and for others to think well of us too. We don't like to admit that we over-ate just because we wanted to, or that we didn't walk today just because we indulged our laziness. Admitting this doesn't make us feel good about ourselves, and we fear others will judge and not accept or like us. It is a lot more comfortable for us to blame it on how we were parented or our busy schedules than it is to admit weakness in ourselves.

Inwardly, these types of rationalizations provide relief. They take the pressure off and help us save face, even with ourselves. This is an indication of faulty thinking and/or denial of what we are doing to ourselves. At a deeper level, these are value statements. *We make time for what we value.* This is true whether what you value is self-defeating or self-affirming. The evidence speaks for itself.

You may have heard that you can tell the values of a person by looking at their checkbook. People spend money on what they value most. The same is true with our time, especially when the patterns are evident. Some people value comfort, so they choose to spend their time doing comfortable things. Some like to work on antique cars, or any number of other hobbies, so they spend their discretionary time on those endeavors. When we want to spend more time on our indulgences we do, and then leave less time for other responsibilities such as exercise, sleep, and relationships.

Our self-defeating values truly are difficult tendencies to confess to ourselves, let alone others. Honesty, vulnerability, authenticity, and understanding your *self* are vital to resolving the underlying issues that currently influence you toward unhealthy behavior. Facing the truth about yourself will result in healing from painful memories and emotions, followed by improved self-esteem. Further, as you address these unresolved emotional issues and begin to heal from them, your thoughts and feelings about yourself will improve, and your behaviors will follow suit.

Dealing with these raw emotions and hurtful memories is very difficult, I grant you. Making these changes is sometimes intimidating and overwhelming. This brings to mind one particular patient who became very upset when she learned that counseling would be necessary to decrease her symptoms of depression before moving forward with bariatric surgery. She explained that she had worked hard to bury her memories of abuse because of her weight, and that with counseling she would be required to dig them out and address them again. I had compassion for this woman. Her memories and experiences carried so much pain. It was more frightening to uncover them than to leave them buried.

So, why is it necessary to dig up these painful emotions? Why can't you just leave these memories safely tucked away in the shadows and get on with the surgery? This is a very good question. Unresolved issues like these can make us uncomfortable at best, and tormented at worst. We don't like thinking about them because they are too painful. There is often a degree of hopelessness because you cannot change the past, so what good would it do to think about these painful emotions?

We try to avoid these memories as best we can by staying busy, anything to stay busy. Getting involved, perhaps too involved, in relationships is a very effective means of keeping the past in the past. Our efforts to anesthetize our painful emotions can propel us toward food. Certain foods taste good to us. Their texture and aroma are pleasing to us, and they are indeed comforting to swallow and have sit in our stomachs for a while. Eating triggers the pleasure center in the brain. Eating is also very effective in helping you to "swallow" your pain and tears.

Perhaps you haven't thought about your painful or difficult memories in a long time, and you are not conscious of them presently, but they are contributing to your deeper feelings of discontentment, low self-worth, and consequential eating patterns. You may not be able to put your finger on it, but for some reason you need comfort, and food is a most convenient and readily available source. The fact that food is a comfort for you implies that there must be something in your life making you feel uncomfortable. Generally speaking, if there is no current source of discomfort in your life, then the source must be in the past or future.

If the source is in the past, you may be experiencing a degree of depression. If the source is something in the future, you may be experiencing a degree of anxiety. In either case, you will need to address this source of depression or anxiety to successfully manage your tendencies toward emotional eating and maintaining the bond between food and external issues.

To the degree that you turn to food for reasons other than physiological, you are putting food into your mouth for more subtle reasons such as cultural, emotional, or environmental. You may eat to give you something to do when you are bored, for companionship when you are lonely, relaxation when you are stressed and overwhelmed, comfort when you are angry, relief when you are hurting or experiencing guilt, or as a pick-me-up when tired, discouraged, or depressed.

Sit down with a pencil and piece of paper and ask yourself "Why do I often feel discontent?" "Why do I need to be comforted?" or "What do I need to be comforted from?" This is an interesting exercise to help you start looking into the shadows at the things that help to keep you overweight. Also, take a look at the exercise in the resources section for a little insight into your personal shadows.

It is important, however, to shine some light into these shadows. It's not healthy to ignore or pretend that your life prior to bariatric surgery didn't exist. It did, and you have to reconcile those emotions. Although you think you have buried or wiped away all that hurt, pain, loneliness, and grief associated with the abuse, disappointment, shame, guilt, and fear of your life as a severely overweight individual, you haven't.

You can ignore it, you can pretend it isn't there, but it is there, and it will continue to adversely affect your decisions and patterns of behavior until you explore it and resolve it for good. Memories and feelings don't go away, but dealing with them effectively changes the links to current emotions, and changes the locus of control these memories and feelings have over your current situation. In the subconscious mind they have control. When brought to the conscious mind they can be controlled.

If you choose to have surgery, you'll undergo a metamorphosis of mind and body that will bring out a more healthy and complete you. This means you'll need to introduce yourself to this newly emerging person and begin to build a relationship.

In discovering who you've grown into being, you should first identify all the parts of you that haven't changed. These are generally things like your morals, your core life values, your principles, who you love, and how much you love them. This will help to ground you, and then you can begin to explore what other things about you have grown, have emerged, or have been freed through this process.

Learning to understand more about your traits, wants, desires, and feelings will help you to become more accepting of yourself. Accepting yourself, with all your faults and strengths, is the key to maintaining your commitment to your new lifestyle and newly found health. Learning to understand your *precious pain* and not giving into it, is also extremely important.

Precious pain is a term used by therapists and counselors to describe the conditions in our lives that we won't leave behind, even though they're painful and destructive, because at least they're familiar, predictable, and less scary than finding out about the alternatives. We see this principle at work when people stay in abusive relationships. They stay not because they like the abuse, but because at least it's a known quantity. The alternative, finding out how to fabricate a whole new and different life, is so scary and overwhelming that it's just easier to stay in the abuse.

Sadly, there are a number of persons who have suffered significant trauma, or physical or sexual abuse in their earlier years. A very common source of comfort and control available to children and adolescents is food. As children or adolescents, many traumatized people turned to food to help cope with painful experiences because they lack appropriate coping skills. As long as the cognitive and emotional wounds are not addressed and healed, these wounds remain in the shadows, sometimes very quietly, but all the while subtly influencing your self-esteem, self-confidence, emotions, and relationships.

These unresolved emotional wounds can have a strong influence on how you use your free time, as well as your degree and type of social activity. If you want to change your behavior, it is imperative that you look at the thoughts and feelings that influence that behavior. Do not fear releasing the precious pain, whether from trauma, physical or sexual abuse, or from the verbal and societal abuse heaped on people who commit the transgression of carrying too much weight.

This last type of precious pain is something the vast majority of overweight people live with every day. The weight, and the circumstances and conditions that surround it and its attendant issues, permeate all aspects of their lives. Thinking about losing the weight and having to find out how to cope with all new situations that don't involve being rejected, being stereotyped, being ridiculed, and assumptions being made about intellect, strength, and character can be a pretty daunting and intimidating task. Patients tell me, "I just don't know how to be thin!" Maybe it's just easier to stay fat? Maybe that's at least safer? Maybe that's how it's really supposed to be? No! It's not!

Surround yourself with people and professionals who will fill in the gaps for you when your coping skills are stretched a little thin. Be prepared to let them help you. If you are deciding to have bariatric surgery you *must* deal with the shadows of your former self that lurk in your psyche. Whatever lurks in the shadows currently, will continue to lurk in the shadows later. If allowed to remain hiding in the shadows after your surgery, these issues will gradually undermine and sabotage your weight loss efforts and long-term success.

Controlling and dealing with your psychological scarring is an important issue, but it doesn't have to be fully completed prior to surgery. For most, the process is begun during the time of the behavioral assessment, and continues throughout the surgery and the following weight loss period. As things begin to change on the outside, you'll have to reorganize and accommodate the change on the inside as well. Julie and Karen are going to talk a little bit more about that in Chapter Nine. Learn to deal with food and pain in a new way.

Let humanity back in to fill the spots formerly held by food. Fill your life with people and experiences, and see food only as a means to keeping you alive and healthy, and maybe for a few pleasant sensations or memories. Mostly, you should remember to negatively associate food with your old life and living in the precious pain. Food kept you anchored there, so cut the line and leave it behind. Accept your new life and know that you are normal, you're good enough for anything and anybody, and you are worthy of a good and healthy life.

Many persons looking for effortless weight loss solutions look to bariatric surgery as being the pinnacle of an effortless cure for obesity. They hope that the surgery will quickly undo or correct the result of years of unhealthy living and give them a new lease on life. What's wrong with wanting more quality and more years in your life? Nothing! In fact, these are pretty normal and healthy life goals, and we all have them. The issue of how to get and maintain them is where problems occur. This is where the value of the *psychological evaluation,* or as I prefer to call it, the *behavioral assessment or interview,* comes in.

The behavioral assessment is an integral part of a more comprehensive assessment, which also includes medical and surgical consultations. The term behavioral includes everything necessary to manage lifestyle. I like to compare it to pre-employment screening, or pre-marriage counseling. It's the "reality check" to help ensure that though your head might be in the clouds, both feet are still planted firmly on the ground regarding assets and liabilities, etc. It's a way to see if this is going to be a good fit all the way around.

The term *behavioral* is an umbrella term that encompasses many different behaviors. Some of these behaviors are obvious, such as eating and exercise behaviors. That's nothing new. But, there are many other more subtle behaviors also under this behavioral umbrella. These include your thoughts, feelings, motives, ambitions, perceptions, attitudes, goals, beliefs, values, and priorities. The list goes on to include your ability to manage your stress, emotions, time, sleep, leisure, relationships, boundaries, and more. All of these subtle behavioral issues will directly influence how consistent you will be with your eating and exercise behaviors. In turn, it is the consistency of your eating and exercise that will directly determine how successful you will be with your weight loss and maintenance.

To be successful in your weight loss endeavors you should be assisting in the behavioral interview by being as forthright and open as possible. To take some of the mystery out of it, the behaviorist should be completing a BEST analysis. A BEST analysis means that the behaviorist is at a minimum looking at:

B - Biological Factors

E - Environmental Factors

S - Social/Psychological Factors

T - Timing Factors

Timing factors include things like examining the current life stressors with which you are dealing. If you've just lost a parent to cancer, changed jobs, and moved, perhaps this is not the best time for you to undertake such a major life change. Additionally, timing factors look at your knowledge of the required behavioral changes, the surgery itself, the other types of issues with which you must deal, readiness to change, etc. In short, pretty much all the stuff that's in this book.

Social/Psychological factors include what you would normally expect a psychologist to be looking for such as addictive behaviors, depression, psychiatric or mental disorders, appropriate mood, suicidal tendencies, suffering from abuse or the effects of abuse, sleep issues, concentration issues, stress issues, and the like. They are looking for factors that might require professional intervention to turn a potential liability into an asset for weight loss success.

Environmental factors include those things that are in and around your daily life such as your work environment, your eating patterns, your rest patterns, commitments to family and other events and functions, support or lack of support of family and friends, ability to commit, ability to be compliant, your financial situation, cultural and ethnic Influences, religious influences, and so on. These environmental factors can often be overlooked as insignificant in relation to biological and social/psychological factors, but they can prove to be some of the most important issues on which weight loss success can turn.

Finally, the behaviorist is looking at biological factors, and this is done, of course, in conjunction with the medical staff. The behaviorist is looking not only at the direct impact of physical and medical issues, but also at the emotional and psychological impact of the biological factors as well. They are looking at the patient's overall health, but are also looking at the emotional toll taken on a person from dealing with say a host of co-morbid conditions such as hypertension, type 2 diabetes, high cholesterol, rheumatoid arthritis, and polycystic ovary syndrome. The patient's emotional state may not be appropriate at the time for bariatric surgery and the patient may need to see a therapist for a while to help them turn that potential liability into an asset before embarking on the bariatric surgery adventure. The biological factors themselves may be resolved by the surgery, but the patient's emotional state may not survive the surgery if it too is not in a state of readiness beforehand.

The BEST analysis is an aptly named process because when performed correctly it really provides the patient and the surgeon with the BEST view of the patient as a current candidate for a successful surgical treatment, and it is designed to put the patient in the BEST possible position to be successful with the treatment plan. The BEST behavioral assessment is not limited, however, to simply asking questions of the patient about these areas, and may include other areas of assessment, and/or standardized assessments and evaluations to further determine a patient's readiness for surgical treatment.

At our center, we usually recommend that your spouse, significant other, or other person who will act as your primary support person accompany you to the behavioral assessment. While we are certainly interested in finding out about you from you, your support person can often be more objective about some things, and therefore provide valuable insight and information. This is another way we gain information that goes into the BEST analysis.

It is also helpful for us to gain a sense of how supportive your support person is. It is not unheard of for a support person to intentionally or unintentionally undermine the patient's efforts to lose weight. There are a variety of causes for this. A partial list might include the support person's insecurity, control, jealousy, or the disruption to their comfort level. When we observe this, we can either delve into it during the behavioral assessment or make a referral to an outside counselor. These relationship issues are vitally important to address before you will effectively manage your weight long-term. Your honesty and integrity throughout the entire assessment process are also essentially important. Many patients are on the verge of desperation to have the surgery and will do almost anything to have it. It is not at all uncommon for patients to minimize their concerns or deny them altogether out of fear they will be denied the surgery. The vast majority of the time, however, covering up their concerns in order to manipulate their way into surgery catches up with them later. They might have been able to squeak through the assessment, gain authorization for the surgery, and have the surgery, but just as they are about to breathe a satisfying sigh of relief, they develop more behavioral problems, or the behavioral problems they covered up previously get worse. Consequently, they are unable to develop any consistency with the lifestyle recommendations and fail to lose the expected amount of weight.

So, although they feel like they won the prize and were able to get the surgery, when they have post-operative complications that won't resolve, or significant frustration because they did not lose the expected amount of weight, they are not exactly sure they really won anything. They almost always inappropriately blame the surgery instead of themselves.

We talk a lot about medical and surgical risks associated with bariatric surgery, but you also need to know that depression is a risk for post-operative bariatric patients. If a person has tendencies toward depression pre-op, there is a greater risk for more, not less, depression post-op. When it is revealed through the behavioral assessment process that patients are struggling with depression, we immediately refer them to counseling, and/or for medical treatment.

The length of counseling will vary from a few weeks to possibly a year or more depending on the severity of the concern. Hearing us say that counseling will be required before moving forward with surgery is very disappointing for patients to hear, especially when they are already depressed. But, we have had countless patients come back later to thank us for prompting them toward counseling, saying how beneficial their counseling was and that they would never have initiated it themselves. After sufficient progress has been made toward the counseling goals, the patient will then be back on track for surgery.

Whether or not counseling is required before surgery, support and insight are most definitely required after surgery. Given the degree and difficulty of change that is necessary, you will need help. Persons who kid themselves and try to accomplish this on their own, fizzle out despite their best intentions and willpower, therefore, a social support network is critically important.

These major life changes are very difficult to maintain over time (remember Barry?). Most people have high motivation going into, and for a time after bariatric surgery, but when the "shine" wears off, and when difficult life circumstances appear, they begin to fizzle out despite the best of intentions. The reason for the dismal long-term weight loss success rate is due to the fact that these lifestyle recommendations are so difficult to maintain over time. Don't be fooled. The same holds true for bariatric surgery patients. You need the loving support and encouragement from those persons in your life who care about you to remain diligent with the eating and exercise plans.

Don't try to go it alone. Social support begins with your family, your spouse, or significant other. They are the ones who know you the best, love you the most, and will be with you through it all. No one wants you to be successful more than those few close persons who love and respect you the most. They are the ones who know you privately. You can fool your co-workers, you can choose to tell your extended family half-truths, but your family, significant other, or spouse knows the whole truth about you. So, include them right from the get-go. From collecting information and learning about the surgery, making the decision to have the surgery, selecting a surgeon, and when to actually make the phone call to schedule your first appointment, include those people who will be your support network. Be sure to include a support person in all the pre-operative assessments. The more your support group knows about the process, the better they will be able to empathize and help you through the process.

After surgery, ask a few of them to call you once in a while to ask how you are doing with specific behaviors with which you know you will have trouble. Throughout this process, you will need a couple of people who care enough about you that when they call and you tell them you have not walked in a few days, they will come over to your house with their walking shoes on and say, "Get up, we're going for a walk."

Gently caution these loved ones, though, that you do not need them to be the food and exercise police. You do not need to be judged for not measuring up or meeting the goal for that day or week. You do not need negative or critical remarks. You do not need sarcastic sighs or facial expressions. There is a fine line between loving encouragement and legalistic monitoring. Loving accountability might be stern, and legalistic condemnation might be given with a smile, but you will still be able to sense the difference.

Another way to surround yourself with support is to commit to consistent participation in a support group. Now I know what some of you are thinking. I don't need no stinking support group! I'm not crazy and I don't need my head shrunk. My weight and my issues are my issues. Well let me clear about what we mean when we talk about support groups. It's support, NOT therapy. The definition of support is as follows: to promote the interests or cause of; to advocate; to assist or help; to maintain.[1] Conversely, the definition of therapy is: an agency (as treatment) designed to deal with a bodily disorder or to bring about social adjustment as with psychotherapy.[2] They are not the same thing.

We are talking about support groups, not group therapy. Weight loss surgery patients should be attending support groups that provide guidance, assistance, tips, tricks, direction, reassurance, skills, information, education, resources, and a lot of laughter. If you are sitting around a circle talking about your feelings and how your parents must have ruined your life and made you fat, you are not at a support meeting. You are at a group therapy session, and not a good one at that.

Support groups should be utilizing *The Total Person Approach* to help patients by dealing with the whole person, not just a particular set of characteristics or qualities possessed by that individual, (like having a weight problem), or a particular issue or portion of a person's very complex life. People play many roles throughout their lives, and indeed, throughout each day. Support group members are more than just weight loss surgery patients, or Lap-Band® patients, or medically managed weight loss patients. They are parents, daughters, engineers, teachers, choir members, students, and more. When they attend support group they will not completely discard all these other roles, or the issues that accompany them.

Similarly, they bring all of their personal aspects with them as well: emotional, intellectual, spiritual, physical, medical, legal, social, cultural, financial, educational, career, and personal lives. Should attention be given only to their psychological or emotional aspects on an ongoing basis? And do all patients need ongoing attention for their emotional and/or psychological issues, or are they often resolved through attention paid to other aspects of their personal selves, or through private counseling? We believe that all aspects of a patient's life need ongoing attention at support groups, and that any patient requiring psychological attention for their unresolved issues needs to seek treatment outside the support group setting.

Support groups should be a safe place to learn the skills and information you need to be successful. Don't be afraid to learn. If you know everything you needed to be successful, and had all the requisite skills, you wouldn't be reading this book and you wouldn't have a weight problem or be considering surgery. Learn all you can and share all you can. Meeting regularly with others who have gone through the same experience reminds you that you are not alone. Some in the group will be further along and will be able to coach you. On the other hand, you will be further along than some, so take the time to coach someone else. You will personally benefit as you encourage and coach them. Sharing in the success of others will encourage them and motivate you. Sharing in the weakness and failures of others will encourage them, while at the same time inspire you. In either case, it will be a win-win situation for you and other group members.

Studies have shown, and it has also been our experience that persons who attend a weight loss support group manage their weight sifnificantly better than those who do not attend a weight loss support group.[3] But, wait! It gets better! Studies have also shown, and we've noted that persons who attend a weight loss support group frequently lose more weight and maintain their weight loss better than persons who attend less frequently.[4] There is a direct correlation between participation in a weight loss support group and successful weight management![5] You will experience not only more personal success, but at the same time, you will also be helping others succeed with their weight loss goals.

Your weight loss goals are perfectly attainable as long as they remain realistic, you explore what's hidden in the shadows of your mind, you modify those behaviors and underlying motivators, you do the work, and stay committed. Always remember that your multi-disciplinary team is there to help you through whatever comes up, and you should not hesitate to ask for help from them, from family, friends, outside counselors, and even religious leaders. There's more support out there than you really imagined to help you deal with the shadows of your former self, and help bring you out of the dark and into the light of your new and vibrant life. Don't be afraid of the dark. Strike the match.

I am not going to limit myself
just because people won't accept the fact
that I can do something else.

DOLLY PARTON

Chapter Eight

~ L I T T L E   V I C T O R I E S ~

Karen J. Sparks
Julie M. Janeway

I specifically wanted to write this chapter because it is very near and dear to my heart. It deals with many of the little things that mean so much to overweight people — things others so easily take for granted. It deals with fear and conquering fear. It deals with balance and perspective. It deals with joy and rebirth. It deals with struggle and perseverance. But most importantly, it deals with triumph.

As I struggled with making the decision whether or not to have this surgery, all the pain and fears of my life stood there plotting to wrestle me for control of the decision — I just didn't think I could take one more disappointment or failure. Among that unruly lot of pain and fears lurked a tremendous dread of undergoing surgery, because I had never experienced that type of thing. I was very scared of possibly dying on the table, as all surgeries that involve general anesthesia have a risk of death (although usually quite low). I was also very frightened that if I died, I would not have a chance to "fix" any of the things in my life that were messed up or delayed because of my weight and the related limitations. What to do? What to do?

In struggling with my fear of the surgical portion of the decision, I attempted to rationalize the facts. I am lucky that I come from healthy Scottish-Irish ancestry. Outside of the normal childhood illnesses, having babies, mom's gallbladder surgery, dad finding out he was allergic to penicillin, one broken arm, and a few emergency room stitches here and there, we are a healthy lot. Being a healthy person (no co-morbitities, although I was on the edge) rationally meant there was no reason to believe that I wouldn't come out of the surgery just fine and dandy. That being said, surgery still scared the beejeezies out of me!

My search for a final decision lead me to Dr. Baker's door. As I worked through building up my courage just to attend the orientation session, Julie shared with me the advice her sister had given her: *you can do anything afraid that you can do unafraid.* I can't tell you how important that was to me. It carried me through the fear and uncertainty of making the decision, right up to being wheeled through the operating room doors, and beyond.

The "beyond" included a substantial fear of losing the weight. Who would I be? How would I look? Would I even know how to be thin? I've never been "not fat" before; will I know how to do it? Can I keep it off? Will it come back no matter what I do? It also included a substantial fear that if I actually lost the weight, would I be able to "get back?"

Would I be able to "get back" to being able to do things that I had once done? Would I be able to "get back" to doing things I'd only done for a brief time in my life? Would I be able to "get back" some of the lost opportunities in my life? Would I be able to "get back" on track with the life plans I'd laid out so long ago?

There were also many things I had spent a lifetime only being able to wish I could do, or didn't think I would ever be able to do. Would I be able to "get back" to a point where I could do them? Would I "get back" the courage to do them? This fear of the unknown gnawed ravenously at what resolve I'd managed to gather.

My resolve was further tested by my awareness that the majority of my weight would take a year or more to come off. As you begin this journey, or you are deciding if it is right for you, a year sounds like a long time. Let's face it: in the past when we thought of losing weight and going on diets, just the thought of how long it would take to lose a pound or two would derail our efforts. So yes, a year seemed like an eternity.

Yet, in some ways it didn't sound long enough to make the kind of changes you know will have to be made. But, in the grand scheme of things, I'd spent this many years living with the pain and limitations of my weight, so what was another year; and what was the difference between another year of the old pain and limitations, or a different set of anxieties? I made the decision, closed my eyes, and prayed for guidance and strength.

Following my surgery, the anxiety shifted to the "waiting." I thought, "Okay, I'm past the hard part, now I wait to see what happens." I waited impatiently to see, to feel, to experience whatever would present itself next. I waited to see if, and what I would "get back." My impatience was quickly rewarded, and the things for which I had waited became a series of events I named my "little victories."

Little victories for me were, and still are, little events that just seem to tug at my emotions as they happen. Little victories are the wound healers in your life. For every emotional memory of something bad that happened in your life as the result of your weight, a little victory makes it all okay; it tells you that it won't happen again. They are the emotional stabilizers you need as you deal with becoming a new person, in dealing with plateaus, body shape issues, and the other issues we'll talk about in the next chapter. Little victories are the happy milemarkers that let you know you are succeeding in your journey towards a new you.

What is truly and amazingly unique about each of your little victories is that they never go away, and they're as wonderful the first time you experience them as the hundredth. They impact you in such a way that you never forget the moment you first realized it was happening.

For those of you who can, you will always remember where you were when you heard President Kennedy had been shot. That day and that moment is indelibly etched in your mind; so too with your personal little victories. They become embroidered on your heart.

I remember fondly the day I first was able to buy a suit all in the same size. I'd never been able to do that before in my whole life. I remember with gratitude the day I got rid of the seatbelt extender in my car. I remember affectionately the day that Julie and I stood in a mall parking lot laughing about the skinny shadows we now cast. I remember vividly the first time after my surgery that I sat in a booth at a restaurant, and found out that I fit. That was an amazing day. I was so overcome with emotion, we sat there for almost an hour before I could concentrate enough to order something.

I happily remember all my little victories, and every time I re-experience them it's like the first time all over again. Every time I walk through the door of my pop-up camper and don't touch the sides, I giggle. Every time I cross my legs and they stay there, I smile and enjoy it all over again. For every bad memory that comes flooding back, or every old wound that re-opens while you're losing the weight, a little victory sneaks in and saps all its power away. They are the steps you take forward to a new life and a new attitude. They are also the wonderful steps you take in "getting back."

Incidentally, you should remember that not all things are really as worth "getting back" to as you might have thought. I "got back" to playing softball. I went and played a whole game, which was truly wonderful to do. I had a blast seeing my old friends, and reliving a snippet of my misspent youth. I also came home with a bruise on my shin where I got nailed with a wicked line drive, and aching muscles I didn't even know I had!

The bruise stayed for a month and half to remind me that I'd "been back," and to reassess whether or not I should ever "go back" again. Little victories help you figure out who you've been, who you were before surgery, who you are now, and who you're going to be. They're not just the milemarkers on the journey, they're the directional signposts as well helping you to determine your future paths, and which paths from your past are worth taking or not worth taking for a visit.

Although little victories can't necessarily give you back missed opportunities from your past, they may afford you replacement opportunities instead. Like many of you, I never had the opportunity to attend my senior prom. I always got to watch my sister get dressed up, be picked up by her date, and go to such events. Will my little victories provide me with an opportunity to go back and attend my senior prom? No, of course not. In fact, now I think the term "senior prom" pretty much means a dance for people 50 and older!!

But what I can do, and what I'm looking forward to doing, is attending my 35th class reunion knowing that I'll look better than I ever have, and enjoying my conversations and time with my former classmates, rather than having it all overshadowed by the specter of my painful high school years.

Little victories give you perspective. They help you to reframe what you want into things that are realistic and do-able, like having a great time at the reunion instead of wallowing in the pain of missed high school proms and dances. Little victories help you to see what's possible and practical now, rather than what you thought you might have wanted all along (like watching my friends play softball, not necessarily having to play softball). They help you to find your inner strength, and give you the patience to wait for the next one (which comes in handy when you're stuck at a particular weight and the scale hasn't moved for a month). When nothing else in your life seems to be going right, little victories keep it all in balance and perspective. In so many ways, little victories are Heaven sent.

We've compiled for your consideration a list of little victories experienced not only by us, but also by many others to whom we've spoken. Men, take note, lots of these will apply to you! We included them to cause you to think about what might balance out your fears and doubts about this surgery.

If you go for it, great! If you decide it's not for you, great too! At least you've made the decision and explored your options. If you've already made the decision to go forward with losing weight and getting your life back (by whatever means you choose), here are just a few of the things that will let you know that the journey is a positive one, and that every step is a wonderful new adventure toward an exciting new life:

- Seeing a picture of yourself and not realizing it is actually you!

- Being in pictures at all!!

- Realizing both you and your 5-year-old nephew fit in the recliner as you read him a book.

- Taking a nap on the couch and having room for the cat(s) too.

- Fitting into the stadium seats at sporting events.

- Not being afraid to walk between people in public because you may rub against them.

- Buttoning and zipping up your skirt at the back, not having to do it up in the front and "spin" it to the back.

- Going through the turnstile at the amusement park like everyone else. Not having to be let in through the "gate" on the side.

- Buying jeans that don't have to be purchased in the "work clothing" section of the department store, or the "big and tall men's" shop.

- No longer being referred to as "big guy."

- Knowing your heart isn't going to explode!

- When doing car repairs, being able to lie down on the creeper cart and roll under the car...all the way.

- Strangers actually holding doors for you, or offering to pick up things you have dropped or knocked over.

➤ Climbing a ladder without fear of it holding you. (Clean those gutters!)

➤ Not feeling invisible.

➤ Not wanting to be invisible.

➤ Strangers acknowledging you with a "hello" who would have never "seen" you before.

➤ Getting diabetes under control.

➤ Putting your legs together and feeling the sensation of your knees and ankles touching each other.

➤ Sitting in the back seat of the car, just because you can.

➤ Hanging your clothes on regular size hangers and they fit properly.

➤ Not wearing out your clothes because they "rub" or "pull" at the seams.

➤ Not wearing out your shoes because you have walked over the sides of them for so long.

➤ Buying "fun" underwear and pajamas! (Not just the two kinds made in your "other" size.)

➤ Noticing you actually have a collarbone!

➤ Getting in the hot tub and not sending a tidal wave of water over the edge.

➤ The towel fits all the way around!

➤ Sitting in an airplane seat, crossing your legs, and the tray table STILL lays flat.

➤ No more racing to the bathroom in complete fear of not making it! (Except maybe for dumping syndrome now...)

➤ Fitting into the ride seats at the amusement park, and the safety bar actually being able to click shut. (Nice to know you won't fall out now when the ride goes upside down...)

➤ Knowing you can skydive if you want to (but why would you want to?...)

- Being set free from the soda pop addiction.

- Smaller size hats.

- No more back pain!

- Being able to dance again.

- Fitting in the chair at the hair salon, and not feeling as though the hairstylist is leaning over too far, or contorting himself just to reach your head!

- Not secretly "pushing up" with your foot under the chair as your hairstylist or barber pumps the chair to a higher position.

- Walking by people who don't recognize you anymore.

- Having a waist.

- Having a shape that doesn't resemble an appliance!

- Finding out you can exercise, and you don't really hate it.

- Wearing a smaller size than you did in high school (or junior high!)

- Not looking like you dwarf other people in pictures.

- Taking a shower and not having the shower curtain constantly touching you.

- Not feeling self-conscious in the locker room.

- Disappearing surgery scars.

- Getting off blood pressure medication.

- Being able to get down on your knees.

- Being able to get up again! By yourself!

- Tying your shoes on the top of the shoe, not the side.

- Hitting your goal size!

- Hitting your goal weight!

- No longer wrestling yourself into your panty hose.

- Going camping and not being afraid of breaking the aluminum lawn chair you brought to sit in.

- Every new size you fit into.

- The growing space between you and the steering wheel.

- Lower cholesterol.

- Climbing more than two stairs without getting winded, and not using the handrails!

- Taking up less space in bed.

- Taking those flying lessons you always dreamed of because now you fit in the cockpit of the plane.

- Not getting wedged in the bath tub — being able to just sit in the bath tub and get out on your own.

- Running around with your kids in the backyard.

- Feeling worthy again.

- Feeling like a life participant.

- Buying a fishing boat and not being afraid of sinking yourself!

- Sharing the porch swing with your honey, knowing it will hold the two of you, and you both fit with room for the pillows!

- Not having to always use the handicap stall in a public restroom.

- Finding out you don't snore anymore!

- Fitting into an airplane seat and having seatbelt length left over!

- Finding out you wear a smaller shoe size, or you don't need wide shoes anymore.

- Feeling proportionate in size to your spouse.

➤ Not feeling like you want to hide when people look at you.

➤ Having people compliment you and not wanting to die.

➤ Feeling you deserve a makeover.

➤ Wearing bright colors.

➤ Joints and bones don't hurt as much.

➤ No more swollen ankles and aching feet.

➤ Being able to get on and ride a motorcycle.

➤ You don't groan in fear at having to pick up dropped items.

➤ No pressure on your bladder.

➤ Not having the arms of a lawn chair (or any other chair) cut into your legs.

➤ Having a BMI that says you're in the "normal" range and you're not "obese" anymore.

➤ Getting a job working with excavating equipment because now you fit in the cab.

➤ Not fearing sliding into a restaurant booth.

➤ Not dripping food on your chest or stomach.

➤ Being able to fit into those little tiny desks or chairs at your kids' school on parent-teacher night!

➤ Going on a date!

➤ Being noticed and appreciated for who you are, not just being noticed for your weight or size.

➤ Actually being able to lean over the sink and brush your teeth.

➤ Fully realizing that you never have to be fat again because you have control of your weight and your life.

- Standing all the way through a presentation instead of searching frantically for a place to sit down.

- Fitting all the way under an umbrella.

- Riding a snowmobile and wearing an actual snowmobile suit!

- Not shopping at the end of the rack (and knowing there's no place else to go...).

- Finding new stores you can shop in.

- Realizing you can actually see your ears when you look at yourself in the mirror.

- Not feeling like you have to make fun of yourself to fit in, or to make the joke about yourself before others do.

- Learning not to celebrate everything with food, and getting other people in your life to accept that as well.

- Climbing the ladder to your son or daughter's tree house.

- Not being exhausted all the time.

- Going ice fishing with your friends and not being afraid of breaking through the ice and drowning the lot of you!

- Being able to physically pick up your kids.

- Finding and fitting into the wedding dress of your dreams.

- Having your kids be able to sit on your lap.

- Having a lap!

- Fitting in the seat of your beloved riding lawn tractor, and not have the steering wheel cut into your stomach.

- Discovering you have hip bones.

- Hugging someone and actually feeling the hug.

- No longer wedging yourself into the "porta-john" on the work site.

- No more insensitive comments or remarks about your weight or your size.

- No fat prejudice at interviews or on dates.

- Feeling like a normal size person and accepting what's normal for you.

- Flirting!!

- Being able to itch places you could never reach before.

- Going on vacation and discovering that you can buy clothes anywhere, even in foreign sizes!

- Waistbands and bra straps not cutting in anymore.

- Being able to take a really deep breath.

- Getting hit on at the bookstore!!

- Climbing up into your 4X4 heavy-duty pickup truck and not needing extra handles and home-built step blocks to get in.

- Passing the junk food aisle in the grocery store and feeling okay about it.

- Knowing you have kicked the fast food habit.

- No cravings/compulsions/obsessions for food.

- Fitting into goal clothing.

- A whole new sex life.

- Feeling good about wearing jewelry.

- Being able to pull into small parking spaces because you don't need to get the car door open as far.

- Being able to buy a scale.

- Not being afraid to get on the scale!

- Riding a bike and not having the seat go up your butt!!

- Fitting into theater and auditorium seating.

- Being able to buy tickets for the "cheap seats" because you know you can make the hike up there.

- Being able to sit in the middle seat on an airplane (but still...why would you want to!).

- Getting your dimples back or discovering you have them.

- Not feeling like you have to apologize for yourself.

- Discovering your fingers have gotten longer and thinner.

- Playing sports again, not just watching it.

- Actually wanting to look in a mirror.

- Being able to get up off low, cushy furniture.

- Breathing properly all through the night (getting rid of sleep apnea).

- Getting down on the floor with your children to play with the slot car track.

- Not feeling self-conscious when walking away from people because they might be getting a rear view.

- Tucking your shirt into your jeans, and feeling good about how you look.

- No longer feeling like you have to wear a jacket because you're self-conscious about your big rear end.

- Taking that cross-country cycling tour.

- Going to the doctor's office and knowing you won't have to deal with any more Fat Nazi doctors!

- Not being agoraphobic anymore.

- Getting on the elevator and not looking at the weight restriction sign.

- Being able to share the armrest with the person next to you.

- Looking down and seeing the shadow of a normal sized person.

- Riding in go-carts!

- Not having to look for the closest parking space anymore, because you can easily walk the distance from the car to the store.

- Being at a size that it becomes noticeable to people when you've only lost 10 pounds.

- Having your honey (or anyone else) be able to get his or her arms more than all the way around you.

- Not having to lie about your weight on your driver's license renewal.

- Being able to "curl up" in your favorite chair and no longer feeling "wedged" into it.

- Slipping "between" the studs on a remodeling job to grab the hammer you left on the other side of the new wall!

- Getting new designer eyeglass frames!

- Wearing a formal gown or a tux for the first time.

- Going to a black tie ball with your honey, feeling like a million bucks, and pretending that it's the prom you missed.

- Walking the dog and not tipping over when you bend down to pick up doggy doo-doo.

- Looking forward to hot summer days and not dreading temperatures over 65°.

- Going swimming again.

- Walking to the gym instead of driving!

Chapter Nine

➤ S E P A R A T I O N   A N X I E T Y ➤

Julie M. Janeway

Karen J. Sparks

As the title might suggest, this chapter will address some of the things you'll be leaving behind along your journey. When Karen and I started this process, we both thought we'd be quite happy to leave behind just about everything (husband, cats, family, and friends not included), in order to craft new lives for ourselves as thin people. What we found was that saying good-bye isn't as easy as one might think — not even saying good-bye to the pounds.

In the beginning, every pound that disappears is like a little gift from Heaven. After all, you have so many more to lose, and isn't that the purpose of all this? At this point you're concentrating on watching the numbers finally go down on the scale (not up anymore!), and on recovering from surgery.

As the pounds come off though, you'll go through periods of shrinkage that are very extreme. Literally you can shrink a size over a weekend. You will have worn a piece of clothing on Monday, then the following Monday, it will be radically too big. It's a very strange phenomenon, and more than a little frustrating. But, more on that later. We call these (appropriately) *shrinks*.

But there comes a time when you go through a shrink, and this time you notice some major difference in yourself. Some drastic change appears, like you can see your ears again when you look at yourself head on in the mirror, or maybe you've shrunk into a piece of goal clothing, or you notice that your hands don't even look like your hands anymore. Maybe it's that your feet have shrunk and you can't keep your shoes on anymore. These realizations are mile-markers along the journey.

So, with each little realization (and there will be many), you're hit squarely in the face with the fact that you're getting thinner, and the fact that you used to be really big (or really, really big as the case may be). All of a sudden you find yourself in an introspective mood, re-examining why and how you got to where you started, where you are now, and where you're going.

This introspection examines each pound you carried around for so long. Each pound came as a result of some rejection, some hurtful remark, or some blow to your self-esteem. In fact, they became part of the insulation that kept you separated from the prickly nature of the world. Many of us wore our weight like a sandwich board that said, "Stay away from me. You can't hurt me anymore."

Of course we also knew, that the louder and more obvious we made that statement, the more the world felt entitled to comment and editorialize — and the more it hurt. It's a vicious cycle. What's a person to do? (And another pizza would bite the dust....)

You begin to re-examine each stage of your life and your weight gain. You examine the pain that accompanied those pounds, and you meet it head on as the pounds drop away. It's not so much the pounds that are hard to lose, but the pieces of the life they represent that really hits you.

Dealing with each pound and its attendant emotional injuries as they come off, you begin the emotional ride of a lifetime. As you shrink into your clothes from days gone past, it brings up a whole new era of painful memories with which to deal. Each compliment about how much "better you look now," seems to be a bittersweet mix of compliment and criticism. The new little victories of everyday life still sit in stark contrast to the memories of failure, rejection, disapproval, self-deprecation, self-doubt, and denial.

But, it's not all bad. Every day there's still elation with another pound gone, and the knowledge that you have dealt with its emotional struggle. Those pounds and those struggles won't control you anymore. The memories will always be there, but with each day comes a strengthened resolve not to succumb to those emotional forces, and an increasing sense of empowerment never to let those weight related emotional injuries happen to you again.

You'll bring the unaddressed pain out of the basement. You'll examine it, try it on, confront its ill-fit, fold it, put it in a box, label it, and tuck it nicely into the attic of your psyche. Some memories and scars are faster and easier to deal with than others, but that's pretty much the process that transpires with each couple of pounds lost.

With each pound lost, and each new change in size comes an exploration and re-examination of *self-perception* and *self-concept*. *Self-perception* is how you see yourself, physically, mentally, and socially. *Self-concept* includes self-perception, but also includes your idea of who you are as person, what you bring to this planet and this existence.

You will struggle with self-perception. It will change many times through the course of this journey. You may have thought of yourself as heavy, but smart. Maybe heavy, but clever. How about heavy, but fun? Maybe creative, or attractive (if not beautiful or handsome), kind, thoughtful, loving, shy, or caring. But always fat, heavy, or overweight. For many people, their self-perception degrades, and they simply think of themselves as "fat, dumb, ugly, stupid, and unacceptable," or some version thereof. This is the problem with self-perception, when one characteristic tends to dictate all others.

As you begin to take away the concepts of "fat," "heavy," and "overweight," you must re-evaluate whether or not you are still "shy," "quiet," or "reserved." Are you still fun? Are you still introverted? Are you really dumb? Are you beautiful or handsome now? This will continue to change and morph as you lose more and more weight. Your self-perception will continue to change along with your entire self-concept.

The famed sociologist Charles Horton Cooley (another Michigander...) said that the concept of *self* is developed from our interaction with others. He coined the term the *looking-glass self*, and summarized the concept with this couplet: "Each to each a looking-glass, Reflects the other that doth pass."[1]

The looking-glass self contains three elements: 1) we imagine how we appear to those around us; 2) we interpret others' reactions; and, 3) we develop a self-concept.[2]

As people insecure about our weight we imagine how we appear to others. We may perceive that if someone is staring at us, it *has* to be because we are fat, not because we are striking, or humorous, or just standing in front of the sign they are trying to read.

As people unhappy because of our weight, we interpret others' reactions or lack of reactions. We may perceive that because no one is looking at us, that it must be a negative thing as well. Our interpretation of thin people getting asked out on dates more often than fat people (or so we surmise) is that we are not acceptable as dating partners, and therefore *everything* about us must be unacceptable.

We interpret many reactions correctly and many incorrectly. And, it's important to note, self-concepts don't have to be based on accurate evaluations, perceptions, or interpretations of what others may think of us, and how they may react. In fact, more times than not, they are incorrect, and based on our own self-doubts and insecurities — like being overweight.

Whether they were right or wrong, we may have taken the collection of all those interpretations and perceptions of what we thought people were thinking and trying to tell us, and strung them together like beads on a necklace. Our necklaces were then wrapped around our throats and became our self-concepts. For many of us, our negative and inaccurate self-concepts veritably choked us to death. On this journey, that will quickly change.

Your physical change will be drastic, and your self-concept will change drastically as well. If you've always been a stay-at-home parent, partially because of weight, but mostly because of self-concept, then losing the weight will cause you to reassess whether you might want to go out now and get a job. Maybe you will, maybe you won't.

Maybe you'll find that being a stay-at-home parent is okay, but perhaps you'll be inspired to join some parent-teacher groups because you have so many ideas for improving your kids' school, and you have the newfound confidence to promote them.

Similarly, for those who've never ventured far into the dating world because of a series of hurtful reactions and events, many of you have resigned yourselves to the fact that you were just meant to be alone. You've developed a concept of yourself as a single person, and a person for whom intimate personal relationships just aren't in the cards. Well, when you lose the weight, many of those barriers will be gone. You may find yourself in a bookstore or grocery store one day, and someone will be staring or smiling at you, and subtly trying to get your attention. And NO, I'm not talking about the salesperson motioning to get you to move to checkout number five!

You may find that people want to get to know you, or maybe even ask you on a date. Accept if you want to — unless you're married. The challenge for you is to leave the hurt behind. Don't let it control you anymore. Don't drag into your new self-concept the resentment toward those who previously rejected you because of your weight. Don't let it hamper your new life. Learn to live in the moment, and put all the rest behind you. Learn to think of yourself as a renewed and vibrant person worth getting to know, and worthy of being loved. Learn to deal with yourself that way as well.

Learning to value and respect yourself is what we term *self-esteem*. You will see almost daily improvements in your self-esteem, but beware the "fat day." Just because you're losing weight and feeling better, doesn't mean that every time you look in the mirror you're going to love what you see. There will be days that you'll see someone you like much better than the person you saw the day before, and on other days (when you're tired, or stressed, or a little under the weather), you may see someone who's still fat, or lumpy, or misshapen.

Beware of those days. Let the day happen, but don't let it affect your new self-esteem. Tell yourself, "I will feel differently tomorrow." And most likely, you will. (But, if you feel down and depressed for more than a week, you need to call your doctor's office as your high protein, lower carb diet may have caused your serotonin levels to drop too far, and some mild anti-depressants may be required for a short time.)

So, you're going to deal with the excitement of new and improved self-esteem, self-perception, and self-concept — all of which we may collectively refer to as your sense of *self* or sense of *identity*. And it can be a really fun ride. But there are some things about which you should be aware.

At some point your sense of *identity* and *self-concept* may begin to run head on into someone else's idea of your *identity*, or who they think you're supposed to be. This has happened to more people than I care to think about.

I talked to one young woman who told me of her two life-long friends. They'd been friends since kindergarten, and they were coincidentally (or not so coincidentally), all overweight. This young woman decided to have weight loss surgery, much to the consternation and dismay of her two friends. Despite the fact that she was one of those surgery mill cases I talked about in the first chapter, she still managed to lose the weight.

As she shrunk through her second size in about 6 weeks, one of her two friends completely stopped speaking to her. When asked why, the friend stated that the young woman losing the weight thought she was better than the other two now. When asked how she came to this conclusion, the angry friend said it was obvious because the young woman who had surgery wouldn't go out to eat with them anymore, and she was just a "little too happy" about wearing a smaller size than they did. And so, a friendship was lost because one person could not accept or keep up with the other person's rapidly changing lifestyle, self-esteem, and self-concept.

It's happened to Karen and me as well: family members who don't know how to deal with you because you've changed; co-workers who are finding that they can't dump all the overtime work on you anymore because you actually have a life to attend to now; and, friends who can't deal with the fact that you're not at their beck and call to solve all their problems for them. It's a whole new deal. There's actually a name for this: it's called *role exit*, and it comes from a sociological theory developed by a man named Erving Goffman.

Erving Goffman created a theory he called *dramaturgy,* to explain interactions between human beings. All the dramaturgy theory says is that life is like a play. We're either on stage (out there interacting with people), or we're off stage (doing things in private).[3]

If we're on stage, we've adopted roles like student, wife, lawyer, sister, father, Aunt, friend, teacher, boss, store clerk, or whatever. With these roles come props to use, and a costume or series of costumes to wear. In other words we dress the part in addition to acting the part. What also comes with our roles is a determined way of interacting with other people in their roles.

If you've seen a play or movie ten times, you always expect the characters to dress the same way, say the same lines, and interact the same way. You're very uncomfortable when you see a remake of the play or movie, and it's radically different. (Ask Leonardo DiCaprio about "Romeo and Juliet"....)

Imagine a remake of "Casablanca" with Chris Rock in Humphrey Bogart's role, or "The Phantom of the Opera" starring Jackie Chan as a martial arts blazing Phantom, or even Kathy Bates starring as Rizzo in a reprisal of "Grease." Get it? Not that it can't or shouldn't be done, but it is really outside of what you expect, and what is comfortable for you. Because it's not comfortable, you'll naturally resist, or even become angry, and want things to be the way "they should be!"

So it is with real life. We adopt for ourselves particular roles — Rock of Gibraltar for everyone, white knight and rescuer, fixer of all things, single person, confessor and confidante, home-body, the one who's always prepared and can/will handle everything, frumpy introvert, or maybe even "doormat." Others adopt their roles accordingly, and they expect that if their roles don't change, neither should ours. We should continue to interact as we always have. They just don't understand why we can't get with the program!!

But that's not what happens. As your self-perception and self-concept change, so do your limitations, fears, and doubts. One by one, the roles you've chosen for yourself based on your weight, limitations, fears, and doubts, begin to fall away. New roles are adopted in their place because interaction with the world changes and increases, and that puts you "on stage" more than you were before.

Our new roles involve taking care of ourselves a little more. Our new roles involve doing the things we couldn't before. Our new roles often involve making up for lost time, if possible. What they don't involve is loving the people in our lives any less. They don't involve a change in our basic values, beliefs, and personal ethics. They don't involve a change in our core being.

But often others can't see that, and conflict arises. This conflict arises from *role exit*. You're leaving a particular role either to play a different role in the same play, or a different role in a whole new play. You may take on a whole new role within your family, for example, as leader and visionary instead of follower and workhorse. That's taking on a new role, but staying in the same play.

Quitting your job because you realize you don't deserve, and no longer have to accept the abuse that is heaped on you day after day, is an example of adopting a new role and moving to a new play. Both are hard, and be prepared for the conflict. Oh, the crying, wailing, and gnashing of teeth that will go on!!

Taking on a new role and staying in the same play (or drama, as the case may be), is especially hard if that play happens to be your family. Your role in the family has been determined over a lot of years. Your role may be as the "fixer of all things." That may be your role because when you were heavy you didn't have much of a life, and you were always expected to be around to fix everyone's problems. Maybe that expectation didn't come from others, but instead you wanted to be the fixer because in your mind it gave people something to love about you, and a reason to be wanted and needed.

Maybe you were the "Ann Landers" of the family, as my mother would say. You might be expected to be everyone's therapist, and we all know therapists aren't supposed to bring their own problems to the proverbial couch. Whatever the role, you may find yourself changing it in favor of roles you've always wanted to play, and that's okay, no matter how others may whine about it. They have two choices — deal with it or don't. Let them choose.

This process is all about dealing with your own stuff. And, as we've said many times in this book, this is a journey that is wholly selfish, and just for you. So, it necessitates you leaving (even temporarily) roles like this, and boy others may not be happy about it!! The trick is to keep reassuring them that you don't love them any less, and that you aren't becoming a whole new person on the inside, just the outside. (You're just changing a little on the inside; tidying things up a bit, if you will.) You need to assure them that you just want to experience life a little more, and they're more than welcome to join you.

Let them know that this is hard for you too, as you're very accustomed to the roles you've played. Also, let them know that part of the reason you adopted the roles in the first place was because of those limitations, fears, and doubts associated with your weight. Maybe they'll understand that the weight is really the driving force here.

Discuss with them how much weight has affected every facet of your life. Let them know that it is still going to affect every facet of your life until you're finally comfortable with yourself. Then you'll decide what roles you want to play in the long-term, and things will settle down a bit. Let them know that the flux and frustration is not permanent.

And flux and frustration there will be. Not only are you going through separation anxiety from the old you to the new you, but you will go through other forms of separation anxiety as well; forms such as separating from celebrating all events with food. That's a hard one because our culture, and in fact so many of the world's cultures celebrate with food.

It's not that you can't ever be in the room with a birthday cake again, or you have to skip Christmas dinner. What you do need to change is celebrating your favorite sports team's regular season win against the last ranked team, by going out for pizza and beer. Similarly, the 80% off shoe sale at the mall is not cause for cookies at Mrs. Fields®!

Although you'll be able to make this change fairly easily (because you'll probably experience dumping as a result of these indulgences), others in your life may have a harder time. They need to understand that you're not imposing on them any sort of penalty for your new lifestyle. They're welcome to continue celebrating whatever they need to, in the manner to which they've become accustomed, and you'll be happy to participate — just not in eating inappropriate food. Sounds easy, doesn't it? Yeah, well… wait until you try this for the first time.…

You may find family members or others who are very insulted that you chose not to eat a piece of birthday cake or a particular dish they made. Or you may find that people want to change all the holiday dishes to make sure you can eat them. Although that's nice and very well meaning, it's not necessary.

Tell them not to change the traditional holiday meal (or any meal) to accommodate you. You'll pick around, and find what you can and can't eat. Everything should remain the same for everyone else's sake, as well as yours. Tell them, "Just don't bug me to eat more, or harass me about what I am eating, or how long it takes to eat it." We hope for your sake, they'll understand. Some will, some won't.

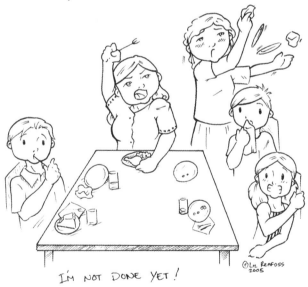

I'M NOT DONE YET !

Remember the story we told you previously of the young woman and her two life-long friends? After her surgery she still hung out with them, and did everything she used to do. She just wouldn't be their eating partner anymore. She went with them to restaurants at first, but she found it boring and annoying to sit there while they ate food she knew she (and they), shouldn't be eating.

She finally stopped going out to the restaurants, but she still wanted to continue hanging out and doing other things together. The one friend simply could not accept that. It was the friend's problem entirely, but instead of dealing with it, she dumped it back on the young woman who was trying to change her life and eating habits. Not cool. But that's the kind of stuff that happens. You just have to realize whose problem it really is, and don't take responsibility for other people's issues. You'll have enough issues to deal with on your own. Trust us on that.

Similarly, here's something that is a constant battle in my house. My husband, Matt, is 6'3" tall, about 200 lbs., and he's built like a swimmer. The man has the metabolism of a hummingbird, and he has to eat like an elephant to keep weight on, let alone increase his weight. (Man, that always just ticked me right off...) Karen calls him the "ten-toed stomach."

Matt is a very hard worker, and one of those people who can never sit down. He's always working at something, so when he wants to eat, he wants to EAT! He, like most other men, is on the see-food diet. He sees it, he eats it. And usually, he'll eat all, or the better part of all of it. The man can eat an entire package of Oreos® in one sitting if he has enough milk to dip them in, and a good movie or a car race to watch!

The problem arises when Matt decides to eat everything that is readily available or microwaveable (the man simply WILL NOT cook), and then he absent-mindedly starts in on the few things that I know I can eat successfully. It is at this point that the battle lines are drawn.

Because I can't eat very much in one sitting, things will either go in the refrigerator for another meal, or go back in the cupboard as the case may be; at least that's the theory. When I make dinner, I'll serve my portion, and then Matt will come in later and get his. The issue is that when I have cooked what I think is enough for at least two more meals after the night's dinner, Matt simply thinks the rest *is* his dinner! One night I cooked 6 pork chops. I ate one, and thought there'd be at least two left over for me to eat as other meals. Matt thought otherwise. He ate all 5 pork chops. (Sigh!... they don't call them Man-imals for nothing....)

Now I can hear what you're saying: "Serve yours and his at the same time, and then he'll know how much he can eat." Duh!!! I tried that! It didn't work. He just went back and got more until it was gone! So you say, "Then serve the plates, and put the rest away before you hand him his." Duh, again!!! He went to the fridge, got it out, and threw the rest in the microwave. If I could figure out how to cook exactly the right amount, and not leave one of the two of us hungry, I'd be golden. I have scientists at MIT working on it....

Maybe he always ate like that. Maybe I just never noticed until now because my food portions are so much smaller. I don't know. If I buy bananas, I can only eat one every couple of days. I might get one out of the whole bunch because Matt decides that over the course of one day, he needs to eat three. I can't keep up with that, nor can I go banana, or grocery shopping every two days!

All I know is that I now have to stash food like a pack rat around the house so I can be assured of getting just *some* of the food I know I can eat (apples behind my computer, granola bars in my underwear drawer, bananas in my briefcase. I haven't quite figured out where to stash cooked chicken breasts though, so they remain vulnerable to Matt-attack in the refrigerator).

I've explained to him that I just can't keep up with that level of food intake, and that I have to know that certain types of foods are there when I need them. He understands, but then he gets very upset when I catch him absent-mindedly delving into my box of low-fat granola bars, my celery sticks, or my fruit, and ask him to stop eating my food! He feels I don't share and I need a day back in kindergarten to learn that skill over again! I can't win for losing here. I can't even imagine what it would be like if I had Matt and children on top of it! I'd starve to death....

So you see, there's a form of separation anxiety that occurs with the food in your house as well. You used to take for granted that you'd get your share, or at least it would be there when you wanted it. Say good-bye to getting your share. Heck, for a long time you won't even be sure what your share should be!

Like I said, I don't know whether he always ate like that, or I'm just noticing now because my food portions are smaller. Maybe it's because food controls me now more than it ever did. Food and its purpose in keeping me alive and healthy are always at the forefront of my thoughts. I'm not a person who likes to cook or bake (a genetic anomaly according to my sister and my father the chef), and in a way I'm glad, because if I were a person whose life and enjoyment centered around making elaborate food, I don't know how I'd cope.

Although Karen doesn't necessarily make elaborate food, she can if she wants to. She really enjoys cooking, baking, and even candy making, and she's incredibly good at it. She reported that she found it strange, and a little difficult her first Christmas when she and her nephew went on their traditional all-day cookie baking and candy making binge.

Now, you have to understand, we're talking Mrs. Claus, North Pole level setup here — 30-40 dozen cookies in 6 varieties, 15 lbs. of peanut brittle, chocolates, and a host of other (killer) goodies. Previously, she'd always enjoyed snacking on her own handiwork as she made it. This particular year she simply made it. She and her nephew still had fun, but only he got to lick the spoons. What she normally would have kept for herself, she boxed up and gave to friends. (The rest appears on Christmas Day at their big family get-together, as a gift from the elves. Isn't that cute? The kids love it. They're such a Norman Rockwell family.)

She didn't really say that the experience wasn't fun, but I think some of the fun came from eating all the good things she'd made. Certainly, her memories were now different from the actual experience, and she had to think about whether or not that was a good or bad thing. That phenomenon is called *cognitive dissonance,* in case you care.[4] These are the types of separations from your previous life that you begin to notice, and some cause more anxiety than others.

I'll tell you what else you may notice (and for a while you may have a hard time with it for some reason): how much other people eat, and wondering where they put it. I never saw this one coming, because frankly I was always so involved in my own eating, I never stopped long enough to notice other people. Now I do, and it's a little disconcerting.

One day, my husband was starving (what else is new?), and he wanted to stop off at his favorite all-you-can-eat buffet restaurant (translation: grazing station). We went in, and I didn't bother ordering anything, because after this surgery there is no possible way you can get your $11.99 worth of food out of the place. You'd have to stay for a week, and pack food in a suitcase to go. (This goes for Mother's Day buffets, Easter Sunday buffets, Thanksgiving, cruises, and any other event or situation that includes gargantuan amounts of available food.)

I sat there while he stuffed his lean frame full of food, and strangely it didn't bother me that I wasn't eating with him. But what did bother me was watching all the other people. They had unbelievably enormous amounts of food in front of them. I watched them go back for three, four, five trips to the buffet.

I couldn't believe how much they put in their mouths at one time. Each forkful was about half of what my entire meal would be now! Did I used to do that? Sadly, yes. How is it that I didn't just explode? How is it that they don't just explode? It's the weirdest thing, and it still bothers me.

I would never in a million years say anything to anyone, but I can't help watching people eat every time I'm out. It fascinates me. Karen too. And everyone else we've talked to as well. We're all enthralled with North America's eating.

It's hard to deal with the fact that you used to eat this way; that you would stuff as much salad in your mouth in one forkful, as you now eat in total with your entire meal. That's very hard to get your head around. Some days you'll be very grateful that's not you anymore, and on other days it will just be depressing. It's hard to separate yourself from all that, and stop mulling it over every time you watch people eat — or every time you eat.

Case in point: If you're wondering how we came to determine that the all-you-can-eat buffet is no longer a cost-efficient, or practical night out, well, let us tell you about our little experience with that.

Karen and I were at yet another conference, this time in Ann Arbor. We'd broken out of the conference, and hit the ground running at all the local discount stores. At one point, later in the afternoon, we determined that we simply had to stop to eat. Protein rules your life. So, we decided that the best thing to do was to go somewhere that the food was already made so we could save time and get back to big-game bargain hunting, and "important-woman-business." Fast food is generally out unless it's a true emergency because the choices are limited, and you have to do too much dismantling. Then we spied "the buffet."

Fond thoughts of being able to eat yourself into a stupor at "the buffet" came flooding back to both of us. All reason was temporarily suspended. We pulled in, quickly paid our $11.99 each, and headed for the steam tables. So many kinds of protein to choose from! And other goodies too like vegetables, and salad, and potatoes. We didn't even give a thought to the desserts or the fried stuff, so I guess not ALL rational thought had flown out the window, but certainly our eyes were bigger than our teeny weeny little stomachs. Our emotional eating memories were taking over.

We each grabbed some baked chicken, and roast beef, and ham, and whatever else looked like it had protein in it. We grabbed some iced tea, veritably raced for the table, and dug in. Now, let's just stop right there. There is just so much wrong with this picture, I don't even know where to start. What were we thinking???

First, we'd taken too much food. Second, it was all covered in gravy or sauce. Third, we were mesmerized by the food, and were eating on memory. Fourth, we were eating too fast. Fifth, we weren't chewing enough. Sixth, we were drinking while eating. And seventh, we'd paid $11.99 each, and we still thought we could get our money's worth. FOOLS!!!

We both ploughed through the first ten bites or so of our respective plates, and then it hit. Auto Eject!! We both made ourselves so sick, we actually laid down on the seats in the booth. (The good news being we'd lost enough weight to be able to lay down on the seats of the booth!)

Oh, and it was a bad one too. I don't know which one of us was greener, but Kermit had nothing on either of us! Fortune had smiled, however, in that we had serendipitously chosen a table near the bathroom. Thank God, for small favors. (Unfortunately, they don't keep pillows tucked behind their toilets for people like us.)

It took about an hour and a half before either one of us returned to some normal skin color. I know people were very afraid. You could tell by the odd looks, and the hushed tones that accompanied long sideways stares. I'm sure we weren't exactly a raving endorsement for the restaurant either. I'm surprised they didn't throw us out.

We sat there, and sat there, and sat there. We kept telling each other that we had to eat more because we hadn't yet consumed enough protein (like either one of us cared at that point!). So, we picked a little here, and picked a little there. By that time the food was cold, so we ditched it and got some new stuff that was warm, and not as drowned in gravy or sauce. Amazingly enough, neither of us felt guilty about wasting the food. After all we'd spent $11.99 each, and it was quickly becoming apparent that we weren't going to be able to eat even $2.99 worth of food in total.

We continued to pick a bit here and there. What we found ourselves doing in the meantime, was watching all the other people in the restaurant. They were more than getting their money's worth. Again, we couldn't understand where they were putting it all. Then we'd look at each other and remember when we used to do the same thing, or worse.

Amid watching others consume $35.00 worth of food, and dealing with the fact that we were subsidizing at least six people's dinners, we simply became consumed with how much money we'd wasted. We were determined to remember this experience, and we were determined to get at least most of our money's worth, one way or another.

All in all, we sat there for four and a half hours. We managed to get out of there with two dozen cookies hidden in purses, coat pockets, and one of our calendar portfolios, that we proudly brought home and presented to Matt. We figured that about made the restaurant and us even.

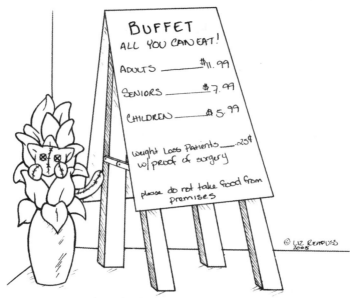

This experience caused us both to examine the fact that we kind of had to separate ourselves from places and events that involved large quantities of food, or inappropriate foods. Drive-thrus, buffets, and sometimes even regular restaurant meals are generally just not worth it.

Fast food drive-thrus are rarely an acceptable choice anymore because even if you order a plain chicken breast, it might still cost you $4.00! Salads are okay, but the dressings generally aren't, and pretty much nothing else is acceptable. Buffets? Well, we've discussed that. Regular meals at restaurants *always* involve bringing at least half home, and then it just dies a cold, lonely death in the fridge before it goes in the garbage. We both had to figure out how to separate from these memories, patterns, and choices, while still living a fairly normal life, and interacting with the world on a social basis.

Making these types of separations is like trying to adapt your personal subculture to living within the dominant culture. You have to live with the big structure of things: restaurants, and food-laden events never go away. But you also have to be true to what you need to do: eat smaller portions, waste less money, and not eat inappropriate food. Separating from one's culture, even a little, is a difficult thing. Ask anyone who's moved halfway around the world.

And speaking of separating from things (or being separated as the case may be...), we now come to the issue of the anxiety associated with giving up material things. By material things we mean, clothes, shoes, and accessories. Now, if you're a man reading this, I would not stop at this point if I were you. We realize that men don't generally have the emotional attachment to their clothing that women do (or, do they...?), but this will apply in part to you as well. You *will* experience some of this stuff. Trust us.

The last thing in the world I expected to be an issue for me, was shrinking out of my clothes. I know Karen echoes these thoughts, because she's sitting here, reading over my shoulder, nodding her head. If you'd asked either one of us what we were most looking forward to, one of the top five answers was wearing a smaller size, and getting rid of my "fat clothes." Oh, how we were both looking forward to that!

Well, we're here to testify that it can be every bit as glorious an experience as you've ever imagined it to be, and more. The celebrations we've had! The happy dances we've done in stores! The hooting and hollering that has gone on in dressing rooms! My, my, my, what fools we've made of ourselves! But here's the ugly side of it.

Because weight loss surgery causes you to lose a large amount of weight very quickly, more quickly than you've ever experienced, you cannot prepare for the pace at which you will shrink. You will have "shrinks" at the strangest times (for women most likely right after your monthly cycle, but any other time your body feels like it too), and you won't necessarily shrink evenly.

You may find that one day your clothes fit fine, and two days later you put on the same clothes and the top or bottom is now too big. Think about it. You're losing between 15 and 30 lbs. a month for the first 6 months or so. That's a lot of weight to drop, and what remains then has to shift around, and get resituated.

Additionally, with fat it's kind of a last on, first off sort of thing. Wherever you put the weight on last is generally where it will come off first. So for Karen and me, we shrank more and faster on the top than on the bottom (typical for many women), and when you are shrinking unevenly in the top and bottom, it's hard to keep up, and hard to know what size you really are.

So the moral of the story here is, "shrinks," although appreciated and the purpose of the entire process, are unpredictable, and they can cause some pretty serious clothing crises. Let me give you a few examples:

I had several sizes of clothes to shrink into. Problem: I hit each particular size during a time of year for which I had no appropriate clothing. Let me explain. I shrank into a size 24, but the last time I was a size 24, it was winter, so the majority of my clothes were winter clothes. When I shrunk into size 24, it was unfortunately, spring. I shrunk past an entire wardrobe of clothes I never got to wear. So, I had to go out and find clothes that fit me. $Cha-ching!$

I bought some clothes, and when I shrunk into a size 22, I had a few spring and summer pieces I could wear, thank goodness. What I didn't have was a pair of navy pants. Navy pants were particularly difficult to find during the summer of 2004 (why???), and it wasn't until about July that I finally found a pair (now in size 20), and a bargain at only $14.00 too!

I bought them on a Sunday (that's important to the story). They were clam diggers so that meant I couldn't wear them to work, but I was looking forward to wearing them the following weekend. The following Saturday I put the pants on and let out one horrific scream. My husband came running. "What's wrong? What's the matter?" he stammered. I was so hopping mad, I couldn't even get words out. Finally, I hissed, "These stupid pants are too big!" I'd shrunk during the week, and the pants were now almost three inches too big in the waist. I was so ticked off!

My husband was trying to be supportive, and of course he missed the point entirely. He said, "Well, isn't that what you wanted? To lose the weight?" Well, duh!! But, I hunted all Spring and Summer for these pants! They were a phenomenal bargain! I love them! I never even got to wear them, and now they have to go back to the store!! Don't you get it???? Of course, he didn't.

That scene has repeated so many times at my house, I've lost count. It happened virtually the same way one day with a belt. The belt fit a week before, and that day, because I was in a hurry, the belt was now two and a half inches past the last hole. I went screaming into the living room, bellowing for Matt. He came in dazed and bewildered at my freak-out over a belt. Again, he simply thought I should be thrilled I'd shrunk again. He plainly didn't realize that once again, it was at an inconvenient time.

Now don't get me wrong. I was grateful for each of those shrinks, and I celebrated those losses appropriately. But, I'm telling you, they do come at the most annoying times sometimes. So, that's one type of separation anxiety over clothes, and here's another: separating from clothes with emotional attachments.

I started weeding my closet about every 2 weeks once I started losing the weight. I figured, once I'm out of it, I'm out of it for good. There's no going back, baby. Of course, I kept a few things to go to the tailor to be resized. If you don't you'll simply end up naked. But then there were things to which I had an emotional attachment, and I didn't want to let them go. One of those things was the long velvet jacket my mother bought me for Christmas, 2001.

I'd barely been out of the hospital after my accident, and my mom bought me this beautiful velvet jacket with rhinestone buttons as a Christmas present. I so loved it, and I know it cost her more money than she really had to spend. More importantly, I felt thin in it. (I *wasn't* thin in it, but I felt thin!)

But those weren't the only reasons I didn't want to get rid of it. The biggest reason was because that was what I was wearing on New Year's Eve, when Matt asked me to marry him. I took it and had it cut down twice, but then it simply got to a point that it couldn't be cut down anymore. It's a size 20 now, and I'm a 12/14. I'll never be able to wear it again. Yet, I still can't let it go.

Similarly, and maybe worse, I couldn't even bring myself to look at my wedding dress. I was a size 28 by the time I got married, and although I designed my dress, and it was beautiful, it wasn't really the dress of my dreams because I wasn't the size I wanted to be. Now, I'm actually the size I always wanted to be when I got married. A couple of months ago, I decided to take the dress out and brave the tears. It was shocking. I could have got myself in that dress twice. In fact, I could have got both Matt and me in that dress at the same time! But more shocking than that was the fact that the detachable train of my dress that only went across the back of the dress from side seam to side seam, now fits all the way around me like a strapless sheath dress! There's no saving anything from the dress except a lot of really expensive fabric, but I can have the train made into a very chic evening gown, so it's not a total loss I guess.

It doesn't have to be clothing that has life changing memories attached though, it can just be things you've really enjoyed. Karen and I both have many pieces that we just loved that have gone by the wayside. They were mainly pieces we'd hunted so very hard to find (being in plus-sizes and all), and we actually liked them, felt good in them, and felt just a little bit like normal people in them. It's hard to say good-bye to something that made you feel good, even just for a short while.

It's hard to say good-bye to your favorite shoes when your feet shrink. It's hard to say good-bye to clothes that seem too long now, because you've shrunk enough that the proportions of plus-size clothes are just all wrong. It's hard to say good-bye to your favorite jeans because they're all "broken in" in just the right places. It's hard to say good-bye to jewelry that appears enormous now, when it was such a treasured find, and important piece of your wardrobe before.

And the sad part is that you don't just say good-bye once. You keep doing it over and over again as you shrink through the sizes. You may shrink into a pair of jeans you've had for ten years. Getting those goal jeans on is what you've been waiting for. They finally fit, and life is just grand. Then three weeks later, they're too big, and you only got to wear them twice. Say good-bye again.

Maybe you've bought yourself something new, maybe even something you've always wanted. Wear it quickly, because you'll have to say good-bye soon enough. This is very hard stuff!!! Especially, when you never get to wear something! Karen and I have just too many things that still have the tags attached; thus the garage sale mentioned in Chapter Two.

Each of us has things we value and cherish, whether it be a wedding dress, a beloved college t-shirt, or a tattered and torn pair of comfy sneakers. Each of you will go through the separation anxiety that comes with saying good-bye to your favorite articles of clothing, shoes, and accessories. You may not think you have any attachments, but mark our words — you do.

When you make changes in your life as extreme as the ones that result from weight loss surgery, you begin to examine all the things in life to which you are attached. We've told you before that this process involves learning new skills, one of which is living a different lifestyle. But another is learning new coping strategies, and facing emotional issues with strength and courage. And on that note, we'd like to discuss another form of separation anxiety. This form has been hastily, recklessly, and irresponsibly termed "addiction transference."

Addiction transference is not a recognized or authoritative medical, scientific, or psychological term. There exists no body of research on the subject as it relates to post-surgical weight loss patients. It is a term that was willy-nilly applied by someone who strung together a series of what looked like related events, without applying proper empirical processes to appropriately research and examine the events to determine the facts and any possible relationship to each other.

The types of events we're talking about here involve some post-surgical bariatric patients who have begun ingesting larger amounts of alcohol, and/or claim to have become dependent on alcohol. In response to varying reports from patients about an increased use of alcohol, a particular medical provider jumped to the absurd conclusion that bariatric surgery must cause patients to become alcoholics!! Brilliant!!!! What an earth-shattering scientific breakthrough that is!!! Of course bariatric surgery DOES NOT cause people to become alcoholics any more than having your appendix out causes alcoholism!!!

This particular medical provider seemed to think that this was some sort of revelation and decided to share the idea with some colleagues. Unfortunately, the media got a hold of this little tidbit, and they ran with it as they do with anything they can find to discredit the treatment of obesity because the prevailing thought is that obese people really don't deserve treatment. Society and the media like us believing that obese people are ill and diseased because they eat too much, are too lazy, have no will power, no self-discipline, and that we basically deserve what we get in life. We certainly are not worthy of having money, time, resources, research, and manpower spent on treating a disease we brought on our lazy, no-good selves. Thus, the ballyhoo about addiction transference was born.

To help you understand what all the sound and fury is about, however, we will try and explain to you how this came about and what issues may be deserving of research. While most bariatric patients do not come to the table with a diagnosed or even undiagnosed food addiction, they may come with inappropriate coping skills that cause them to turn to food in times of stress, anger, depression, fear, etc. Some people just really like food. Some people find comfort in food. Some may even have what has been scientifically described as a fat-sugar addiction. But very few actually have an addiction to *food*.

As for other addictions, or the propensity for addiction, hopefully the behaviorist conducting the pre-surgical assessment has determined whether the patient has these characteristics, and has dealt with them appropriately. Patients who smoke or drink are required to have quit for at least six months prior to surgery, but that is a tip-off that they may have an addictive nature in their personality make-up. But just because one has an addiction to one thing does not make one automatically predisposed to be addicted to another. All smokers are not alcoholics, and all alcoholics are not drug addicted. Similarly, the term *alcoholic,* is not the same as having a lack of control with alcohol, mismanaging alcohol, being irresponsible with alcohol use, or having an issue with alcohol. Patients have reported all of these conditions, yet someone decided to lump them all into the term *alcoholic* and declare a state of emergency.

Now, hopefully you have read Dr. Buffington's prologue, as well the portion of Chapter Five about alcohol. Maybe you've even read the piece on alcohol in the resources section. If so, good for you. It's important to understand at this point that the post-surgical bypass patient has a drastically altered metabolism when it comes to alcohol. It's virtually like mainlining it, and the high is very quick. The pleasure center of the brain is very quickly stimulated. Post-surgical patients can definitely encounter problems with alcohol use as Dr. Buffington has so clearly related.

Patients should be counseled and informed of this before surgery, and again afterward. We firmly believe in such a practice. "I've been warning my patients about this for 20 years," said Dr. Neil Hutcher, a past president of the ASMBS. However, it does not automatically follow that patients now are in danger of becoming alcoholics or any other kind of addict. Dr. Hutcher does warn his patients, especially adolescents, that thanks to their improved self-esteem they might find themselves in new social situations that involve drinking, and "not to make bad decisions due to the bad effects of alcohol."[5] In other words, be responsible in your alcohol use.

We also believe that there is a group of patients out there who are abusing alcohol, who are mismanaging alcohol use, and who may have issues with alcohol use. There may even be alcoholics out there as that term is clinically defined. What we do not *know* is exactly what is happening, at what rate it is happening, to whom it is happening, and why it is happening. With all those unknowns, how can anyone jump to the conclusion that bariatric surgery causes alcoholism, or that patients who may not have any addiction coming in are somehow transferring that non-addiction to alcohol?

The term *addiction transference* presupposes that every patient has some addiction that can be transferred to alcohol or to another addiction. Even if this were true, which we know it not to be, then why are we only seeing this phenomena being reported with regard to alcohol? Why not sex, or prescription drugs, or shopping? Lord knows, I've come pretty close to becoming a compulsive shopper on occasion (or at least looking like one) when replacing everything I owned several times over.

Perhaps there is a commonality between all of these things. All of them, and indeed all compulsions or addictions involve an issue with impulse control to one extent or another. So, if this were true, then under-developed impulse control skills might be a more common unifying factor among bariatric patients, and thus may be a more logical cause of increased alcohol usage.

Similarly, many patients have under-developed coping skills for which eating and food have become a replacement. When that is taken away, and the patient undergoes all of the various stressors that come with such a total life change, then perhaps alcohol becomes a replacement coping mechanism. That too may be a plausible explanation, but it still does not rise to the level of addiction or necessarily to alcoholism.

Perhaps patients undergoing all of the physical changes that the body experiences suffer from a chemical imbalance that causes them to seek out something that stimulates the pleasure center of the brain. Could this be the cause? Chemical and other imbalances in the system are causing the pre-surgical patient to become increasingly obese despite their best efforts, so why not?

The point of all this speculation is to drive home the fact that the phenomena has been drastically overstated, and the alarmist media frenzy should, as usual, not be taken to heart. We believe that there is in fact an issue here that needs to be examined and researched. It needs to be dissected and put under the microscope, and for the good of all the current patients and those to come, we need to find out what is really going on. Fortunately, that research is now underway, and we will have some empirical data from which to draw logical and rational conclusions.

We and the other responsible and progressive members of the bariatric community will continue to counsel patients about the issues surrounding alcohol and medication modifications post-surgery (see Chapter Twelve), and we will continue to study and define the phenomena that present themselves in the patient experience, but we will do it properly, correctly, responsibly, and scientifically. After all, if we continue to let irresponsible individuals and the media just start making up terms to apply to patients based on a set of phenomena that purportedly occurs in a percentage of the patient population, then I guess we'll soon be labeled as being "flatulence control impaired" because we have a lot of gas, or "disfigured" because we may have scars, or "severely nutrient intake challenged" because we can't eat as much or may get a stricture. How silly is this? This comes right under the heading of dealing with whatever may come your way and using your resources to help you through.

If you are separating from things in your old life, and you are using alcohol, drugs, sex, gambling, or any other type of repeated behavior that is negatively affecting your life, then seek help. It doesn't mean you are a bad person. Your separation anxiety may simply have gotten the best of you in this one instance. You are not a failure. You just don't have all the assets you need for this one job, so seek out those who can increase your assets and decrease your liabilities in this particular circumstance. Remember that your team can help you through. You don't have to be labeled as anything anymore, and you should certainly never willingly wear the label of *addiction transfer victim.* Don't let anyone hang that bogus term on you.

Well, we hope that letting you in on some of the situations we've encountered will provide you with a little more strength and courage to face your own. Know that separation anxiety is really just a bunch of funky growing pains. Let yourself grow. Become who you always wanted to be. You can. You should. You will. We know.

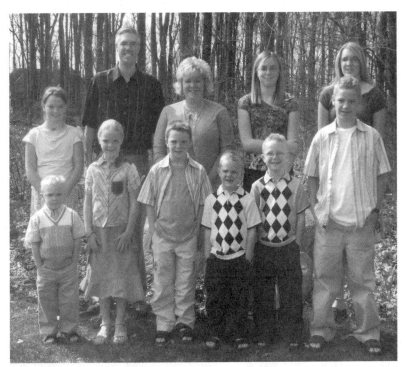

Dr. Randal S. Baker and his family

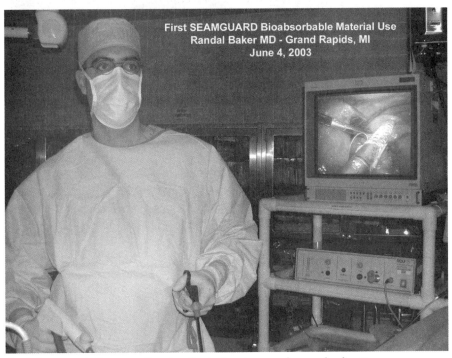

First SEAMGUARD Bioabsorbable Material Use
Randal Baker MD - Grand Rapids, MI
June 4, 2003

Dr. Baker using the Seamguard® product for the first time anywhere on the planet!

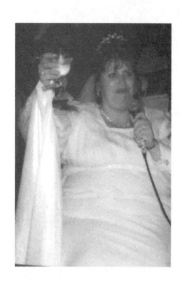

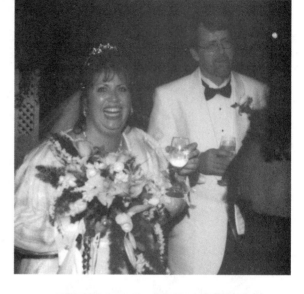

Julie's "before & after" pictures

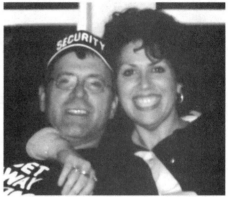

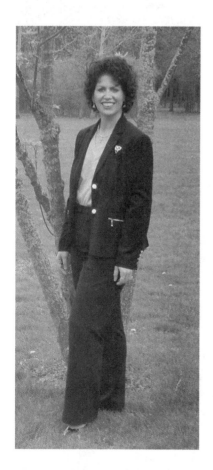

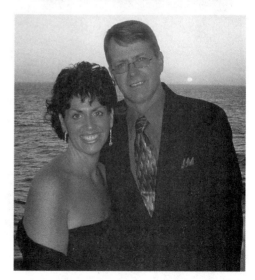

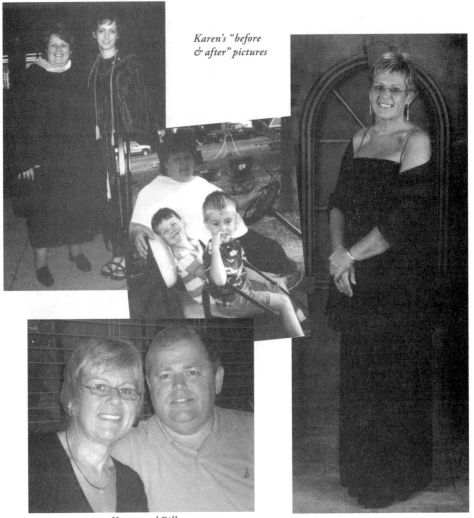

Karen's "before & after" pictures

Karen and Bill

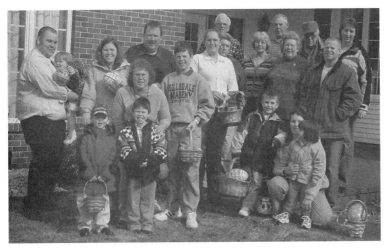

Karen's family

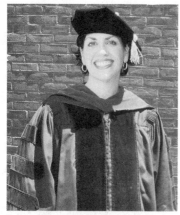

Julie in her doctoral robes

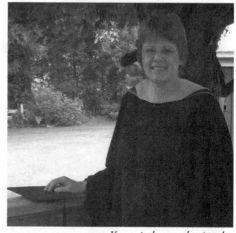

Karen in her academic robes

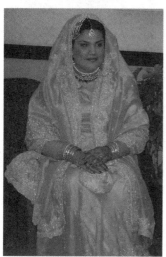

Nabila at her wedding

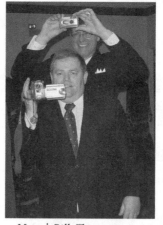

Matt & Bill: The camera crew

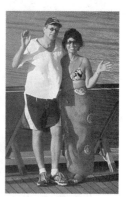

Cruising...

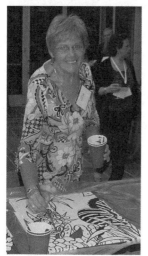

Starving artist?

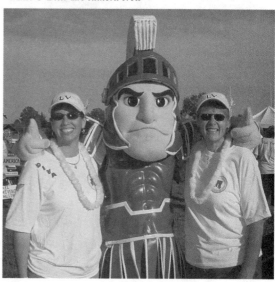

Us with Sparty. Go MSU!

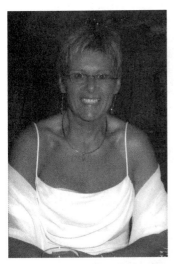

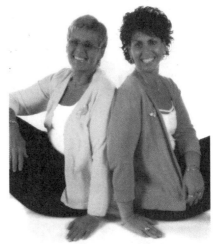

Push-mePull-you

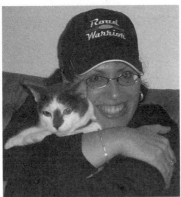

Julie and Nabs' Kitty Moto

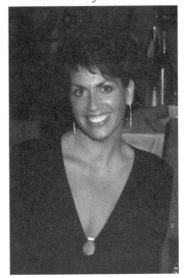

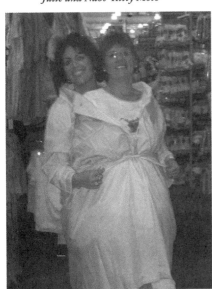

US in one XXXL robe

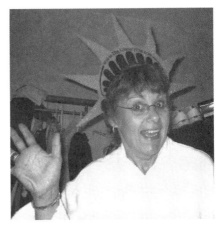

Hi Mom, from NY!

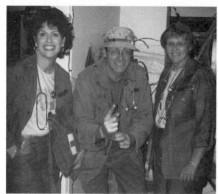

Enuff said...

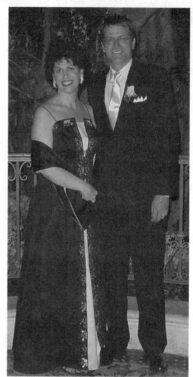

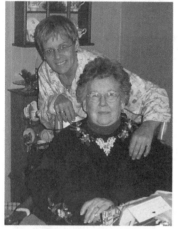

Karen and her mom

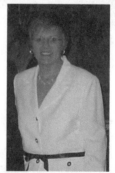

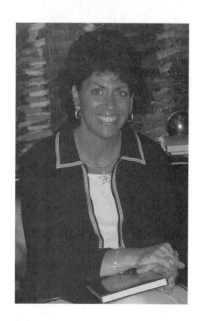

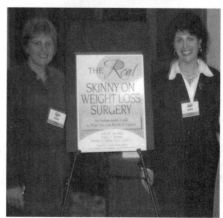

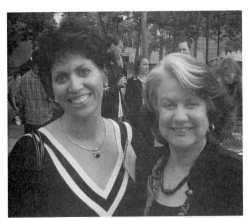

Julie and Dr. Buffington

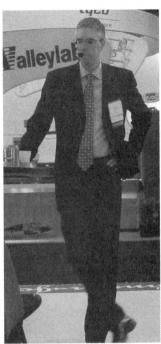

Doc Baker teaching other docs

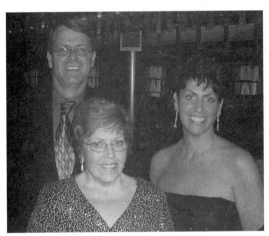

Julie, Matt, and Julie's mom

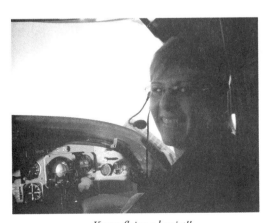

Karen flying a learjet!!

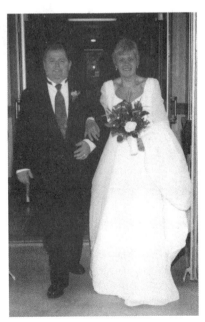

Karen and Bill's Wedding!

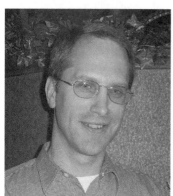

Scott H. Glass, MS, MA, LLP

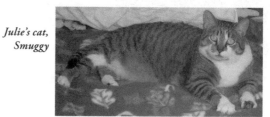

Julie's cat, Smuggy

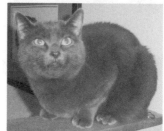

Julie's cat, Smudgie

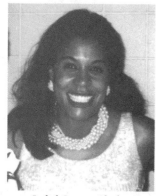

Judith Brown-Clarke

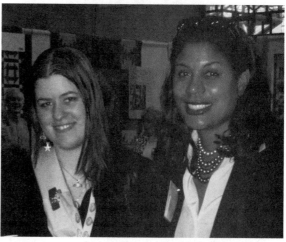

Liz our illustrator and Judi

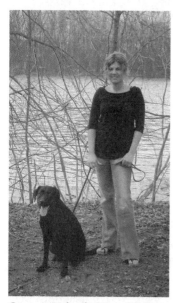

Carrie A. Liebrock, RD and Willow

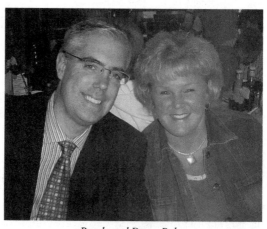

Randy and Dawn Baker

Chapter Ten

⟍ NO GIRLS ALLOWED! ⟍

Randal S. Baker MD, FACS
Julie M. Janeway
Karen J. Sparks

More and more men are having this surgery these days, and we thought it was about time to bring the issues that men deal with out into the light. The vast majority of information lurking around out there deals with women who are choosing to have the surgery, and so this chapter is dedicated to the guys and the difficulties they encounter by virtue of the fact they were born male (and no, that is not a character flaw). This is not a new millennium version of the "he-man woman-haters club," but let's just say you have to have a "Y" chromosome to join.

We interviewed a number of male weight loss surgery patients, both from my practice and from other medical institutions as well. Some recently had their surgery, and some were as far as 5 years out. Some were young, and some were older, some married and some single. They shared their experiences, their stories, their insights, and their lives with us, and we appreciate that immensely. The story of what men experience as weight loss patients has never really been studied or told, and we're proud to be one of the first to draw attention to the special needs of male bariatric patients, and bring this knowledge to the general public.

The men we talked to were not afraid to tell us that they were afraid. Some had a fear of dying from the procedure, but they also had a fear of dying without it. All but one had a fear of having a big open incision scar, and that one fellow didn't really have the fear because he was never given the option for a laparoscopic procedure by his surgeon. He was a candidate, but it was never even discussed or offered.

Others had very real fears of dealing with dumping syndrome, and strangely very few of them really had it. They also feared the procedure not working and the weight staying put, or they feared the needles and the band fills with a Lap-Band® procedure. That fear was the hardest to work through before going into surgery, and most said they didn't really get rid of it until they'd lost about 50 lbs. We believe one of our interviewees, Scott, said it best: "I couldn't try it on to see if it was going to fit!"

To Scott, as to many of the other men we talked to, the fear of the drastic life change was daunting, at best. They feared not knowing what they would be able to eat (or drink!), and they feared things just being "different." It's a well known fact that men fear change more than women (as a general rule), and these men were no exception.

Almost all said they had to deal with fears about other complications as well, and for the men who had their surgeries at a non-multi-disciplinary practice, the fears of complications were amplified because complications like pulmonary embolism, hernia, gallbladder disease, leaks, erosions, slippage, infections, and obstructions were never defined nor discussed. Having said that, not one of them expressed a fear of having a stricture or a gallbladder issue.

Complication rates for men versus women have not yet been studied extensively. A Vanderbilt University study performed in 2005, however, did produce some interesting results that are being taken very seriously by bariatric medical professionals. This study of 54,878 patients, both male and female, studied risk factors for post-operative mortality following bariatric surgery. The study concluded that men over the age of 39 who were Medicare patients with a need for re-operation due to a surgical complication, had the greatest chance of dying.[1] The chance of dying, however, was still very low.

Several other studies have also been performed, although none from such a large patient population. Each of them attempted to determine a different piece of the puzzle. The results when looked at together, give us a better picture of what men should be considering when thinking about weight loss surgery, and what medical professionals should be considering when caring for male bariatric patients.

A 2005 study conducted at the University of Pittsburgh Medical Center sought to determine whether advanced age or gender had any effect on adverse outcomes following bariatric surgery. The results of this study were that males have a slightly higher incidence of mortality from a surgical complication (not an underlying co-morbid condition like a heart problem or high blood pressure). The difference was 1.2% for males, versus 0.47% for females.[2] These are still pretty small percentages when you look at the general scheme of things, and when you consider that all surgeries, no matter how simple or common, can result in a complication causing death.

The two studies we just referenced dealt with gastric bypass patients. This next study dealt with adjustable gastric banding patients. Swiss researchers looked at 404 post-surgery gastric banding patients in 2005. They were attempting to determine the impact of age, sex, and body mass index on outcomes at four years after gastric banding surgery. What this study noted was that during the four years after surgery, men had more band leaks than women (7% for men, 1.9% women), and older men had more band slippages than younger men (8.4% versus 0%). Patients with a BMI greater than 50 were less likely to experience gastric complications from the banding surgery than were patients with a BMI between 35 and 50, but were more likely to experience port and tube complications that required a second surgical procedure to correct.[3] Mortality rates were not reported in this study.

The last two studies that yielded some important information include a 2006 study from the State University of New York – Albany that looked at predictors of in-hospital post-operative complications among adults undergoing bariatric procedures. The study examined 7,868 patients in New York state who underwent a bariatric procedure during 2003. Among other findings the study concluded that men 50 or older, of Hispanic ethnicity, and who had congestive heart failure, cardiac arrhythmia, neurological disorders, and/or peptic ulcers were more prone to immediate complications while still in the hospital following a bariatric surgical procedure.[4]

This study followed on the heels of a 2004 study that found that men with sleep apnea or metabolic syndrome were more likely to have a prolonged hospital stay following open or laparoscopic bariatric surgery.[5] Again, the studies did not look at mortality rates, but rather complication rates, or predictors of extended hospital stays.

So what it comes down to is that men have an ever so slightly larger chance of having a complication either from surgery or from an underlying co-morbid condition. Take this into account when you are making a decision about bariatric surgery, but don't let it be your only consideration. Remember to take into account that you have a disease that will result in death at some point. Take into account the chances of living and having a happier, healthier, and probably longer life are around 98% or better. Take all that into account and discuss it all with your bariatric surgeon before you make your final decision.

Also remember that complication rates as referenced in these studies can mean anything from a pulmonary embolism to a stricture or a little infection of one of the port sites. The use of the word "complication" doesn't have to mean that they were all life-threatening complications. Several of the men we interviewed for this chapter had what is considered a post-operative complication. Two of the men we talked to did have strictures, and one had it three times, just like Julie had. He didn't have quite as bad a time with it, and he too survived the stricture fairy. One of the patients had a post-operative gallbladder issue like Karen had, for which I prescribed medication, and it resolved itself without surgical intervention. Another patient experienced a more serious complication: the bowel was not working at all for a few days after surgery, but fortunately it spontaneously resolved itself.

That was about it as far as complications went, and as for after-effects I was surprised to hear how many of these men had "scramps," to use little Meghan's word. They spoke of severe cramping in both their legs and their diaphragms/abdomens, and strangely described it exactly as Julie and Karen had described it to me months before. Two of the patients also told us, almost sheepishly, that they had this weird sneezing response to eating heavier foods, carbohydrates, or anything that got stuck. Karen was vindicated and she let out a whoop that could be heard in south Florida!

Speaking of whoops, all of these patients were extremely happy to report that they had gone into the surgery with a variety of the most basic types of co-morbidities, and all but one man had every co-morbidity completely resolved. That one patient had five medications for high blood pressure cut back to only one. In addition to high blood pressure, these patients had high cholesterol, sleep apnea (including having it so bad as to require a machine to help breathing at night), insulin dependent diabetes, joint issues, circulation issues, back problems, and gastroesophageal reflux (chronic heartburn). These patients have seen an almost 100% resolution of their co-morbidities, with the exception of the high blood pressure patient mentioned above. The men were more than eager and excited to detail those stories for us in the interviews.

One of the topics they were not so eager to talk about, however, was their behavior modification as it relates to food. The men all said that they still had food issues with which they grapple, and they were surprised to find that to be very normal. The biggest complaints were dealing with not drinking during meals, staying away from bad foods, chewing their food well enough, getting their water requirement in, and maintaining appropriate portion sizes. They said those things were daily struggles. The biggest one, however, was slowing down their eating. Every one of them said that was an issue on some level, and they still found themselves in "shovel" mode (eating too fast) when eating.

Other food issues included forgetting to pack food with them when they go out, and difficulty finding appropriate food and protein sources when at work or anywhere outside the home. Most of the patients confessed to being seduced on a regular basis by restaurants and fast food joints, and reported tremendous difficulties with avoiding these temptations. Luckily they also reported that the majority of the time they are able to avoid the siren call of the fast food vendors, and make good and healthy food choices.

For many men, cooking is an issue. Lots of guys just don't really know how to cook, and that's part of the reason they put on weight in the first place; pizza, fast food, restaurant food, and vending machine type snacks will do it to you every time. Some of the men we talked to knew how to cook, but rarely did. They informed us that they have taken over more of the cooking duties now (albeit mostly grilling), and that has helped with keeping up with their protein. For two others, cooking has been a newly acquired skill, and they are still attempting to master the culinary art.

We asked our patient participants about another newly acquired skill, and that was life without alcohol. One man said that he rarely drank anything anymore, maybe a small glass of wine with dinner on occasion. He said that his friends didn't like that aspect of his new life, as they used to include alcohol in many of their activities. Many others, however, said that it was really no big deal to give up drinking.

The beer drinkers either gave it up completely or switched to a non-alcoholic brew (which the bypass patients found still had some effect, although greatly reduced). Yet another said he still had an occasional drink when hanging out with buddies just to keep the ribbing down to a bare minimum. He said he experienced a radically quicker response to the alcohol, and it gave him quite a bit of gas, but no dumping unless he drank it too fast. He said nursing one beer along through an entire football game was the way to go.

The fear of dumping, combined with the intensified effect of the alcohol was the main reason most of these men chose to avoid drinking. We were surprised to learn, however, that the second biggest reason for avoiding alcohol was the empty calories that would go primarily right to fat. It was rewarding to know that we had instilled those rationales deep enough to be applied in any food situation including situations that involve choosing or not choosing alcohol.

Several of the men reported that alcohol causes bloating, a phenomenon they never noticed when they were heavier. Many also stated that they were surprised to find that they could gain and lose between 3 and 5 pounds in water weight as well.

They all said they didn't know men could carry water weight. In fact, all humans can carry water weight. When the body becomes dehydrated it attempts to conserve as much water as possible, rather than keeping it flushing through the system.

Many of the guys we spoke with also expected to have a major surge of energy immediately following surgery, or shortly thereafter. They were surprised to learn that it took a little longer than that, but eventually that surge kicked in, and now they're clicking on all cylinders. Although some of our guys were getting regular exercise, most of them reported that it was still very difficult, as they had long established patterns of inactivity that they were finding very hard to break. We were informed by one patient, and asked to remind the public at large that "not all men are genetically encoded to be sports fanatics, whether watching or playing them."

Whether they exercised or not, most of the men we talked to told us that they had lost a significant amount of weight — off their rear ends! Now I imagine that to many female readers this sounds like a very positive thing, but as we found out, it is more of a problem than we thought for male patients. The male patients who discussed losing weight off their buttocks, all recounted to us that the biggest problem is pain when sitting. It simply hurts to be sitting right on the pelvic bones. They said that the discomfort doesn't take long to set in either, and many are now avoiding situations in which they might have to sit for long periods of time.

In fact, bariatric reconstructive plastic surgeons are seeing an increase in male patients who are seeking not only "butt implants" but also pectoral implants, face lifts, and body lifts. Men are finding that they benefit equally as much as women from the improved body image and acceptance, as well as the effect on the libido and sex life. They report being happier with the way they look in clothes, as well as in the way they fit. Plastic surgery, although not a requirement, can be helpful to some male patients and should be considered when and if it becomes necessary after bariatric surgery. Until then, you might just have to put up with baggy pants and a tighter belt, or shirts that are cut a little closer in the tummy.

One of the patients said that he was seriously considering getting buttock implants, not for the vanity of having a very nicely shaped butt, rather for the cushioning, and to fill out the seat of all his "baggy-butt" pants. For those of you who may be unfamiliar with "butt implants," the procedure is basically the same as the breast implant procedure, only the implants enhance the buttocks region of the body. They all stated that they were very self-conscious of their now flattened posteriors, and fitting clothes was hard enough without having to constantly have the seats of their pants taken in.

The clothing issues were a big sore spot with the majority of our male interviewees as well. Several of the guys said that they still had a terrible time finding clothes to fit because of their new proportions. Men's clothes are all based on inches, and specifically men's pants are all based on waist inches and inseam inches with the waist generally being larger than the inseam. For several of these guys, however, their inseams are actually the same as, or longer than their waist sizes, and that makes pants that fit properly very hard to find.

The other issues raised about clothes included the fact that men don't generally share or trade clothes like women do, primarily because of the waist/inseam combinations, so getting clothes from a buddy isn't really an option. Other men complained of the price of replacing business clothes, and the fact that they found that suits can only be tailored down two sizes. They found that to be expensive, and said they weren't prepared for the cost. For the most part, the men did say that they would attend a clothing swap even if it meant only picking up a few smaller shirts or suits for a minimal price.

Several of the men asked Julie and Karen if they had any shopping tips on where to find clothes. Being the big-game bargain hunters that they are, they informed the men that they should be shopping at discounters and liquidators. These types of stores tend to carry unusual or off sizes, and sell at seriously discounted prices which helps the budget out a little too. Garage sales, thrift stores, and consignment shops are also good bets for very inexpensive replacement clothes, including suits and ties (remember, you'll probably have to replace the ties too as the big and tall men's ties will end up being too long).

Several of the guys told us that it was very hard to get a perspective on their new sizes as they shrank, because they would go back to the big and tall men's store, and the sales people there would, of course, sell them things. One of the men said, "The sales people still see you as a big guy, so they point you toward big clothes. I still start in the big clothes and then have to work my way down. Inevitably I end up coming out with something that is still too big, or becomes too big a week later."

We suggest a cheaper alternative: get someone to take some digital or Polaroid shots of you before you shop. Have them taken full length, and have them taken in the same spot, next to the same things every time. This will help to give you perspective, and let you see what's really there, and what really isn't anymore. It should also help you to start trying on clothes closer to your actual size.

Julie and Karen suggest that if you're still in the active shrink phase, then don't buy clothes that fit unless you are wearing it out of the store. Buy clothes a little bit snug so they'll fit longer. You'll shrink into it, have no fear. Also, check out Tips From the Tailor in the resources section. And men, there is no shame in buying goal clothing — something you hang there and shrink into. Whether it's an Armani suit or a pair of Levis you wore in high school, set some goal clothing and celebrate when you fit into it. Nobody else has to know but you.

If you have weight loss surgery, the shrinking you will so come to cherish and despise is greatly facilitated by the ingestion of your daily vitamins. We asked the guys about the vitamin issue, and we got responses that were all over the map. The men who did not have surgery at a multi-disciplinary practice were not prescribed vitamins of any sort, and in fact, one man was told he could never take vitamins again, which is totally false, misleading, and dangerous.

Most of the guys admitted to skipping their vitamins about half the time, and when asked why, answered that they just felt stupid taking vitamins. Vitamins are nutritional supplements only. They augment your food intake to keep your body functioning at a better efficiency level. They are not for "wussies," nor are they unmanly. Take your vitamins! You'll have more stamina to get through the day...or through the night....

Speaking of stamina, that brings us to probably the biggest issue for men in having this surgery: their sex lives. We know that obesity has a profound effect on the sexual quality of life for both men and women. In fact, a really good study on this ws done with 500 patients in Durham, North Carolina in 2006. That study reported that obesity is associated with lack of enjoyment of sexual activity, lack of sexual desire, difficulties with sexual perfrormance, and avoidance of sexual encounters.[6] Additionally, we know it has a profound effect on opportunity for sexual encounters for single individuals as well.

Researchers in Italy studied men who had undergone bariatric surgery and found that before surgery most of the patients had subnormal testosterone levels, and other hormone levels were equally out of whack. This resulted in a condition called *hypogonadism,* in which hormone irregularities in men affect stimulation of the testicles that inhibit sperm production.

Excess fat actually causes the male hormone, testosterone, to be converted into estrogen, and those estrogens decrease testicle stimulation. Researchers from Reproductive Biology Associates (RBA) in Atlanta, Georgia, report that a high BMI in men correlates with reduced testosterone levels. RBA reports that overweight men tend to have testosterone levels 24% lower than men of normal weight, and obese men tend to have levels 26% lower. Men with high BMIs typically are found to have an abnormal semen analysis as well.[7] The Italian study reported that following surgery, testosterone and other hormone levels all returned to normal. Subjective improvement in sexual performance was reported by 80% of the patients studied.[8]

All of the men we talked to reported having a significantly improved sex drive. They stated that their sexual encounters were more sustained, more frequent, and their stamina was markedly improved. The men told us that they felt more desirable and attractive as they lost weight. As their self-images improved, so did their outlook on sex. Many said that it was much more enjoyable, varied, and not as laborious as before surgery. One man simply said, "It's not uncomfortable anymore."

Also associated with obesity is male infertility as a result of the lowered testosterone and other hormones. Studies conducted at the U.S. National Institute of Environmental Health Sciences (NIEHS) are confirming that men with increased body mass indexes (BMI) are significantly more likely to be infertile than normal-weight men. The NIEHS data suggests that a 3 unit BMI increase, or a 20 lb. increase in a man's weight may increase the chance of infertility by about 10%.[9] Reduction in BMI can reverse the infertility if there are no other causal factors present.

Post-bariatric surgery patients, however, also have to be extremely careful about nutritional deficiencies. Another Italian study found that bariatric surgery in men did not correct infertility or raise testosterone levels in all men. Some men who had nutritional deficiencies developed secondary male factor infertility.[10] So, if you are going to consider having bariatric surgery, you really want to make sure that you can deal with taking those vitamins and eating that good food. Building Blocks® vitamins can help, but only you can eat the foods that will keep you healthy, both generally and sexually.

Male patients report that they are happier overall with the quality of their sex lives. In fact, many report that since their weight loss, their penis size is bigger. Now we have no proof of that, and there have been no studies, but we presume that it does *appear* to be bigger because the weight at the base of the penis is no longer pushing skin down and making it look shorter. In other words, the entire length of the penis is now uncovered.

Maybe you care about this, and maybe you don't but we thought we'd tell you anyway. Maybe it will have a positive psychological effect on you and/or your partner. Maybe it will help improve your sex life. Maybe not...

The men who were in relationships told us that the weight loss had improved their view of themselves, and combined with their improved sex lives, lead to stronger and more intimate relationships. The closer the relationships became the more communication was occurring, and the less the men found themselves withdrawing from their partners. Several of the men told us that before surgery they were just pulling away, and closing others out because of how badly they felt about themselves. Now they report being fully committed and engaged in their relationships again, and they attribute most of that change to the change within themselves.

The changes in how they viewed themselves also affected other relationships as well. Those men with children stated that they had far more interaction with their children now, and enjoyed being able to participate in activities with them. One man, Brian, told us that it meant the world to him that his thirteen year old daughter was proud of him. We're proud of you too Brian.

Other men also told us about issues that arose with friends and relatives who were not so supportive. Karl told us that many of his friends and family were worried that he had simply taken the easy way out. They were worried that he was going to die because he so drastically cut down his eating. They unknowingly attempted to undermine his efforts out of sheer worry, fear, and lack of understanding. He said he simply wasn't prepared for that, but dealt with it appropriately.

Another man told us that he wasn't prepared for his other overweight friends to shun him because they could no longer relate to him as a result of his changed eating behaviors. On a similar note, other interviewees talked to us about how the dynamics changed with their friends because of changing size.

Apparently for several of these guys, there was an unwritten understanding that with size went proportional strength. In other words, Jeff's buddies assumed that if Jeff was "big" he must also be very strong. When Jeff began to lose weight, and despite packing on at least 20 lbs. of muscle, the assumption became that Jeff was now much weaker. This assumption was confirmed in the minds of Jeff's friends when one of them went to punch him in the arm in a friendly gesture of greeting, and virtually knocked Jeff to the ground. The "old" Jeff wouldn't have budged, while the new Jeff was a push over. Jeff wasn't expecting the male friendship dynamics to change in that way. Neither were we, frankly.

In exploring that a little further, we found that increased respect for self does change the dynamics of all relationships for men, whether they be intimate, familial, social, or work related. To get to the point of self respect and increased self-esteem, the emotional work that has to be done during this process was also very unexpected to most of these men.

Like the average "Joe," most of these guys thought that they had no emotional issues with which to deal. To their profound dismay, they found that they did have some emotional baggage from years of being heavy, and it had to be unloaded along with the weight. They found that in order to ditch some of this baggage, they had to turn to the women in their lives for support, because most of their male friends were not equipped or inclined to really help. Most of the women they turned to (and a few men) were other patients they met at support groups. Some of the men we interviewed went to support groups, but they were men who had their surgeries at multi-disciplinary practices. The men who did not attend support groups all came from surgical programs that did not provide a multi-disciplinary care and follow-up program, thus the concept of support groups was foreign to them. In fact, they all seemed to be under the same misconception about the function and purpose of support groups.

As we've said earlier in the book, support groups are not places for group therapy. They are not places for therapy at all. What they should be is a place for patients and the members of their personal support circles to congregate, share information, become educated, share tips and stratgies, provide resources, motivate each other, celebrate each other's little victories, and learn new skills to be successful in the long-term. They should be fun and enjoyable, and *all* men who have surgery should attend support groups for the rest of their lives.

When the men we interviewed said that they turned to women to help them ditch some of their baggage, they all meant that often the act of simply knowing that they were not alone in their feelings and perceptions helped them to get past them. Additionally, others would provide assistance in ways to deal with certain issues of situations that helped our guys move through whatever needed to be moved through. Support groups should be a place you want to go, and that you value yourself, your health, and your success enough to make time to attend. It is not unmanly or a "sissy" endeavor.

For those who attended support groups, the men told us that they turned to women for help, understanding, and insight because men just don't turn to other men for emotional support. It was hard for them because they were often turning to virtually total strangers for validation of their emotional issues and constantly changing experiences, and yet they could only feel comfortable turning to unfamiliar women rather than unfamiliar men. We were a bit surprised and made special note of the emotional privacy issue.

Men seemed to have an inordinate sensitivity to keeping the fact of their surgeries quite private as well. Many said they just don't tell people they had surgery "because it's none of their business." Some said that they don't tell people because of the prevailing misconception that it's the easy way out, and you're just lazy and want a quick fix. They said they get tired of defending their decisions to have surgery (we hear that a lot), so they just don't admit to it to prevent being seen as weak.

The unanimous view of these men after surgery, however, is that they are anything but weak. They are stronger, leaner, healthier, and happier now. Although they are men, their experiences are not completely dissimilar from female bariatric patients. The men told us that they all enjoyed being able to get around easier, fitting into places and things they couldn't before, and being able to participate in physical activities.

Like other weight loss surgery patients, they found it hard to go back and look at "before" pictures, they could get life insurance now where before they couldn't, and food no longer controlled them. Interestingly, several of the men said that it disturbed them deeply to watch other people eating in a restaurant as it brought up too many painful reminders of their own self-abuse with food.

The bypass patients told us that they avoid like the plague any foods that will cause dumping, and all chase their protein requirements every day like an elusive fox on an English hunt. Our interviewees reported no after-effects that concentrated in any one area over another. Brian did tell us that the air in his abdomen after surgery (the beach ball effect) felt like an "internal wedgie." We thought that was pretty funny, and Karen and Julie both said it was a rather accurate statement.

Despite the possibility of a very short term internal wedgie, all of these men expressed to us that they had no regrets at all about having this surgery, including the ones who were not cared for at a multi-disciplinary practice. When asked what they would tell other men who were considering surgery, here's some of what they had to say:

"Don't do it for vanity, do it to save your life."

"Just do it. It will help in more ways than you can imagine."

"This is not the easy way out. It's hard work and sometimes frustrating, but consider what your quality of life is like right now. Could it be any worse?"

"Don't hesitate because you're a tough guy or being macho. Do it, and do it now."

"It wasn't just a lack of willpower that got you fat, so don't just rely on willpower to get it off. Get the help you need."

"Really learn about this surgery, then explain all the potential problems and benefits to your family, including your kids. Make sure they understand. Tell them in an age appropriate way. Include them in the decision process."

"Don't listen to all the media hype on the mortality rate of this surgery. Find out your own facts and don't let the media make the decision for you. They don't have your life in mind when they run those stories for ratings and advertising dollars."

"If you're freaked out by the bypass then look seriously at the Lap-Band®. It's not easier than bypass, but if it gets you where you want to be, then go for it."

"Be afraid, but do it anyway."

We couldn't have said it better ourselves! We hope that we've shed a little light on what men experience with this surgery and metamorphosis. If you're a man thinking about weight loss surgery, our advice is to talk to other men who've had the surgery, and to really discuss the subject with your doctor. Take a really hard look at the risks, benefits, alternatives, and complications of both obesity and weight loss surgery, and compare them side by side with your doctor. Make an informed decision, and whatever path you choose, make a plan to become healthy, lose the weight, and live a better quality of life. No matter the choice, here's to you finding a multi-disciplinary medical and support team who'll be behind you all the way.

On those days when you think this is hard...

remember... it's supposed to be,

or everyone would be doing it...

that's what makes it so great.

ANONYMOUS

Chapter Eleven

F E N G   S H U I
➤ F O R   T H E   B O D Y ➤
A N D   M I N D

Carrie A. Liebrock, RD

Scott H. Glass, MS, MA, LLP

Hi. It's us again, Julie and Karen. We're back. We thought we needed to make an introductory statement or two for this chapter, so we're butting in on Carrie and Scott. We feel we must apologize from the start about the dog story in this chapter. It's gross, but it's funny, so we voted to keep it. Okay, with that done we'll get down to business.

We've entitled this chapter "Feng Shui for the Body and Mind" not to endorse or educate you about the ancient Chinese practice of Feng Shui (pronounced "Fung Shway"), but to use it as an analogy for taking care of the environment in which you travel through life. The reason it's such a good analogy is because the real practice of Feng Shui is about creating a healthy flow of life energy, or "chi" within the space where we spend most of our time.

We all may think that we spend most of our time at work, or at home, or maybe even in the car. But, the truth is we spend the most time (indeed all of our time) in one place: our bodies. So if we are to learn from the analogy, we must look at finding a way to create a healthy life force, or "chi" in our own bodies, and that is exactly what this chapter is about.

Feng Shui is considered a metaphysical science in which one learns to recognize and tap into the "chi" to help achieve many life endeavors. We all know that we feel better, do more, achieve more, and believe in ourselves more when we are healthy, and look and feel good about ourselves. So being healthy certainly aids us in achieving our many life endeavors.

Now, according to ancient Chinese belief, all true life changing power lies in working with the rules of nature. What more basic rule of nature is there than eating natural foods in a moderate amount for the purpose of nourishing the body, and moving the muscles of the body in such a way as to keep it running and in good working order? That's the definition of how we stay alive! What's more natural and basic than that, right?

So, by following this basic rule of nature and being healthy, it naturally follows that we will increase the life force within ourselves, feel better about ourselves, interact with the rest of the world more, and thus achieve many life endeavors.

We've examined the facts, and proven true the assertion that "life changing power lies in working with the rules of nature." If we eat healthy, and live in a healthy body, other things in our lives work out a little better for us too. Okay! Is it that easy? No. So, let's move on to the next step.

The ancient tradition is also about following the rules of nature, and about finding some harmony between all the varying elements of your life. So what are we trying to harmonize? Well, we're trying to harmonize health, good nutrition, movement, sensory satisfaction, variety, and minimize pain, discomfort, and distaste. That's just the attempt at "harmonizing" your mind regarding food choices and eating properly, as well as in trying to get your carcass off the couch to move for five minutes! You are constantly "assessing" all the options, and trying to "harmonize" the options to create the best possible, least offensive outcome for yourself.

Feng Shui is also considered to be the art of "assessing." It is about "assessing" quality of life through observations and analysis of a person's living environment. Again, we come back to the fact that your primary living environment is your body. As overweight people, we know far too well that the quality of your life is dictated by your weight and self-esteem, both of which are part of your primary living environment — your body. So we must assess through observation and analysis how to change the primary living environment in order to positively affect the life force within, and the quality of life we seek. Okay. So how do you do that? Glad you asked.

The first step taken in Feng Shui is to change the living environment. (We're usually talking about your house here.) This step is called *space clearing*. Space clearing is defined as a technique that will cleanse your living environment of the negative energy that naturally accumulates over time. Well I don't know about you, but our bodies and lives have certainly accumulated some "negative energy" over time in the form of poor self-esteem, extra pounds, toxins, and emotional baggage from both. So by choosing to lose weight, you're starting your space clearing right off the bat.

To properly perform your space clearing, you'll need the help of a behaviorist (emotional and habit cleaning), a dietitian and an exercise physiologist (extra pounds, toxins, and self-esteem cleaning). You will deal with and dispose of much of the emotional baggage and bad habits, and will learn to take care of your primary living environment in a natural and healthy way. In so doing, many (but not all) of the other issues and difficulties in your life may seem to clear away, or at least become more manageable.

Feng Shui theorizes that by combining space clearing with the elimination of unnecessary clutter, and a commitment to keeping your living environment as clean and functional as possible, you can begin to make real and lasting changes in your life. We wholeheartedly agree with this theory.

This chapter will provide you with many of the tools to make real and lasting changes in your life, even if you don't choose to have surgery. It's not the same old tired speech you've heard about the food pyramid, and exercising until you drop. We think you'll be pleasantly surprised at the information and advice Carrie and Scott are going to give you. So read on. You'll be glad you did.

And again, sorry about the dog part, but we're still laughing. Take it away, Carrie.

THE CARE AND FEEDING OF YOUR "CHI"

Hi. I'm Carrie Liebrock, the registered dietitian they nabbed for this project. Though my family will often lovingly refer to me as the "food police" when I attempt to lovingly encourage them to eat a little healthier, I can assure you that I have never attended any sort of food policing academy, nor is it my goal in life to incriminate those for what they choose to eat. The reason that I chose to major in dietetics rather than criminal justice was to in some way help everyone I meet become a little healthier. I just wasn't feeling that vibe in criminal justice. Call me crazy, but I prefer non-violent client interaction, and an office, not a jail cell to work in. It's a personal thing.

As a dietitian working with weight loss patients, I've heard it all when the office door closes. There have been confessions of "cheating," frustrations about weight not lost, stories of foods not tolerated, and expressions of anger, happiness, sadness, disappointment, excitement, anxiety, laughter, and even tears (sound familiar, Julie?).

You name it, I've heard it! At times I've even thought of asking the patient if perhaps their appointment was supposed to be with the behaviorist not the dietitian. But, with all of that said, I wouldn't trade what I do for anything, because helping people through those times, good, bad, or as ugly as they might be, is incredibly rewarding for me. Although I work pretty hard, I only wish I could work harder and do more for my patients.

Since it would be illegal, and let's face it, a little scary, to have myself cloned so that I could be a shadow to each of my patients as they leave my office, (more than one of me? Yikes!…), the next best thing I can do is educate them. So given the fact that they haven't yet invented the home cloning kit, let's begin by learning a little bit about the practical side of nutrition.

We'll start with nutrients. A person's daily nutrient requirements should be met through the foods they eat whenever possible. Nutrients are categorized into two different groups: macronutrients and micronutrients. Macronutrients include carbohydrates, protein, fat, and water. Micronutrients include vitamins and minerals. First, I'll chat a bit about the micronutrients, and get them out of the way.

Micronutrients

Micronutrients consist of vitamins and minerals. Vitamins and minerals, (as pure substances, not as commercial products), do not contain any calories, and are ideally obtained through the foods we eat. Supplementation is necessary for bariatric patients, (including Lap-Band® patients!), because of the malabsorptive and/or restrictive components of the surgery. Dr. Baker has talked quite a bit about the necessity of vitamin supplements in Chapter Three, so I hope you've taken that information to heart.

So, let's think about the word *supplement* and what it means; it means *to add to,* not replace. Supplements add to the diet, *they do not replace foods,* mainly because they do not contain the macronutrients our bodies need. I'll explain that in a minute. Additionally, folic acid, vitamin B1, B12, iron, D3, and calcium aren't absorbed as well following gastric bypass surgery because of the malabsorptive component, and because patients are limited in the amount of food they can eat. Many necessary micronutrients are not being absorbed in quantities adequate for the body's needs, and, therefore, supplementation is recommended pre and post-operatively to ensure patients get their requisite nutrients. In short: take your Building Blocks® bariatric vitamins! They have even formulated a special vitamin regimen specifically for Lap-Band® patients' needs, so no excuses!!!

Patients not only develop vitamin deficiencies after surgery, but a good number of patients actually come in the door with nutritional deficiencies as well. In fact, a significant portion of the western world, even those who aren't overweight or obese, are suffering from various nutritional deficiencies simply because of our processed foods, our lifestyle, and sometimes where we live and our accessibility to particular types of foods. Even dietitians!! So, by learning about your possible deficiencies you're not really adding in a new medical condition, you're just finally treating one you already had and preventing it from getting worse.

It is becoming an industry standard today for bariatric practices to perform pre-operative nutritional testing. If your surgeon's office doesn't want to draw blood to test for nutritional status then perhaps you should suggest such an evaluation, or maybe find a new surgeon's office. It is extremely helpful for the dietitian to know whether you are chronically low in iron, have a zinc deficiency, or have low potassium levels. Incidentally, many practices do complete blood counts (CBC) tests, but may not get an accurate iron level for you from this test. Instead they should be doing the newer, more accurate *serum ferritin* test which reveals the amount of iron blood cells have stored. This will give a better evaluation of iron levels or deficiencies in your system both before and after surgery.

By testing both pre-operatively and post-operatively the dietitian and physician can help you to maintain maximum weight loss potential by keeping all the body's systems supplied with the fuel they need to work effectively and efficiently. So get tested regularly, eat healthy, take those vitamins, and have a look at the nutrition related charts in the resources section of this book. Hopefully nutritional deficiencies will not be a major part of your health and future!

Two of the nutrient deficiencies in those charts we would like to warn you about are the B1/thiamine deficiency, and various deficiencies that can result in a condition called Pica (Pie-ka). First off it is imperative that you get enough of the B1 vitamin in your system after surgery. Most people do not get enough from their food sources so you must take a bariatric vitamin that contains appropriate amounts of B1/thiamine. Thiamine deficiencies can cause fatigue, confusion, loss of short-term memory, cardiovascular disease, loss of sensation in hands and feet, nerve damage, brain damage, and even death. Also, drinking heavy amounts of alcohol severely depletes thiamine stores and interferes with thiamine efficiency. Don't play with this issue when all you have to do is pop a couple of bariatric vitamins in your mouth every day. It's much easier than steering a wheelchair around or living on a respirator every day.

The second condition is called Pica and it can be caused by a number of nutritional deficiencies, but the most common is an iron deficiency. Iron deficiency Pica is most often manifested in bariatric surgery patients by a compulsion to eat ice. Again, very easily treated by simply taking the iron recommended by your surgeon or dietitian. Other forms of Pica also exist that manifest themselves in strange compulsions to eat even stranger things like dirt, hair, and newspaper. In fact, the best Pica story we ever heard was when our dear friend Dr. Steven Hendrick of Henry Ford Hospital Wayndotte Campus floored us by reporting that a particular patient of his developed a compulsion to eat a whole roll of toilet paper every day!!! Those types of Pica may require a little more involved treatment, but if you find yourself wanting to chew on ice, contact your surgeon's office and ask for a serum ferritin test, and remember *not* to take your iron and your calcium within an hour and a half of each other.

Well, that's about it for micronutrients, so on to macronutrients.

Macronutrients

This is the stuff we generally call "food," including protein, water, fat, and carbohydrates. We'll tackle these in reverse order, starting with carbs.

Carbohydrates

Carbohydrates are the main energy source for our bodies, and they contain approximately 4 calories per gram. Once eaten, carbohydrates turn into glucose, which is our body's form of sugar. Eating too many carbohydrates causes excess glucose in the body, which is stored in the liver or muscles, and converted to fat. From there it is stored as nasty body fat that causes us to hate the fat, but amazingly, not the carbohydrates.

So…do carbohydrates make us fat? If eaten in excess, yes. Are carbohydrates bad? No. Repeat after me, CARBOHYDRATES ARE NOT BAD! Anything consumed in excess is not good, whether carbohydrates, cheesecake, or too much Chardonnay on a Saturday night. Too much is just not good. M-O-D-E-R-A-T-I-O-N is the key. Easier said than done, but true nonetheless. You need to eat at a minimum 50g of carbs a day, and no less. I hope all of the low-carbohydrate dieters, and carbohydrate Nazis have heard me loud and clear. I proudly proclaim: "I eat carbs!"

I like to look at foods not as good or bad, but as some being better for you than others. The better carbohydrates to choose are the complex carbohydrates, which include fruits, whole grains, legumes, and vegetables. Complex carbohydrates provide us with vitamins, minerals, fiber, and of course energy.

Fiber, incidentally, is a wondrous thing. Fiber helps to keep us fuller longer, it can lower cholesterol, keep us regular, and since our bodies have to work harder to digest it, it can also increase our metabolism. Because of this slower digestion process, carbohydrates are turned into glucose less quickly. So, what I like to tell my patients is to eat everything in its most natural state, or "closer to God and nature" as my dear dietitian friend and mentor, Bunee' Morrison likes to say.

High fiber foods sometimes "talk behind your back" as one of my patients refers to it, so proceed with caution when adding these foods back into the diet. Gas, bloating, and cramping can occur if too much fiber is consumed. On the other hand, fiber might be just what the dietitian ordered for that common constipation problem that can occur after surgery. It'll make your body do the work it is supposed to do.

Also, make your body do the work of processing the foods, rather than buying foods such as white bread, white rice, or white pasta, where the processing has already been done. These processed, refined carbohydrates turn into sugar faster in our bodies, making us hungry sooner, and they offer little nutritional value. Instead, choose whole-wheat bread, whole-wheat pasta, brown or wild rice, dried beans, fresh fruits, and vegetables.

It can often be difficult for post-surgery patients to consume carbohydrates. Many of the carbohydrate containing foods, *i.e.*, breads, rice, and noodles, are often hard for patients to tolerate. They can swell up, and become gummy if not processed, prepared, or cooked well. Patients complain that they sit heavy, and often there isn't room for them after eating the protein first.

In contrast, however, be aware that other carbohydrate containing foods, such as crackers, chips, corn chips, and the like seem to go down just fine for most patients that I see. These foods are crunchy, and can be chewed to a very fine consistency with no problem. Unfortunately, they are usually of low nutritive value, so limit your intake of these foods. That brings us now to simple carbs.

Sweets are considered simple carbohydrates. Foods such as fruit, milk, and yogurt contain natural sugars, and are good for you. Cakes, candies, cookies, and ice cream are processed sugars that are high in calories, and usually fat. They are not good for you. In addition, sweets can sometimes cause *dumping syndrome* after surgery.

Do not in any way, however, count on sugar or dumping syndrome as your sweet tooth cure, because some patients are able to tolerate sweets after surgery. On the other hand, some patients completely lose their desire for sweets of any kind. Most patients that I see can tolerate a small amount (meaning one cookie, not three), on occasion. Those that push the envelope usually end up on "auto eject," and running for the restroom.

Avoiding sweets all together would be best, although maybe not realistic. Keep in mind that sugar-free does not mean calorie-free, and some sugar-free foods contain sugar alcohols, a derivative of sugar that when eaten in excess can cause gas, bloating, and diarrhea. Sugars can easily be identified in the ingredient list by words ending in "ose" — glucose, sucrose, dextrose, lactose. Sugar alcohols can easily be identified by words ending in "tol" — sorbitol, malitol, xylitol. Sugar alcohols can cause serious gas and flatulence issues along with diarrhea if too much is ingested. Other sugars, especially processed sugars can just cause dumping. So, even though we want you to get lots of exercise, running to the bathroom is not what we had in mind, and I'm sure not what you had in mind either. Well, that's about all for carbs, so on to fat.

Fat

Fat offers 9 calories per gram. The word "fat" has a negative connotation to it, some of which is warranted, but let's not forget that it is an important nutrient that our bodies require. Fat is a source of energy, it's our body's insulation, it regulates hormones, it aids in the production of prostaglandins that protect the lining of the pouch and the intestines, and it protects our other organs from injury. Fat aids in the absorption of certain vitamins such as vitamins A, D, E, and K. It adds flavor and texture to foods, and since it is the last to be digested, it keeps us fuller, longer.

Too much fat obviously makes us fat, and it can lead to heart disease; and that brings us back to that word "moderation" again. The amount of fat a person should have in their diet varies depending upon age, gender, height, and weight. For successful weight loss, bariatric patients should typically try to limit their overall fat intake to less than 30g of fat per day.

The majority of fat in the diet should come from monounsaturated fat sources. These foods are generally liquid at room temperature, and come from plant or vegetable origins such as olive or canola oil, avocados, natural peanut butter, nuts, and olives. The monounsaturated fats help to lower our bad cholesterol (LDL cholesterol), and raise our good cholesterol (HDL cholesterol). This good cholesterol helps to clean out the bad cholesterol in our bodies, so having a higher HDL level is important.

Another type of fat, polyunsaturated fat also comes from plant or vegetable origins such as safflower or sunflower oil, and some seeds and nuts. Though these foods help to lower overall cholesterol, they do tend to lower the HDL cholesterol as well. Eating less polyunsaturated fat, and more monounsaturated fat is advised.

Polyunsaturated Omega-3 fats, however, are considered good fats. These are found in deep ocean fish, such as salmon and tuna, as well as nuts, flaxseed, and flaxseed oil. These fats are often referred to as "brain fats." They help to lower triglycerides, prevent stroke, and in some studies have been shown to help with depression.

The bad guys, or saturated fats, are generally solid at room temperature, and come from animal sources such as bacon, butter, lard, ice cream, 2% and whole milk, regular cheese, and regular sour cream. Saturated fats raise our cholesterol, and clog our arteries putting us at risk for heart disease.

Our bodies need almost no saturated fats, so limit the intake of these foods. Unless you are under the age of two, in need of gaining weight, or are a baby cow, there is no need to be drinking 2% or whole milk. Instead, choose 1%, ½%, skim, or soymilk. Choose low fat cheeses, and low fat sour cream instead of the regular, full fat versions to help limit your saturated fat intake.

Worse than saturated fats, however, are hydrogenated fats or trans fats. Once a "hidden" fat found in foods such as crackers and many low fat snacks and sweets, trans fats are now being listed on the nutrition facts food labels. And thank goodness, as hydrogenated or trans fats are pesky little fat-makers.

Hydrogenation is a chemical process in which foods are made more solid (like saturated fats), giving them the texture and taste many people like. Hydrogenation also aids in food preservation, allowing foods to sit on the shelf for as long as year. So, again, I will remind you to eat foods in their most natural state, not a chemically made state. If the ingredient list is as long as this chapter, it cannot be good for you.

In addition to processed foods, the bariatric patient should avoid fatty, greasy, and fried foods. Though I like a french fry as much as the next person (especially if it has cheese all over it), fried foods eaten in excess make all of us gain weight. Because fat stays in our stomachs the longest, and is the last to be digested, it can cause acid reflux, and nobody likes that.

Cramping, bloating, and diarrhea, or dumping syndrome can also occur if the patient consumes these types of foods. I've had patients who removed the breading from fried fish before eating it, and still became ill from the grease that had seeped through to the meat of the fish. So, be careful, and ask yourself: will those foods help me to lose weight? No. So why eat them? Have a glass of water instead.

Water

Ahh, water. Can anything be more natural? How fabulous can it be? It has no calories, suppresses the appetite, hydrates us, helps to breakdown fat, relieves fluid retention, helps maintain muscle tone, flushes waste and toxins out of our bodies, and helps keep us regular. What more do you need?

Bariatric patients should consume a minimum of 64 oz. of non-carbonated, non-sugared, caffeine-free fluids per day. Water is the best choice. If you don't recall why it's the best choice re-read the previous paragraph. If patients don't want to consume all 64 oz. as water, they should absolutely consume at least half, or 32 oz. as water. An avid water drinker myself (at least 64 oz. per day), I highly recommend and encourage my patients to drink all 64 oz. as water.

Patients should avoid drinking with their meals following surgery, as this can cause nausea and vomiting. Not only does it cause nausea and vomiting, it washes food out of the pouch twice as fast. Patients then lose some of the protein they ate, and they become hungry sooner. If patients do not avoid drinking with their meals, or do not wait to drink for an extended period of time after meals, they increase their chances for weight gain after surgery. That's a scary thought.

More water is also needed if patients are suffering from vomiting, diarrhea, and/or constipation. If you're experiencing one of these things, sucking down a glass of water is generally not the first thing on your mind, but it will help. Vomiting and diarrhea deplete the body's supply of water, and constipation is caused in part by a lack of it. Hydrating the body helps all the way around.

It is imperative that patients keep themselves hydrated before and after surgery, and avoiding caffeine is one way to do that. Because caffeine is a diuretic it can dehydrate us, which, hello! is the exact opposite of what we want! Caffeine is also a gastric stimulant and can make us hungrier — just what you want when you are trying to lose weight, right? Wrong! Caffeine, along with some acids (like those in soda pop), also leach calcium from our bones, which can cause osteoporosis down the road. When you consider that calcium is not absorbed as efficiently after weight loss surgery, don't add insult to injury by consuming caffeine or soda pop. Skip the caffeine and take your calcium citrate supplements.

Speaking of pop, carbonation can be painful and bloat patients after surgery. If you have stopped drinking caffeine and carbonated beverages before surgery, by all means do not return to consuming them after surgery.

Our society drinks way too much pop as it is. This includes all kinds of pop, including the clear ones. The acid in pop is just barely below lethal. With every mouthful, it so drastically alters the pH level of your body that your body then has to cough up some hard mineral to balance it out again in order to keep you breathing. The first thing it coughs up is calcium (which you are having a hard time getting enough of to begin with!), and it gets it directly from your bones.

Don't believe me? Do some research on the web. Many physicians have written about the dangers of soda pop. There is nothing good for you in pop, unless of course you think all those chemicals in pop are preserving you somehow for the next century! Chemicals and sugar are the least of your worries. In fact, if you're a weight loss surgery patient, the carbonation will probably get you before anything else will. I refer you again to Julie and Karen's treatise on air bubbles in Chapter Four.

Soda pop causes dehydration, and another thing that can cause dehydration after surgery is alcohol. I will again say that if you did not consume alcohol prior to surgery, please do not start after. Alcohol provides 7 "empty" calories per gram. They're empty because there is no nutritional value to alcohol, and for bariatric surgery patients it causes other problems as well.

After surgery alcohol passes through the new pouch directly into the second portion of the small intestine, known as the jejunum. The jejunum has a large surface area that readily and rapidly absorbs the alcohol, making patients "cheap drunks" after surgery. I believe Julie has already related to you her experience with alcohol. If I had a nickel for every time I heard one of those stories…. As you can see, bottled, or even tap water is the way to go. So drink up, and drink plenty!

Protein

The last macronutrient that I want to talk about is protein. The reason I saved protein for last is because it is probably the most important nutrient that the bariatric patient can consume. In its purest form protein provides 4 calories per gram, and it is the basic structural material of all cells. From the protein we eat the body synthesizes hormones, structural molecules, enzymes, immune system components, helps regulate fluid and acid-base balance in the body, and much more. It helps to build and repair new tissues, aids in wound healing, provides satiety, prevents hair loss, and it preserves muscle tissue. Protein gives red blood cells their structure, and it helps antibodies function properly. It also helps in the regulation of enzymes and hormones.

Protein chains are created through a combination of amino acids, most of which we should be getting from our food sources. Amino acids are the building blocks of protein, and basically they are either "essential," or "non-essential." Our body makes the non-essential amino acids we need, but the essential amino acids must come from the foods we eat.

Essential amino acids found in the proteins we eat are either "complete," or "incomplete." The complete proteins, also known as "high biological value" proteins, come primarily from animal sources, and they contain all 9 essential amino acids that our bodies need. Cheese, meat, eggs, milk, yogurt, and soy are examples of these. Eggs, incidentally, especially egg whites, are considered the standard against which all other proteins are measured because it has an amino acid pattern that is highly compatible with human nutritional needs.

Incomplete proteins, such as beans, grains, nuts, and vegetables, lack one or more of the essential amino acids. Therefore, two incomplete proteins, or an incomplete and complete protein must be combined to make the protein more useful to the body. An example would be beans and rice. Together they make a complete protein, but they don't necessarily have to be eaten at the same meal. Overall, foods with higher proportions of essential amino acids are generally better for your health. That basically means protein sources that are meat and dairy rather than plant based, but it doesn't mean you should leave out the plant based foods as we are aiming for a balanced diet here and they often offer other benefits as well such as fiber and other nutrients.

For bariatric patients, protein is emphasized right from the start. Approximately 2 weeks prior to surgery patients are put on a high protein diet, which should not be confused with some of those popular high protein, low carbohydrate, high fat diets out there. Having been vegetarian for nearly 13 years now, I'm certainly not an advocate of the Atkins® diet, and in fact, would love to de-Atkinize most of the world. But, I will jump off my anti-Atkins® soapbox and move on.…

Patients are generally placed on a high protein *fast* prior to surgery. *Fast*, meaning patients are starved before surgery? Heavens no. Though the term *fast* does mean to abstain from food, we do not starve patients. Patients may feel as though they are starving, considering what most were eating prior to the fast, but they do survive (is that Gloria Gaynor I hear??). What we are aiming for is to nutritionally prepare the patient for surgery as Dr. Baker stated in Chapter Three.

Patients are generally placed on a two week supplemented fast prior to surgery, during which they consume specially formulated, high protein products that contain little sugar or fat, and are low in calories. The protein fast is approximately 800 calories per day, and anywhere from 75-150g of protein per day. I've had patients tell me that some of the medical protein products they've taken in other physician's offices taste like something you'd eat on Fear Factor®. We use Bariatrix' SmartForme products that taste really good, offer a huge product line, and the vast majority of people can handle it. I suggest checking with the dietitian in your surgeon's office for more information on the products they use, what they taste like, and the related nutritional values. If they don't use SmartForme have them check into it for you.

Incidentally, protein supplements are not all the same. There are lots of protein drinks out there that originate from many sources including soy, milk, whey, and collagen. They also like to use words like *isolate, concentrates,* and *hydrolized.* These are manufacturing and processing terms. The term *isolate* generally refers to a filtering process used with milk and whey solids that removes the fat, lactose (milk sugar), and minerals from the base material to give it better mixability and taste, and get more protein in a smaller serving size. The isolates are very low in lactose, and most lactose intolerant people can generally tolerate them just fine, but do not assume that they are lactose-free unless the packaging states as much. Of all of the protein sources *casein* has the lowest lactose content. For soy and other vegetable proteins, isolates tend to remove much of the carb content which can also reduce the gasiness that can accompany them when they are in their vegetable state. Finally, hydrolized proteins are sort of somewhat pre-digested meaning that they are already broken into smaller protein bits so it may make digestion easier if other protein forms are not tolerated well. Bariatrix' SmartForme products are casein isolate based (from Ireland, the best quality casein in the world), although the spaghetti and the chili use high quality protein concentrates. The flavors are amazing because patients from all over the world help them develop the products. So, hopefully you will survive your fast and your post-surgical first phase protocol very well with the huge variety of drinks, soups, meals, bars, puddings, gelatins, snacks, and other offerings from Bariatrix' SmartForme line.

After surgery, the first phase protocol for patients is generally a liquid protein diet for anywhere from 2-4 weeks, and Julie and Karen have told you a little bit about that. The next step is transitioning to soft foods, such as low fat cottage cheese, cream soups made with skim milk, sugar-free pudding, soft eggs, deli meats, and low fat cheeses, supplemented as necessary with the protein products.

Patients look forward to seeing the dietitian on this day. In fact, this is usually the day that I love my job most. I'm no longer the food police. I'm no longer that "thin, mean, food lady." I am the patient's best friend. I've even had patients profess their love for me at this visit!

As you can tell, patients are usually more than ready to transition at this point. Some have even tried to eat the fake food models on my desk! And, Julie's right, they are pathetic! I've had patients tell me that their cat was even starting to look good to them! Poor Kitty! But, as you read in Chapter Six, and will read about in a different context in a following chapter, getting enough protein in after surgery can be somewhat of a challenge for patients.

One reason for this is that patients generally do not feel hungry again until about 6 months after surgery. Therefore, patients often have to force themselves to eat after surgery, which is a concept hard to imagine for most people. I tell my patients to think of eating their protein like medicine, you have to get it in if you want to heal, if you like your hair, if you want to preserve your muscles, and if you want to have optimal weight loss. So, unless you want to be bald, skinny, flabby, and have a lot of atrophy, I suggest getting the protein in whatever way you can!

Another reason it can be challenging to get in the necessary protein after surgery is the size of the new stomach, or "pouch." It is approximately 1-2 oz. after surgery. Not a lot of room. So, patients have to eat small meals three times a day in order to get in all of their protein. Ideally, we'd like to see 80 or more grams of protein a day for patients, but it's often difficult for them to get in the minimum of 60 that we recommend. The generally recognized formula for protein intake is 1.5g of protein for every kg of *ideal* body weight in order to maintain nitrogen balance in the body. Your dietitian can figure out this protein level for you if you're curious or don't want to do the math.

After patients have been on the soft protein choices for a few weeks, they then gradually advance to more solid foods such as meats, fruit, grains, and (sparingly) nuts. Because of their "roughage," raw veggies and salads are last to be added back to the diet. Patients who follow the lists given to them, do not transition themselves early to foods, follow the rules of the pouch tool, and get some form of exercise, will be the most successful. Until you start memorizing those protein values for various foods (and you will…), here's a quick little way to remember about how much protein is in what you're eating. It's called the 5-10-15-25 rule:

- 5g protein for each egg or handful of nuts or seeds
- 10g protein for a cup of milk or yogurt
- 15g protein for a measured cup of beans, cup of cottage cheese, or 3 oz. of tofu
- 25g protein for a 3-4 oz. serving of meat, chicken, or fish

Now, these aren't exact of course, as milk has 1g of protein per oz., so it really comes out to about 8g not 10g, but then this is why you learn to read labels and remember protein values. The 5-10-15-25 rule may help when you can't read a label though, like when you're at someone else's house for dinner, or at a restaurant. At least you'll have a handle on approximately how much protein you're getting into you, so you know where you stand for the day and whether you'll need a supplement or not.

Living on protein drinks and protein products after surgery is not recommended if patients are able to eat regular foods. When hunger returns you want to fill the pouch with good quality, solid foods so that you stay full for as long as you can. Protein drinks, or any liquids with calories such as milk, juice, and thin soups go through the pouch twice as fast, slowing weight loss, and in some cases, causing weight gain. Protein supplements should only be used in cases where patients are having a difficult time getting all of their protein in natural sources. They are supplements!

Protein bars, which are more solid than protein drinks, are an acceptable snack after surgery. Beware though, that many of the protein bars on the market are practically glorified candy bars. Look for protein bars that are 200 calories or less, contain less than 10g of fat, and at a minimum 10g of protein per serving. Too much sugar means it tastes yummy, but you might end up in the bathroom in auto eject mode. Bariatrix' SmartForme products have 6 great tasting nutritionally responsible bars that are properly portioned and have 15g of protein. Give them a try instead.

The most common dietary complications seen after surgery are nausea and vomiting. If patients eat too fast, if they drink while they eat, if they don't chew their food well enough, or if they eat more than their pouch can comfortably hold, they can get sick. The surgical *tool* is designed to restrict the amount of food a patient can eat. Old habits die hard, however, and just about every patient gets sick at least once.

In fact, I've heard more than I ever cared to about patients vomiting. I've heard about dry heaves. I've heard about the gagging. I've heard about the color, the consistency, and the texture of their vomit. I've even heard about a patient getting sick outside, and the dog eating it! Ewwww!!!! Heck, I've even had a patient vomit in my office! It comes with the territory, and at this point, nothing phases me.

My point is, many patients learn the hard way. And, if you were a fast eater prior to surgery, you will likely be one of those that learn the hard way because you just have to slow down. Food should be chewed 25-40 times before swallowing, and patients should take 30-45 minutes to eat each of their meals. If not, your dog could be in for something he didn't count on for dinner....

While we are on the subject, let's talk about pets for a minute. Because patients cannot eat the quantities they used to, I'm told by many of my patients that their pets are being fattened up with what is left on the plates, otherwise they are cooking for two: themselves and the garbage disposal. Being the animal lover that I am, I cringe at all these scraps being given to pets, and can't help but envision gastric bypass for animals in the near future.

Please don't feed all your extra food to your pets. Learn to cook smaller portions, or get some plastic food saver tubs. You know how bad you feel physically as an overweight person? They can get all the same aches, pains, and related health conditions you can, only they can't choose to lose the weight. For all those overweight pets out there, I just hope their owners are becoming more active, and taking them on more walks....

Well, I hope you have learned a little about weight loss surgery and nutrition after reading this, and that you don't feed the junk you shouldn't eat to your pet. Keep in mind that surgery is not a miracle cure, and you have to truly be ready to change your old behaviors into new behaviors.

The surgeon will do her job, the behaviorist will do his or her job, and the dietitian will do his job, but unless you do your part, the surgery will only be another failed weight loss attempt. We are here to help you, and to give you the tools you need to be successful; it's up to you to use these tools to their maximum potential. We know you can. You're worth it.

Now I'll hand you over to Scott who's going to make you get up and walk around while you read this part of the chapter.

THE FUNCTIONAL LIVING ENVIRONMENT

Movement

Hello. It's Scott Glass again. You're friendly neighborhood behaviorist/exercise physiologist from Chapter Seven, remember? Good. Nice to see you again too. Now, we've let you avoid it as long as we can, but I promise I'll make this information as painless as possible. If you would rather clean your bathroom than exercise, you are not alone. I'm hoping to change your mindset on that. I'll bet I can, so take a deep breath and stay with me.

For many overweight people, exercise represents more aches and pains, more discouragement, more discomfort, more awkwardness, more social rejection, and more self-loathing. Who in their right mind would go out of their way for more pain? I hope that by the time you get to the end of this chapter, your attitude toward exercise will shift, even just a little. So forge ahead and keep an open mind. I believe you will find that exercise, or "movement" is not as bad as you think, and yes, you can do it.

As patients with serious weight issues, we know that your excess weight results in muscle soreness and joint pain. We know you become short of breath quickly. We understand that you are not in good physical condition. We empathize with your discouragement and hopelessness from failed exercise attempts in the past, so we are not asking you to do very much. Are you doing okay so far? Read on, it gets better!

There are three dimensions, if you will, that exercise physiologists consider when writing or evaluating an exercise plan. It helps to use an acronym, F.I.T. (Hey, at least it's not F.A.T.)

"F" is for frequency, or the number of times you do an activity in a given week. Do you walk several days a week? Ride the bike 3 days a week? Go get the mail everyday?

"I" is for intensity, or how hard you push yourself while doing that activity. With walking, the intensity would be your walking speed. With stationary bicycle riding, the intensity is your pedaling speed and the tension at which you have your bicycle set. With weight training, the intensity is the amount of weight you are lifting.

"T" is for time. How long, or how many minutes you do that activity each session constitutes your time interval.

If you have not had weight loss surgery yet, the most important dimension for you is frequency. Neither intensity, nor length of time is important for you right now. Although your mind may tell you to push yourself harder or longer, your body cannot handle that kind of physical stress at this point. That is what the surgery is for: to help you lose the excess body weight resulting in less stress on your muscles and joints, so you will not be so quickly short of breath, and so that you will be able to enjoy more strenuous activity. The most important goal for you at this point is for you to get into a pattern of daily activity.

Developing a healthy habit and changing your style of living requires repetition — doing it over and over, repeatedly and consistently. Remember, it doesn't have to be a lot. Just do some form of physical activity, or movement, over and above your normal daily activity in oxygen, a minimum of 4 days per week. If you can do it 5 or 6 days a week, that would be even better. Setting your goal at 7 days per week is probably unrealistic, and may result in frustration, more discouragement, and ultimately fizzling out. Don't worry yet about how long you have to do this "onerous" thing, I'll get to that in just a minute.

Thirty minutes of aerobic exercise is the medical recommendation for healthy living. Starting at 30 minutes, however, is not realistic for many people. Many patients have difficulty walking from one bench to the next bench in the mall, and are unable to walk for 5 minutes, let alone 30 minutes! These people see one half hour of continuous walking as out of reach. It seems like too much. It's just not something they're able to do, and once again, they are defeated before they start.

Instead, wouldn't it be a lot easier to simply start where you already are? The main reason people fizzle out on their exercise program is most often due to starting out far too fast. After their first walk or work out, they drag themselves into their easy chair and lament, "You've got to be kidding?! Do I need to do this again tomorrow?" This person is already defeated in their attitude after their first day of moving.

Contrast this with another scenario. You go for a short, leisurely walk, and you stop when you get short of breath or your knees start to ache. You have a little pep in your step, and you feel good that you did it. You say to yourself, "That wasn't too bad. I can do this again tomorrow!"

The best and safest way to start is slow and easy. Don't push it. If you were training for a competition of some sort, a beauty contest or an athletic event, you would really need to push yourself to be ready to go by a certain date. But, we are not in any contest. Weight management is not a competition. There is no end date. There's no deadline. Weight management is a process; it is a style of living.

As you improve your style of living, the weight will come off, and as you maintain your new, healthier style of living, you will maintain your weight loss. So there is no hurry here. It is a life-long process. Get rid of all those old notions, and listen to what I'm telling you now. To quote Hans and Franz from that Saturday night show, "hear me now, and believe me later! We're here to pump (clap!) you up!"

Eating less and exercising more until you reached your goal weight, was the old mindset of dieting that we are trying to get away from. It doesn't work, right? You end up gaining all the weight back and then some. Just start with small changes, one at a time. These should be changes that are small enough to make you feel confident, and to help you be consistent for the long-term.

Begin with any physical activity that will get your heart rate up a little and do it only as long as you are comfortable. If you decide to begin walking, and you get short of breath after 15 minutes of leisurely walking, STOP. Call it good. Do not push yourself.

You will be thinking that you should really walk further than this. You will be thinking that you could do so much more when you were younger, but that was the past, and many pounds ago. Don't allow guilt or shame to make you do more than you are able. Do what you can, and the rest will follow.

A little bit each day is the key. I would rather have a person walk for 5 minutes, 5 days per week, than have them walk one half hour once on the weekend. Even though this works out to 25 minutes compared with 30 minutes, it is the repetition that will prove to be most effective in the long run.

Give it 2, 3, or even 4 weeks to get comfortable, and then bump up your time a little bit. Don't feel compelled to increase your time by 10, or even 5 minutes. If you feel comfortable with a 2 or 3 minute increase every other week, that would be fantastic! Remember, you are not in a race, and there is no pressure. You have the rest of your life to get your movement program where you want it. This is about life style.

There are many who will read this chapter who cannot walk for 2 minutes due to severe muscle weakness, severe joint pain, or excessive weight. Just do what you can. We're behind you, and we understand. I had a patient who was nearly 700 lbs., and he spent most of the day in bed. Getting out of bed was too much for him. He still had a positive attitude though, evidenced by the fact that he did leg lifts, and arm exercises in bed. We're okay with that. It's a start, and it's what he could do, and do consistently.

Many patients will start by standing up at each television commercial, walking to the kitchen, getting a drink of water, and sitting back down again. Some will simply walk in place when commercials come on. You don't have to lift your feet high, just move.

Another woman was walking the length of her 10 ft. hallway in her one-bedroom efficiency apartment 4 times a day, over and above her normal daily activity. Don't do more than you should, but don't do less than you can either. As you lose weight and become more fit, you can do more, and you should. Worry about it when that time gets here.

Getting more physical activity is as much an attitude, as it is an activity. Do you like the direction your weight and health are going right now? If you picked up this book, probably not. Are there important things you are missing out on due to your weight? If so, then there are no alternatives. You must get up and move.

One lady stands in her kitchen leaning on the counter with stiff arms so the counter bears much of her weight, and does leg swings to the side and to the back. It's not a lot, but she has started! She is doing a little bit every day, and SO CAN YOU!

When you begin moving, and you don't set yourself up for failure by expecting to do more than your reasonably can, you will develop a better attitude about yourself, and see yourself as more in control of the situation. You will feel less like a victim. Exercise and movement have a very positive effect on attitude, self-esteem, self-worth, and overall emotional health. Everyone on the planet can benefit from movement of some sort.

Yes, everyone! Even those who have physical disabilities. There are many exercise physiologists and physical therapists who specialize in patients with disabilities. Julie had disabilities from her car accident. She had a terrible time just walking to get from one place to another, let alone walking for exercise. We sat down with her, and we found various "movements" she could do as she lost weight, and became physically stronger. Now she's walking all over the place, and we can't keep up with her! We've created a monster!

Don't worry if you have physical limitations. We understand that. We can work with it, or around it. The important thing to know is that you can do it, and it doesn't have to be painful or onerous. As you lose the weight, your body will react differently, and your weight loss surgeon's office will have an exercise physiologist there to make sure that your movement program is keeping up with your new capabilities. It shouldn't be designed to push you, but it should be designed to determine what you are capable of doing, and therefore should be doing. Don't resist the change. Call it "progress."

Movement doesn't have to be boring either. You'll be shocked at what fun things we can come up with, and still call it exercise! Virtually any movement has some benefit to it. So, if you can add a few more sustained movements in every day, you're well on your way to creating a better and healthier life. Just don't forget to rest.

Rest is very important, and incidentally plays a vital role in weight gain and loss. The body needs to revitalize itself as much as it needs to move. That's how we are designed, and since we really can't do too much about redesigning our genetic blueprint, we just have to go with that. So move when you can and how you can, drink plenty of water, and get your sleep. That's my professional recommendation. So let's get started!

To help you remember all of the good stuff in this chapter that you need to use on a daily basis, memorize this one little word: LEARN.

L - Lifestyle

E - Exercise (movement!)

A - Attitude (choose a positive one)

R - Relationship (to food and to others)

N - Nutrition

No one else has the ability to get you up and moving, to choose healthy foods for you, to adopt a positive attitude, to create healthy relationships with food and with people in your life, or to change your lifestyle for good. So, what are you going to do? You must take responsibility and ownership for your condition. You can begin to change the direction things have been going. You can do it! It is not too late! You are valuable! You are significant and important! You are loved! You are worth it!

Whether or not you decide to have weight loss surgery, please take the first step, no matter how small, toward a healthier life. Remember: every wondrous journey begins with just one step. Stand up and take yours.

Avoiding the phrase
"I don't have time...!,"
will soon help you to realize
that you do have the time needed
for just about anything you choose
to accomplish in life.

BO BENNETT

Chapter Twelve

MEDICATION
➤ MISADVENTURES: ➤
HOW TO AVOID THEM!!

Nabila Ahmed-Sarwar, PharmD, BCPS, CDE
Assistant Professor of Clinical Pharmacy, Ferris State University

By now you've heard about the possible complications and after-effects, but one thing you may not have thought about, (and to be honest about it neither did I until I met Julie and Karen) is how your totally re-arranged gastrointestinal tract is going to affect the medications you may need to take. Well, this chapter is going to discuss some of the discoveries we have made through the hundreds of questions that have come my way, and no, they are not all from Julie and Karen.

I'm going to share a little secret with you. After countless hours of research to answer the questions from patients, nurses, dietitians, primary care physicians, bariatric surgeons, and my own colleagues and pharmacists, I've come to realize that there is a significant deficiency in the research in this area. A great deal of the information was gathered from going back to the basics of pharmacy education and applying what we know about nutrient absorption to formulate some general guidelines.

Hence, before I go on, Julie is going to interrupt for a moment to give you the legal disclaimer for the information in this chapter:

All disclaimers and legal notices previously mentioned, stated, or reported at the commencement or anywhere else in this or previous editions of this book, do hereby apply, attach, and are incorporated by reference, for the purposes of this chapter, its information, opinions, suppositions, jokes, lame attempts at humor, potentially boring stories, science lessons, and all other data and text, Signed: The Legal Staff.

Okay, now that the lawyers' needs have been met, let's hope that what you'll discover in this chapter will help you avoid having your own personal "medication misadventures."

I want you to take a moment and think about the last commercial you saw on TV for a medication. Do you recall the disclaimer they run towards the end, the one that the announcer whips through really fast so he/she sounds like a used car dealer? It kind of goes like this:

"This medication may cause some common side-effects including; headache, sedation, confusion, itching, insomnia, lethargy, blurred vision, nausea, vomiting, stomach pain, cold or flu like symptoms, diarrhea, gas, urinary retention, muscle weakness, irritability. Serious side-effects can include kidney and liver failure, unusual bleeding, irregular heart beats, stroke, and seizures. Use this medication only under the direct care of a physician, if your symptoms do not improve, or get worse contact your doctor immediately. Make sure your doctor knows if you are pregnant, may become pregnant, or are breast feeding."

Now, you must be wondering where I'm going with this. I'm sure one day after you've had your surgery, or if you've already had surgery, you may find yourself wondering why 9 out of 10 times one of those side effects they rattle off at the end of the commercial always seems to happen to you. Hmmmmmm......

Maybe it's worse than that though. You may come to discover that all of a sudden the allergy medication you used to take for years is just not working any more, or the Tylenol® you used to take for aches and pains now makes you feel like you can't keep your head off the desk, the pillow, or the kitchen counter. Maybe you're trying to figure out who decided to name you as the poster child for medication side-effects because you seem to have gone from no side-effects before surgery, to just about all of them after! Well, stay tuned to this chapter for more info on that.

Now before we get to explaining the increased potential for side-effects thingy, we can't forget about "medication separation anxiety" either. Out of nowhere your physician may instruct you to stop taking the diabetes and blood pressure medications you've taken for the past ten years. The reality is that regardless of what procedure you've had, the changes in your gastrointestinal tract affect almost all the medications you have, or will take orally, whether it's increased or decreased side-effects, reduced or increased dosages, or being taken off some meds entirely and cold turkey. So, let's get into why all these medication related changes occur, shall we? I promise not to make this a tenth grade chemistry or biology class.....

Medication Absorption Basics

The journey oral medications take through the body is very similar to that of food, and Dr. Baker has already explained all that in Chapter Three. I won't bore you with the details again, but if you can't remember, or it's been a while since you've read Chapter Three, I highly recommend skimming through it again before reading on!

The key to a medication's ability to provide its intended effect is that it must enter the blood stream, hence it must be absorbed. Medications can be absorbed through injections, through the skin via a patch or cream, and the not-so-friendly suppository route, just to name a few. Unfortunately, the one route that will be most affected by your surgery is the one most commonly used — oral ingestion.

Patients that undergo Lap-Band® procedures may not experience significant issues with medication absorption due to the fact that their entire gastrointestinal tract is still fully functioning. Being a Lap-Band® patient, however, doesn't mean that you can skip this chapter altogether. Nooooo.....!! Remember: a "misadventure" can happen to anyone, so keep reading Lap-Banders as there is more information that pertains to you later in the chapter.

The absorption of oral medications is highly dependent on three factors: medication characteristics, location of absorption, and transit contact time through the gastrointestinal tract. Each medication is unique, kind of like a snowflake (being Canadian, I've had an opportunity to inspect a snowflake or two...). All snowflakes serve the same purpose, and may look the same at first glance, but when you look closely they all have unique characteristics that makes each one different. Take for example allergy medications. We've got Claritin®, Allegra®, and Zyrtec®, and they all work the same way in the body. But, when you look at them closely, there may be one or two slight differences in their chemical structures that affect where they may be absorbed in the gastrointestinal tract, or the potential to cause a particular side-effect. Bottom line, the chemical structure of the medication dictates the type of environment required for it to be absorbed.

Naturally, when medications are taken orally they end up in your stomach (or the small portion of it known as the pouch after bariatric surgery). They then make the journey through the various parts of your intestines and out the other end...and you know exactly which end I'm talking about. The majority of oral medications are absorbed through the stomach and small intestine. The environment of the stomach and the intestines are where the characteristics of the medications have to play nice in order to make this absorption thing happen.

For non-bariatric surgery people, the stomach, which is a naturally acidic environment, does a great job absorbing medications that are weakly acidic, and those that are fat soluble. The greater the surface area available and amount of time spent in the stomach, the better the absorption. Hopefully you can see where I'm going with this....

As you already know the pouch is a fraction of the size of what the stomach used to be, and things travel through the pouch fairly quickly. So, medications that were once freely absorbed in the stomach may not be absorbed as much, hence you may not be getting the full effects of a medication that previously worked wonders for you. To top it all off, the acidity of the pouch is very, very low, in comparison to a full sized stomach, and the acid in the remainder stomach decreases and sends less acid down the pipe to meet up later with the food or medication to break them down. So, special coatings on medications to protect the stomach (now pouch) may not work as well anymore. We'll explain this further a little later in the chapter.

Now that we've got a handle on the stomach, let's move on to the intestines as a site for absorption. This is where all the action takes place. The majority of medications are absorbed in the small intestine, specifically in the duodenum and jejunum. As you already know, the functioning portions of these specific areas of your gut are rearranged, and the length of it all is reduced after surgery, thus affecting how the medications work. The main concern here is that a shorter intestine with low acidity to begin with, equals less contact time for the medications to be fully absorbed.

Well, just to add another "kink" in the intestine... (lame joke, I know!), as luck would have it, the area of the intestine that is bypassed, the duodenum, is not only responsible for absorption of medications that travel directly through it, including important nutrients such as calcium, but also medications that undergo the *first-pass effect*....and yes, this is a real medical term, not just something I made up. I'm sure by this point you're just DYING to hear about the *first-pass effect!!* Well, your wait is over....here it is.

The *first-pass* is a common pathway many medications take before they are ready to provide their effects. To make a long story short, medications that have this effect go into your mouth, into your stomach (or pouch), get absorbed through the stomach or intestines (depending on the characteristics of the medication), and enter the blood stream. They then go for a ride through the body, and visit the liver to get kind of broken down and cleaned up a bit, hence the name *first-pass*. (Maybe they should call it the *I-got-distracted-and-went-for-a-tour-and-a-spa-treatment-first effect.…*) They are then released back into the duodenum before they are re-absorbed in the small intestine to do the job they were intended to do in the first place.

Are you seeing where the dilemma lies? The duodenum is bypassed after surgery (but not with a Lap-Band®) so what happens to the ability of these medications to work??? You got it, they may not work as well. Just as calcium and iron are not being as well absorbed because of the bypassed duodenum, the medications may not be well absorbed either. Big problem. We'll resolve that a little later in the chapter too, so keep reading.

Alright, I'm going to take pity on both of us and change subjects now.…(there is just so much chemistry even I can take at one time!.…)

How to Get the Right Medication for You

If you're expecting to read the next section and be able to miraculously determine which medication would work best for the condition you have, I'm sorry to burst your bubble. But, for being a good sport about staying with me thus far in the chapter, my gift to you is a couple of tips to avoid medications that will *not* be the best choice for you.

We've spent some time talking about how the reduction in the functioning portions of the stomach and intestine decreases the actual amount of time available for medication absorption. An obvious way to get the most out of your medications would be to avoid taking medication formulations that require lots of time to be absorbed. Well, at least you'd think it would be obvious.…

I'd like to take a moment to tell you a story about how I came about this amazing little discovery. One evening, after what was scheduled to be a 30 minute talk to the Little Victories™ bariatric support group, which ultimately turned into a 5 hour discussion on medication concerns, I came home with a voluminous number of medication lists from individuals who had questions regarding their prescriptions. Needless to say, this is where my journey into the world of bariatrics began. I was curious to see what types of medications everyone was taking and the various dosages they were on. I had many of my own questions, but the most frequently asked patient question was "Is it safe to take this high of a dose?"

As I began to evaluate these lists I discovered that a large number of individuals were on fairly high doses of a specific medication. This concerned me. After spending about a week evaluating the absorption characteristics of that particular med, I could not figure out why everyone required such a high dose. It's interesting to note that they all claimed it worked the best on relieving their symptoms after switching between an average of 2-3 other medications for the same condition.

About a week later I was talking to my students about the significant lack of information available on this subject, and how I couldn't get to the bottom of why everyone claimed this medication worked for them but they required such a high dose. One of my students looked directly at me and said, "Dr. Ahmed, doesn't the extended release tablet take longer to dissolve in the stomach? So how can it be completely absorbed?" Duh!!... If that wasn't a Homer Simpson® moment, then what would be! So after feeling like a total idiot, and basically failing to identify something a first year pharmacy student would be able to do in their sleep (I'm hoping), I realized it was all about the basics.

So here's the bottom line: medications that are in a liquid form will be absorbed faster than those that are solids, hence the reasoning behind sending almost everyone home with a prescription for liquid Lortab® elixir for pain management following surgery. Tablets or capsules that have special time related release or other types of coatings to slow down the amount of time needed to become a solution obviously may not have enough time to be completely absorbed. So basically what I'm telling you is when possible, do the following:

- Request your physician write you a prescription for a medication in liquid or solution form when possible. (I bet you never thought you'd be going back to the pink bubble gum flavored antibiotics again.)
- Request your physician write prescriptions for tablets or capsules that are NOT in the following special coating formulations:
- No extended-release
- No sustained-release
- No controlled-release
- No timed-release
- No osmotic pumps

Now, obviously you've read what Julie and Karen had to say about the many after-effects that can potentially occur, and aside from various medication formulations that can cause problems, common sense would dictate that whenever possible one should avoid medications that may exacerbate after-effect conditions. If you didn't pick up the fact that Gas-X® strips (or your choice of any other brand of Simethicone™) will become your new best friends for food related gastrointestinal air issues, be aware that many medications can also have gastrointestinal side-effects.

For example, and as I mentioned earlier, most surgeons will prescribe Lortab® elixir for post-surgical pain management. Okay. It is a liquid. That's a step in the right direction. And, it does not contain any medication that can hurt the integrity of the pouch (more to come on this topic). That's another step in the right direction. Can you believe it? We're actually on the ball!.... Well, not completely... Lortab® contains a Morphine derivative that is known to slow peristalsis, leading to constipation. Now keep in mind, the daily iron and calcium supplements you have to take to prevent deficiencies can also cause constipation. I know what you're thinking.....Oh great, I'm either going to have to suffer in pain, or call 1-800-Roto-Rooter® to have a bowel movement! Not necessarily so, my constipated friends....

Actually, the key is identifying side-effects that can occur....and unfortunately they will... and treating them appropriately. I can say with confidence, for the most part side-effects can be treated. We typically don't like to treat a side-effect from one medication with another medication, but, unfortunately, sometimes you gotta do what you gotta do!

So, the question becomes, "How do you figure out the potential side-effects of a particular medication?" You may think I'm totally insane for saying this, but ... TAKE THE TIME TO ACTUALLY READ THE PAMPHLET ATTACHED TO THE PRESCRIPTION BAG!!! You know, the piece of paper you usually tear off and toss in the circular file when taking your prescription vial out of the bag?? Come on, don't even try to deny it! I know that is exactly what you do with it, because I myself am guilty of not reading it either.

Yes, I am referring to the pamphlet with the micro-sized print that lists every potential side-effect known to human-kind. Now, if that is just too much trouble for you to go through, just check with your local pharmacist. That's what they are trained at graduate school to do. (I figured I needed to include a shameless plug somewhere!) Oh yeah, don't forget to tell them you've undergone bariatric surgery. I apologize if you have to explain the process to them. We are working hard on educating my colleagues along with "all the masses" as Julie would put it, but I'm sure your pharmacist will help you with understanding the side-effects, and determine how likely you are to experience them. (More to come on being a self-advocate. Keep reading!)

Protect Your Pouch

Now if you've basically slept through the chapter thus far....WAKE UP! This includes you Lap-Band® people! This section is *the most important section* in the whole chapter....possibly even in the whole book (in my opinion of course....shhh, don't tell Julie, Karen, or the others I said that). What you learn in this portion of the chapter may potentially help save your own life.

The real educator in me is going to come out in this section. This is going to be all about business because you REALLY NEED TO KNOW this information and take it seriously. No more jokes for the time being.

There are many medications that can be very harmful to you as a weight loss surgery patient, and can cause complications that you really don't want to happen. Believe me! Now that your pouch is about the size of an egg (or smaller depending on your specific surgery and surgeon), some medications can irritate the pouch, and over time, can cause ulceration. This is NOT a good thing. Ulcers are not good, they can bleed, and they can cause a whole lot of problems you don't want to have to deal with. Dr. Baker touched on the subject earlier, but we're going to get into the details of medications to avoid, and other medications that can be taken to prevent this from happening.

There may not be much research available on what happens to the absorption of medications after bariatric surgery, but there are more than enough case-reports (short stories about patients in medical journals) to know that you need to protect your pouch! Think of it this way: if a medication can irritate a regular stomach that holds 1500 mls, just imagine the damage it can do to a pouch that holds 30 mls! Lap-Band® people, this means you too because the band is in essence creating a pouch for you not unlike the one created after bypass. So everyone, PAY ATTENTION!

First and foremost, if you don't walk away with anything, walk away with the fact that NSAIDs (nonsteroidal anti-inflammatory drugs) should be *avoided*. NSAIDs are often prescribed for pain and inflammation. Many of you who have osteoarthritis, joint injuries, rheumatoid arthritis, and other types of persistent owwies have taken or currently take NSAIDs.

This class of meds threatens the integrity of the pouch by two mechanisms; they prevent the production of *prostaglandins* (a natural substance produced in the body) that provides protection for the stomach and pouch linings, and they directly irritate the lining of the pouch. Newer pain medications such as Celebrex® are known to provide better protection than traditional NSAIDs, as they do not affect prostaglandin production, but they still have the potential to directly irritate the pouch.

To help you avoid taking an NSAID, it helps to know what drugs actually are NSAIDs, so we've provided a handy-dandy chart for you. Be sure to tell your pharmacist to note on your file that you should not take any NSAIDs without a protectant. We'll discuss protectants in a minute. Be sure to inform ALL of your physicians, dental professionals, and health care providers that you should not take an NSAID without a protectant.

Point in fact: a great story from Julie. She went to her family physician's office with a sore shoulder from lugging around cases of books (1st edition of the REAL Skinny...) She saw the practice's physician assistant (PA) who has been a PA for almost 30 years. After examining her shoulder, he determined that she had some inflammation, but it was basically just strained muscles. During the entire exam, however, they had been discussing her weight loss, her general health, and the fact that she was not to take NSAIDs without a protectant. They had quite a discussion on that note.

Well, you can guess how the story ends. The PA whipped out his script pad, and absent-mindedly wrote Julie a script for an NSAID with no script for a protectant. Now, luckily Julie has a good understanding of pharmacology and knows her NSAIDs cold. (Hmmmm....I wonder who she has to thank for that??) She was able to correct him on the spot, but most patients aren't able to do that. If another patient had been in the same position, and had not warned the pharmacist (who acts as the last line of defense for patients), then the patient would have been taking an NSAID without a protectant, and would have certainly suffered some level of damage to the pouch. Moral of the story? Tell your docs, tell your pharmacist, tell your bariatric surgeon and his/her staff, and be able to recognize an NSAID when you see one.

NSAID and MEDICATION TIPS

OTC NSAIDs

Aspirin, Ibuprofen (Motrin®, Advil®), Naproxen (Aleve®), Ketaprofen (Orudis KT®)

PRESCRIBED NSAIDs

Ibuprofen (Motrin®), Naproxen (Naprosyn®, Anaprox®), Kertoralac (Toradol®), Etolodac (Lodine®), Prioxicam (Feldene®), Indomethacin (Indocin®), Oxaprozin (Daypro®), Nabumetone (Relafen®, Cataflam®), Diclofenac (Voltaren®), Mobicoxib (Mobic®), Celecoxib (Celebrex®)

BLOOD PRESSURE MEDS

Avoid time release formulas such as:
• Extended • Delayed • Controlled • Sustained

MOOD ENHANCERS/ANTIDEPRESSANTS

Avoid time release formulas such as:
• Extended • Delayed • Controlled • Sustained

THYROID MEDS

DO NOT take with a multi-vitamin that contains IRON (wait at least one hour).

ALLERGY MEDS

Avoid time release formulas such as:
• Extended • Delayed • Controlled • Sustained
Avoid formulas with decongestants (*i.e.* Allegra-D®) as they are extended release. Oral dissolving forms may be the best.

PMS MEDS

Midol®, Premsyn®, Pamprin®

NSAIDs = Non-Steroidal Anti-Inflammatory Drugs
OTC = Over the Counter

DO NOT TAKE NSAIDs WITHOUT ALSO TAKING A PRESCRIPTION FOR CYTOTEC® / MISOPROSTOL

(ASK YOUR DOCTOR OR CALL YOUR BARIATRIC SURGEON'S OFFICE)
Do not take Cytotec® or Misoprostol if you are pregnant, think you are pregnant, or might become pregnant.

OTHER TIPS TO DISCUSS WITH YOUR DOCTOR AND/OR YOUR PHARMACIST:

• Enteric coating on pills – this prevents the medication from being released until it reaches the small intestine.

• Prodrugs – a type of drug that must enter the bloodstream to be "activated" before providing effect.

• Liquid, chewable, or dissolvable formulations.

• Do not take multi-vitamins that contain iron at the same time as calcium. Wait one hour.

• TYLENOL® is NOT an NSAID. It is OKAY to take in limited amounts. Certain nutritional deficiencies can cause Tylenol® toxicity if large amounts are taken. Talk to your doctor or pharmacist.

Now for those of you that are absolutely allergic to every pain medication that is known to man except for NSAIDs, if *absolutely necessary* an NSAID can be taken, but only if taken with a medication that protects the pouch. Multiple studies in patients that have *not* undergone bariatric surgery have proven that administering a gastrointestinal protectant can significantly reduce the occurrence of ulcers. Once again, with the lack of studies in patients post bariatric surgery, the safest practice is to apply the findings of the studies we have at our disposal.

Excess acid production in the stomach in combination with an irritant that disrupts the gastrointestinal lining leads to ulcer production. Proton pump inhibitors (PPIs) protect against ulcer production by preventing acid production, but the fact remains that the pouch and the intestines have very little acid to prevent, so the only thing they may provide in this instance, is a false sense of security. The best protectant medications to help guard against ulcer production are Cytotec® which is basically prostaglandin in a pill form, and Carafate® which coats the stomach.

To make sure we are all crystal clear on this topic, NSAIDs should **always** be used with one of the following medications, preferably one from the *left column* over the right:

PROTECTANTS	PROTON PUMP INHIBITORS (PPIs)
Cytotec® (misoprostal)	Prilosec® (omeprazole)
Carafate® (sucralfate)	Aciphex® (rabeprazole)
	Protonix® (pantoprazole)
	Prevacid® (lansoprazole)
	Nexium® (esomeprazole)
	Zegrid® (omeprazole/sodium bicarbonate)

For those of you that are taking an aspirin everyday to protect your heart health or prevent a stroke, be sure to talk to your physician about weighing the risks vs. the benefits. The recommended dose for heart health is between 81mg and 325mg daily, and the use of *enteric coated* aspirin is encouraged to prevent irritation of the stomach by the aspirin itself.

In a standard patient, the aspirin's enteric coating is designed to dissolve in a lower acid, or more basic environment such as the intestine to release the protectant medication for absorption in the intestine. Now rewind a little bit, and think back to when I told you about how the acidity of the pouch and the stomach decreases after bypass surgery. For gastric bypass patients, there is a good possibility that the enteric coating may dissolve in the low acid pouch and release the aspirin (an NSAID) inside which may possibly irritate the lining of the pouch. The aspirin will eventually make it to the intestine for absorption and do its intended job, but not before possibly irritating the heck out of the pouch. So, say good-bye to that so-called protection!

Can we say with absolute surety that the low-dose aspirin will cause irritation or ulceration of the pouch? No, we can't. Studies in standard patients report that lower doses of aspirin *without* enteric coating *have not* been shown to cause significant ulceration problems, however, we have no studies for post bariatric surgery patients. Moral of the story? Better safe than sorry. Use a protectant medication with your low-dose aspirin for heart health, or talk to your doctor about alternative agents such as Plavix®.

Now, one last thing about NSAIDs: for all my sisters out there who suffer from PMS or PMDD and are taking over-the-counter (OTC) medications such as Midol®, Pamprin®, Premsyn® and the like, be aware that most if not all of these types of medications contain an NSAID. Do not take them without an appropriate protectant. Read ALL OTC MEDICATION PACKAGES for any condition to see if the product contains an NSAID.

Whew! That was exhausting....Let's take a break before we go on............

Okay break time is over. I promise, only a couple more medications you have to be cautious about, and we'll be all done.

Naturally, if non-steroidal medications can irritate the gastric lining, how much do you want to bet steroids can do it too? It's obvious that any medication that has the word steroid in it, or even sounds like the word steroid, should raise some questions, regardless of the route of administration — with one exception: inhaled steroids taken for asthma really don't get into the blood stream to cause any problems, they're okay.

Steroids, like NSAIDs, directly and indirectly damage the gastrointestinal lining and have the potential to cause ulcers. Steroids are often prescribed for respiratory issues, asthma complications, and allergic reactions. They can be prescribed in a pill form, an inhaled form, a cream or topical solution, an injectible form, or even a patch.

In addition to prescribing pills, creams, or patches in non-life threatening situations, steroids are typically administered in injectible form in life threatening circumstances such as asthma attacks, or severe allergic reactions. You know...the kind where your whole face swells up like a tomato on steroids....?? ...okay, I know, another lame joke.... In any steroid situation, emergency or not, take the steroid, but don't forget the gastrointestinal protectant unless you are literally unconscious. Even if they stick a big fat needle into you to get the steroid into your blood stream, you need to protect your pouch from the effects of the steroids!! Okay. Enough about steroids. Moving on.

One would think this last class of medications would only be relevant to women, but MEN LISTEN UP!!!!! Osteoporosis can affect men as well as women!! Especially if you are a gastric bypass patient and you no longer have the same calcium absorption efficiency you used to have.

Bone health is dependent on receiving sufficient calcium intake. The decrease of calcium absorption may increase your risk for developing osteoporosis. Medications commonly used in the treatment and prevention of osteoporosis such as Fosamax®, Actonel®, and Boniva® have the potential to cause gastrointestinal ulceration.

Unfortunately, the addition of a protective medication has not proven to reduce the risk with these medications. There exists no studies to explain why or whether this class of medications can irritate the stomach or pouch lining despite the use of a protectant. To be safe, and if you are at an increased risk for developing osteoporosis, other options exist and should be discussed with your doctor. Alternatives include. injectible versions of these medications, Miacalcin®, Evista® (for women only), or Forteo® for extremely high risk patients with osteoporosis. And don't forget you need to take *calcium citrate* not calcium carbonate if you are a bypass patient. Call Building Blocks®. They'll help you out.

Medication Separation Anxiety

Shortly after your surgery, possibly even as soon as the day you are discharged you may come to realize that half the medications you took prior to surgery (specifically those for diabetes and high blood pressure) are no longer on the medication list they gave you when you were discharged from the hospital. At that point you may find yourself panicked and thinking, "But wait, I've been taking these for years! It really can't be safe for me to stop them cold turkey!"

You really have to take a step back and trust your surgeon; they really do know what they're doing. In addition to the changes your body is going through on the outside, the way it functions on the inside has also significantly changed. The difference is you can't see it or feel it until things go wrong.

Case in point: for those of you that may have type 2 diabetes, it is not uncommon for your surgeon to ask you to stop medications that directly affect insulin levels, or even stop insulin injections immediately or shortly after bypass surgery. Did I hear you ask why???.... Well let me tell you why. All of a sudden your body is secreting hormones that affect metabolism it hasn't seen in years, and it's burning through calories like there's no tomorrow. Wooo! Hooo!....Isn't that kind of what we wanted — a metabolism that's burning on jet fuel, and a cure for diabetes!??

Unfortunately, your diabetes, like your obesity, is not cured. It's controlled, but it's not cured. There is a difference! Your diabetes and your obesity are not cured, so don't be making plans to taste all 31 flavors at Baskin Robbins® any time soon. If you don't continue to respect your diabetic and obesity conditions and treat your body with proper nutrition and movement, then aside from turning multiple shades of green due to dumping, eventually your body will catch up with you, and you'll find yourself back on those medications the weight loss was suppose to help you discard. This goes for any other chronic conditions such as high blood pressure or high cholesterol too.

Respecting your condition *does not* include self-medicating! Continuing to take the medications such as insulin injections or blood pressure medications after your physician has ordered a decrease or a discontinuation can cause your blood sugars or blood pressure and heart rate to drop to dangerously low levels. Do not continue to take prescriptions if the dosage has been raised or lowered just because you still have pills in the bottle. Immediately change to the new dosage unless otherwise instructed by your doctor. If you either continue discontinued meds, or don't change dosages as instructed, it's almost guaranteed that this will win you a free trip right back to the hospital. I know by this point you love all the nurses and the physicians who took care of you at the hospital, but do everyone a favor and just stop by for a visit, don't get admitted! Please follow your physician's instructions and trust that if they got you this far, they know what they are doing with your diabetes, blood pressure, and other medication modifications. If you still have questions, ask your pharmacist.

One last thing….just as you go through "shrinks" with your body, the size of clothes will not be the only thing changing. As you lose body fat, medications that like to hang out in fat tissue will also need to have dosages decreased. Some of the more common classes of fat soluble meds include: some antibiotics, digoxin, and amiodarone. Stay in touch with all of your treating physicians as you lose weight, and be sure to ask each of them, or ask your pharmacist if any of your med dosages are affected by a decrease in body fat. If they are, then stay in touch with your prescribing physician's office on a monthly basis to keep them updated on your current weight. Be patient with this process (no pun intended). On a scale of 1 to 10 for annoyances this ranks about a 2.

How to Become Your Own Best Advocate

By no means am I an expert on speaking up and speaking out. Julie and Karen will back me up on that one. They're still working on developing my I'm-in-control-of-this-classroom teacher voice. Apparently, one of these days I'm supposed to get loud enough that I shouldn't need a microphone to lecture to a hundred or more students… I doubt it.… Anyway, as a post-surgical bariatric patient, one thing you're going to have to learn to do is speak up. Especially when it comes to telling health care providers why they need to know you are a post-surgical patient!

Don't ever assume that just because you told them once, they'll remember. Honestly, you have to be a nag about it. Every time they write you a prescription, ask if there is any potential for that medication to harm you. Basically, become a broken record until you've trained them to voluntarily tell you that the medication will not affect, or be affected by your surgery. Hey, if you're not going to look out for yourself, then who is?

Unfortunately it doesn't end with your primary care physician. Health care providers include your physicians, surgeons, physician assistants, registered nurses, dietitians, nurse practitioners, pharmacists, dentists, chiropractors, podiatrists, ER personnel, ambulance attendants or paramedics, and any one else you might see who can administer treatment or write a prescription. Advertise it loud and clear. The last thing you want is for your dentist to hand you a script for Motrin® following a root canal, or for your chiropractor to give you a script for Relafen® that could result in some very painful problems down the road. Make sure your pharmacist knows! They are your last line of defense!!!

Also, be sure to create a little card to carry in your wallet or purse that lists:
- Your surgeon's name and phone numbers.
- The type of surgery you had and when.
- Your current medications with dosages, who prescribed them, and what they are for.
- Any medication allergies or warnings (*i.e.,* No NSAIDs without a protectant like Cytotec®)
- The name and number of the pharmacy that fills your scripts.

Lastly, but certainly not in the least, be sure to develop a relationship with your pharmacist. Try and have all of your scripts filled at one pharmacy so you can get to know your pharmacists better. They are highly trained and skilled individuals, and it is their job to help you with medication questions and issues. If you are afraid to approach your physician about dosage questions, or anything else, then have your pharmacist do it for you. If you're having a side-effect, ask them if one of your medications could be causing it, and have them help you determine if there are better alternatives for you.

Wrap Up

Okay, so we've gone through a whole lot of stuff here. Let me break it down for you in one easy to reference, simple little chart. Would that help?
- If side-effects appear or increase, consult your doctor or your pharmacist about dosage or other medication options.
- First-pass effect medications may not provide effective absorption at the current dosages. Check dosage or check for alternative medications that do not have first-pass effect.
- Medications that are in a liquid or solution form will be absorbed faster than those that are solids. Check for liquid forms of medications.
- **No** extended-release, sustained-release, controlled-release, timed-release, or osmotic pump medications.
- Many medications can also have gastrointestinal side-effects like gas, diarrhea, constipation, or intestinal cramping.
- Read the pamphlet attached to the prescription bag for potential side-effects.
- You should not take any NSAIDs without a protectant such as Cytotec® or Carafate®. EVER!!
- Be able to recognize an NSAID when you see one.
- Use a protectant if taking daily low-dose aspirin for heart health or to prevent stroke.
- Check all PMS OTC medications for NSAID ingredients.
- Read all OTC medication packaging to check for NSAID ingredients.
- Inhaled steroids for asthma are okay.
- Taking steroids of any kind, even by injection, requires taking a protectant as well.

- Medications commonly used in the treatment and prevention of osteoporosis such as Fosamax®, Actonel®, and Boniva® have the potential to cause gastrointestinal ulceration. Talk to your doctor or pharmacist about alternatives.
- Do not continue to take medications that have been discontinued.
- If dosages have been changed, do not finish out a previous dosage just because it is there. Change the dosage immediately unless instructed otherwise by your doctor.
- Ask your doctor or pharmacist if any of your medications are fat soluble. If so, stay in touch with the prescribing physician and report your current weight every month for possible dosage changes.
- Tell all medical providers about your status as a weight loss surgery patient (you too Lap-Banders!).
- Keep all your scripts at one pharmacy if possible.
- Meet and get to know your local pharmacists. They truly can be invaluable friends.
- Remember to have everyone work as a team for you! You're worth it!

Well, I'm hoping that at this point you've got a better handle on what to expect, and what you need to do to prevent your own "medication misadventures." If it all just seems like the questions, and the combinations, and the dosage issues might be a little too difficult to handle... well... there's always suppositories!

Chapter Thirteen

— T H E   P R O T E I N   S A F A R I —

Julie M. Janeway

Karen J. Sparks

Ah, Protein! The building block of life! By now, we hope you've read Chapter Eleven, and you've learned all about how important protein is to your body, and your life. We're not going to re-iterate that information here, but what we are going to do is discuss the many facets of living a life in search of protein.

We have named this daily quest the protein "safari," rather than the protein hunt, the protein pursuit, or the protein chase, because "safari" says it best: the adventure of hunting big-game!!

Every day is an adventure too! What you ate yesterday, may not sit well today. Your busy schedule may take you to places that give you limited opportunities to find protein, or limited time to eat. No two days are ever the same. The only constant is that you must continue to get the protein in whatever way you can.

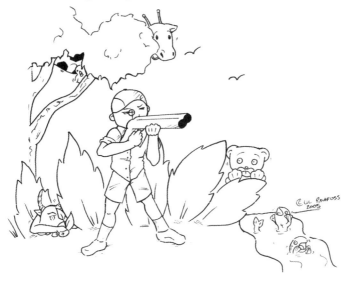

Getting enough protein, however, is often the problem. As we've mentioned several times in this book, when you come home from the hospital you simply don't feel like putting anything in your "stomach." That's generally true no matter what type of surgery you might have (and trust me, I am a living expert on surgeries after 23 of them!) Despite the natural inclination not to eat, "if at first you don't eat, try, try again."

When I had the stricture, I couldn't get anything in. I was in bad shape. My nurse friend Judy was determined, however, to find me something I could tolerate because she knows the importance of getting enough protein every day. Judy left the college one day (basically because I looked so bad and could barely hold my head up), and came back about an hour later with $50.00 worth of protein drinks from the health food store.

At that time, what she brought helped to save my life. It was a water based whey protein drink (as opposed to milk or juice based), and a 16 oz. bottle contained 15g of protein. Now it's wasn't exactly Kool-Aid®, but then it wasn't supposed to be. It is generally designed to be a nutritional supplement for the general public as opposed to bariatric surgery patients, but for me it was the difference between survival and dehydration. Shortly thereafter, however, we were introduced to Bariatrix' SmartForme products and they made all the difference.

You must make eating the requisite amount of protein one of the most important things you do each day. Now, we'd be lying if we said that either one of us managed to get all of our protein in every day. In fact, even when you've given it your best try, there are days that you simply don't get anywhere near your goal.

Being tired or stressed will certainly affect your ability to get and keep food in at all. Your body just seems to reject food because it doesn't want to waste the energy processing it. I guess all your energy must be going to keeping you awake, or keep you from throwing yourself off a bridge, depending on your sleep deprivation or stress load.

Speaking of being stressed, or stressing others as the case may be, diminished protein levels also affect your hormones (men have them too!) which can make you one cranky baby! Take pity on those around you, and don't purposefully turn yourself into a psychotic hormone-ravaged lunatic by perpetually evading your protein needs. We can't tell you what to do about any other hormone issues you might have, but just don't add to the problem by missing your protein.

When you do eat, you will learn to eat the protein first. Sounds simple enough, right? Wrong! You've spent a lifetime going for the starches and carbs first, and using the meat or other protein based foods simply to stuff the other food down to make more room! A lifetime habit like that doesn't go away over night.

But, you will learn to eat the protein first because after you've eaten the potatoes or the veggies, or even some salad, and you find there's simply no room left for the chicken or the fish, you figure out that you probably should have eaten the protein first. It's just like a safari: you aim, you shoot, and you miss. But, the more you aim and shoot, the more likely it is that you will eventually hit something. It just takes some people longer to learn to hit the target.

In case you're one of these slow learners, this means that you may not be figuring out that you need the protein to go in before the other foods until something drastic happens, like your hair begins to fall out. That will most certainly get your attention, and tell you to put down the fork, and step away from the potatoes.

Putting down the potatoes or veggies in favor of the meat or fish will help with something else as well: getting your protein in bigger doses. When you eat the non-protein foods first, you fill your pouch/stomach and leave less room for protein. When you are full, you're full, and you must now wait at least 4-5 more hours to eat again. But now you've got yourself worried that you are behind in getting that all important 80-90g of protein in for the day. So what happens? You graze.

Grazing means that you try to make it up in between meals with a little protein here, and a little there; but grazing leads to more calories, and a reinforcement of your previous eating habits. Grazing is not good because it is generally contrary to what your behaviorist, doctor, and dietitian are trying to help you learn. When you eat you should try to eat your protein in big doses (20-30g at a time). It sounds like it would be a huge amount of meat, fish, or what-have-you, but really it isn't. It's just about the size of the palm of your hand.

Eating your 20-30g per meal doesn't mean you can't have the other foods too. In fact, you should be learning to eat balanced meals, and if you skip the veggies too much, you'll begin to sort of crave them. But you should base the meal around the protein, which means learning to read labels and memorize protein values to determine how much protein, fat, and carbs you're combining in a meal.

It's not really a conscious thing, you just kind of start doing it. You don't really want to waste what little room you have in there on foods that don't get you where you need to go as far as your daily required intake. After a while, you'll be reading food labels as closely as a prenuptial agreement! Once you start doing this, you'll find protein in a number of unexpected places, and your meals won't just consist of a chicken breast (20-30g depending on size), a scoop of veggies (1-2 g depending on veggie), and maybe a small spoonful of potatoes. Soon you'll be having wonderful meals, and your family will love them too.

There are many high protein oriented cookbooks on the market, and even a number of cookbooks for people who've had weight loss surgery. I, however, do not like to cook, and never have liked to cook. I can do it when necessary, but I don't enjoy it. To me cookbooks and cooking are only useful if I'm having a party and have to lull people into thinking I'm really a Susie-homemaker. I cook only when I feel guilty because my husband is on his eighth PB&J in two days, or because I spent too much money shopping. Hate it! Hate it! Hate it!!!

Karen loves to cook, but she's forever on the go. Both of us have had to learn some tricks, and learn to adapt our lives in order to get our required protein every day, and thus keep our hair and lose our fat. The first of these tricks is learning to dismantle food.

If you must eat out, whether at a restaurant, someone else's house, or even the cafeteria at work, then learn to dismantle food. Look first for items that have a probable high protein content, and then look to see if things can be left off, or taken off in order to lower the calories, fat, carbs, and most of all bulk of the food. An example is a grilled chicken sandwich. You can ditch the bun, leave off the sauce or mayo, eat the lettuce and tomato, and if it needs a little something, dip it in a spot of regular mustard. That's dismantling your food.

If you're at someone's home for dinner, then skip the rolls, leave the gravy off the meat, or pick out what you can eat from the casserole. If you let someone know ahead of time that it's not their cooking, that you simply have a limited range of foods you can eat, people generally aren't offended. If you don't tell them, however, they tend to think it must be something they did, or maybe you're just rude or ungrateful.

If you're not comfortable with telling someone that you've had weight loss surgery and can only eat certain foods, and a small amount of food at that, there are other ways you can get around this. I've often quietly told people that I have food allergies, or a gastrointestinal disorder that prevents me from eating many foods.

There are many such disorders that exist like Celiac disease, or a carbohydrate malabsorption disorder. You don't have to name what disorder you're claiming to have, simply know that many types exist that cause all kinds of people to have food issues similar to yours. It's really not all that uncommon.

The moral of the story here is: do whatever you have to do to effectively dismantle food when you're in situations that don't afford you control over what's offered or available to eat.

Second to dismantling is substituting. If you go to restaurants like Bennigans® or TGIFridays® you'll find protein friendly menu items. The problem is they often sell them with a side of broccoli. That sounds all well and good, especially if you like broccoli, but I suspect you might find that broccoli gives you terrible gas and air bubble problems. Not a plan.

If you tell the waitperson that you have a gastrointestinal disorder and can't tolerate broccoli, they'll generally substitute another vegetable without charge. These two restaurants will do that anyway, but that's just a little lawyer/daughter of a restauranteur tip for you for the restaurants that want to charge you for substitutions. Generally, if they think they could end up getting sued for feeding you something they are now on notice will make you sick, they'll suck up the 15 cents it may cost them in substituting the food.

The foregoing is just general information. Do not construe this as personal legal advice. This is an express disclaimer of all responsibility for liability claimed or incurred as a result of the previous statement. (Sorry — occupational hazard....)

Another tip for finding your protein if you hate to cook or don't have time, concerns what we affectionately call "plastic food." Plastic food is the high protein, low-fat, low-carb frozen entrée made by the brand name of your choosing. Plastic food can be a lifesaver. Men: this will appeal to many of you.

First off, you have to choose the regular size ones — "hungry-guy" dinners are no longer an option. If you choose the regular size ones, they are generally about the right amount of food, and they help teach you what proper portions should look like. They'll give you some variety in your diet, and they give you a protein count that is pretty close to what it will say on the box (give or take a half ounce or so of meat).

Plastic food also gives you a calorie count so you can keep track, and provides a decent balance of foods. Finally, they're portable, so almost anywhere you go you can have some reasonable protein available to eat, and they don't require cooking! Just slap it in the microwave, and you've got an edible pile of protein, and no dishes!

The portability of plastic food has helped Karen and me so much. We have crazy class schedules as professors, and add to that our consulting and presentation schedules, and we're just never near home cooking (unless I'm feeling guilty over shopping…) You simply can't live in restaurants or fast food joints. Not acceptable.

Restaurants get old so fast because the food has to be dismantled, and it costs an arm and a leg. You can only eat about a third of it, and the rest goes home to the styrofoam jungle until it rots and goes in the garbage. (My mom, who was raised in the "clean your plate, there are starving children in Africa" era, thinks that throwing away food is just awful. She calls it the pagan ritual of feeding the garbage-god.)

Karen and I got so sick of restaurants and trying to find foods we could eat, that we took to ordering one entrée (with appropriate substitutions and deletions) and sharing it. People look at us kind of funny, but it works out a lot better. Also, we figured out that sometimes sharing an appetizer is the way to go; like those little appetizer rib things. Protein filled, and not too much. Sometimes you have to ask if they can send things out without the sauce, or simply put it on the side. Dipping is okay, swimming in it is not.

Planning ahead and taking food with you becomes a skill you acquire. Karen and I have to travel to a lot of conferences and other speaking engagements. We plan what we're taking to eat, before we plan what we're taking to wear. Heck! We plan our food for the conference, before we plan what we're going to say in our presentation at the conference!

We take low-fat cheese sticks or cheese cubes, fat-free yogurt, small apples, bananas, peanuts (Karen likes them — I say yuck), deli shaved turkey breast, a few veggies, and of course some of Bariatrix' SmartForme protein supplements. We don't even go shopping, or to teach classes without planning and packing food now. You simply can't be caught without it; not if you want to keep losing weight, and keep your hair!

Now in an absolute emergency, you may be forced to stop at a fast food place to find your protein. Do not make this a habit!!! Weight loss surgery will have freed you from the heinous grasp of the fast food demon. Do not let it get its sharp little claws into you again, or all this will have been for naught! Be as careful in going to fast food joints as you would be in walking near quicksand — or a trial lawyer. (I'm allowed to poke fun at my own kind.…)

There are a few acceptable alternatives at some of these places, but for the most part they're off limits. If necessary, however, a *grilled* chicken breast sandwich minus bun and other stuff is okay, albeit expensive. Wendy's® 99 cent chili isn't bad, and the nutrition information can be found at the company's web site. Some of the salads at various places are good, but be very careful of the content of the salad dressings. You can get great salad dressings in to-go packages from Bariatrix' SmartForme products. See the back of the book for contact information.

Does this mean you can never have even one french fry? No, it doesn't, but trust me on this, you won't be able to eat many. Again, I've suffered so you don't have to.

Of course avoid all the fried foods, and the hamburgers of every type and description; you just can't get the fat out of them.

Some Asian food is okay, but beware the oils in which it is cooked as they contain a lot of fat, and may cause dumping syndrome. Some Mexican food is okay, but again beware what it has been cooked in, how spicy it might be, and watch the rice content as it will just keep expanding in your poor little pouch/stomach until you feel like you're going to pop! Basically, you just have to use your common sense, and watch your step when it comes to being on the daily protein safari.

To help you with what I sense to be your growing angst over the adventures involved in the daily protein safari, I suggest (and so will your dietitian and doctor I suspect) that you make a daily list or record of the protein you've consumed, the other foods consumed, your water intake, and the approximate fat, calorie, and carb counts for the day as well. Tracking the times you eat, and where you eat also helps to remind you what worked for you and what didn't. Eventually you'll be able to do all this in your head.

If you have one of those stressed or tired days that you just really can't eat, then write down what you did eat, and put the day behind you. Look at your protein totals for the whole week. Don't stress out over missing your goal (even if it's by a mile) on one particular day. This is a long haul, big-picture thing. Don't look at the snapshot, look at the whole roll of film.

Looking at things in the aggregate helps you to remain in control instead of letting the food issues control you. Isn't that kind of how you ended up fat in the first place? — emotional eating, boredom eating, stress eating? Oh, and don't forget eating without awareness.

Eating without awareness is the phenomenon that occurred when you sat in front of the boob-tube and simply stuffed potato chip after potato chip (or substitute donut, cookie, cracker, pizza slice, etc.) into your mouth until, without even noticing, you'd finished off the entire bag or box. We all did that. Nobody gets to the point of considering weight loss surgery without having experienced eating without awareness.

Although you've pretty much got the eating without awareness thing licked (no pun intended), the other food issues are still there skulking around in the back of your emotional vortex waiting to strike. Be vigilant! Lock, bolt, bar, block, barricade, impede, hinder, and blockade the door behind which these food issues prowl, and never again let them through!

Take care because they will lie in wait, ready to attack when your defenses are low. They're prone to strike right before your monthly cycle, after an argument with your spouse, while watching the Sopranos, or anytime during the entire boring basketball season. Opportunities abound....

To beat back these insidious little food assailants, I suggest taking a tip from the people who teach self-defense against sinister human assailants. (I do this and it really works!) When you feel some unexplainable need to stuff food in your mouth, and you know you shouldn't be, say firmly, or even forcefully, "NO!"

Now it doesn't work if you only say it in your head. We know this to be the case because if it worked by saying it in your head, I wouldn't be writing this book, and you wouldn't be reading it. You have to actually say it out loud! Say it with me. NO! If it doesn't work on the first try, say it out loud again. Usually, by the third time I've said NO!, the food fixation goes away. I don't really know why it works — don't care. It works.

Another tip is one that was given to me by a nurse who helped me in my recovery following my accident. She liked to analyze the little food predators by using the HATTS method. HATTS stands for Hungry, Angry, Thirsty, Tired, Stressed. At the moment the gnawing need to have a snack creeps up on you, ask yourself whether you are hungry, angry, thirsty, tired, or stressed. If you're one or more of those things at that moment, attempt to relieve the condition by a more appropriate method than eating, and the food yearning should go away. If it doesn't, start yelling, "NO! NO! NO! NO!" at the top of your lungs, and then run for about a block. That may not help either, but it at least got you a block away from the food!

Now running from food is not what you want to be doing very often. You need to learn to control the food, and to control your actual "need" for food. The only real control food should have over you is the fact that it keeps you alive, keeps your weight moving down, and keeps your hair in your head.

But the brain is a funny and complex thing, and it likes to play horrible tricks on us. You will grapple for a long time with getting your eyes and brain to communicate with your pouch/stomach as to the proper amount of food it will hold. Your "eyes being too big for your stomach" will be something that is hard to equalize.

In the beginning you will not want any food. Then you'll only want a little food, which isn't enough. Then when you can really eat food, and you're getting the hang of what foods work, you get a bit complacent, and you start eating like a normal person again. Not eating like you used to, just eating like a normal person.

You're not a normal person though. You're plumbed differently. You need to eat less than normal people. You will often just take too much food, and figure out you can't eat it. Case in point: the buffet story in Chapter Nine. Karen and I still take too much food on occasion. Inevitably one asks the other, "Exactly what were you thinking when you did that?" Then, if at all possible, we feed the rest to my husband Matt. (Why feed the garbage-god when you can feed the human garbage disposal?)

Anyway, you deal with it and move on. But here's a tip that might help: when I am eating at home (and not eating plastic food), I have learned to eat my food on a salad plate rather than a dinner plate. I can't fill it up as much, and it still looks full.

Now I know many of you have tried this trick in the past, but it didn't work then because you still had room in your stomach. You simply went back and filled up the salad plate again (and maybe again). But it works now because of the limited amount of space in your pouch/stomach.

The problem in my house became that as soon as I started using the salad plates all the time, so did my husband for some stupid reason! What the heck?! Did I start a new fad or something? So I went out and bought a box of eight cheap, clear glass salad plates, and that kind of kept the supply healthy in between running the dishwasher and Matt's four PB&J sandwiches per day.

If you have lapses in putting the proper amount of food on your plate, and you have no human garbage disposal spouse or growing child to feed it to, just stick it in a container and call it leftovers. At least it will be easy pickin's for another day's protein safari.

Living a life on the protein safari is simply a matter of trial, error, and environmental adaptation. It's like moving to a big city, or a new country: you simply have to live there a while, grumble a bit about how different things are, and then figure out how to make it work for you in order to get you what you need, and where you need to go. Adjust.

So, in conclusion, the protein safari, like everything else in your life after weight loss surgery, it has an annoyance and an amusement factor. The trick is making the amusement factor outweigh the annoyance factor. Any time you think the annoyance factor is winning, sit down and review your personal list of little victories. That will put it all in perspective for you, and prepare you for another fun-filled day of tracking big-game on the safari.

Happy hunting!

P.S. If you have decided to have surgery or join a physician's medically managed weight loss program, and you have become the patient of a bariatric surgeon or a bariatric physician, you can try Bariatrix' SmartForme products for free. Simply go to the web site www.smartforme.com, or call 1-877-895-3511 and request a free sample of the products you'd like to try. Only one sample of each product per customer though, and you must be a confirmed patient of a bariatric physician or surgeon. This way you can try the products before you buy. Mention the LVP-MI code when you do order and receive an additional 10% off your order!

Chapter Fourteen

— THE JUNK DRAWER —

Julie M. Janeway

Karen J. Sparks

This chapter is the book's junk drawer. Everybody has a junk drawer, right? It's the place where you put the stuff that doesn't really have any other place to live. Shoelaces, ticket stubs, odd batteries, tape, rubber bands, your old glasses, loose change, etc., are the kinds of things you find in the junk drawer. Most of them are useful for you or someone else, but they are all unrelated items residing in one space.

So, that's what we put in this chapter: all the things that had no other place to go, are useful to you or someone else, and are basically unrelated to each other. They're now all sharing one space, so if this chapter seems a bit messy and disconnected, that's what it was designed to be. Please bear with us as we've basically just tossed in all this information that has no other home. It will just sit here until you need it, minding it's own business. But, when you're looking for it later, hopefully you'll remember to check the junk drawer first.

Hidden Costs Related to Weight Loss

Where to start? Well maybe from the bottom up? Let's start with shoes. When you lose a tremendous amount of weight, as you should with bariatric surgery, your feet get smaller. So, you may find that you move from wide width shoes to regular width shoes. You will just wake up one day, and when you put your shoes on, you'll walk right out of them because they're too big.

Now that's a bit of a tick-off when they are your favorite shoes! But this is kind of the cost of doing business: you will have to start replacing your shoes. But wait, there's more! Not only may your feet shrink from wide width to regular width, but the length of your feet may actually change as well! No, really!

I've worn a size 10 medium shoe all my life — since I was in fifth grade. I rarely had to wear wide shoes, but I always needed a 10 for the length. By the time I lost about 100 lbs., I noticed that all of my size 10 shoes were starting to just sort of flop around on my feet. It wasn't that they were too wide, it was that they were too long, and I was walking out of them.

Now I wear a size 9 or 9½ shoe. Go figure! I've had to begin replacing my shoes because the 10s just won't stay on. That was an expense I hadn't counted on. Few people do.

And here's another one you might not see coming: socks and hosiery. You shrink out of all that too. Socks maybe only once or twice, but with hosiery you'll shrink down several sizes, so don't buy in bulk, because you'll either shrink through and not wear them, or you'll be stuck wearing hose with baggy "elephant" ankles. Don't waste the money. Buy as you go.

This next one is really more for the women reading this than the men because it deals with underwear. We know it to be an undisputed fact that men will not buy new underwear no matter what the conditions or circumstances. Men will tie their underwear on with a shoelace, or tape it on with duct tape before they'll buy new underwear.

Women, however, will need to buy new undies at least two or three times during the weight loss period. Now the undies you can handle unless you're addicted to expensive undies from the "lady with the secret" store, but the real kicker is replacing your bras. That gets expensive. You don't realize how that adds up until you've replaced them for the third (or more) time. Again, it's also a real drag because we always have our favorite bra, the one that doesn't pinch, bind, or pull, and you will hate having to say good-bye to it. Not only does it not pinch, bind, or pull, it doesn't lift, shape, or separate anymore either. We can only hope it has a twin in a smaller size.

Related to underwear are bathing suits. Nobody really thinks about this one, unless you live in a climate in which you can wear a bathing suit all year 'round. In Michigan, we only have summer for about 10 minutes each year (somewhere in July), so we don't spend much time in bathing suits. So when you have one on in July, and then you don't have it on again until next July, and you've lost 150 lbs. over the year, the bathing suit has to be replaced.

If you live in a climate that is conducive to year 'round bathing suit wearing, then you'll probably have to replace this item more than once as you shrink. You may have more sunshine and warm weather year 'round, but we can spend less money on replacing bathing suits, so there!

When you get out of the pool in your bathing suit, or you get out of the shower, you put on your...what? ROBE. That's right. Yes, you'll have to replace your robe too. When you are actually wrapping it around and it's meeting in the back, no belt in the world is going to hold it in place. Your favorite, comfy, squishy, warm robe will have to go in the pile of too big garments with all your other favorite things. Again, this tidbit is only for women, as we know men will not buy a new robe, EVER, assuming they own one in the first place.

If you've had your swim, and you've had your shower, maybe now you'd like to put on your jammies and go to bed. Oh...but wait...they're too big too. So now you'll have to replace your pajamas. The good news ladies, is that you can make your nightgowns last quite a while, but at some point they'll get so big you'll actually squirm out of the neck of them during the night. Also, when the sleepwear gets really big, the significant other isn't finding it quite so attractive and alluring, if you know what I mean.

Now this little problem is no problem at all if you sleep in the buff, but you'll have to buy at least one sleepwear item to keep in your stash in case you're ever in a hotel and it catches on fire. Everyone (men too), needs to own a set of "hotel fire" jammies. Speaking of hotel fires, when you see them on T.V., there's always people who didn't bring their hotel fire jammies, and have to stand around with their coat on (or someone else's coat on), so they don't have to hide behind a bush while the fire is being put out. That brings us to the next thing that costs money: coats.

Coats have to be replaced as well. I had a most favorite coat, that I affectionately called my "teddy" coat. It was a suede coat in the shearling style, but it was completely lined (pockets too) in the softest fake fur you've ever felt. It's the kind of fur they use to make teddy bears for newborn babies. I bought it two weeks before my surgery, because I didn't know I'd be having surgery that soon. If I'd known I'd have to give it up so soon after adopting it, I would have saved myself the grief and sorrow.

I just adored that coat. It was the warmest, most cuddly coat I'd ever owned, even though it was a size 4x. I had my surgery on October 29, 2003, and by March of 2004, I could wrap the coat around me and tuck each side underneath the opposite arm. I absolutely did not want to give up my teddy coat. I searched and searched, and to this day have not been able to find another one exactly like it. Finally, in April of 2004, as the ice was beginning to melt and a hint of spring was in the air, I found the courage to part with my beloved teddy coat.

In the fall of 2004, however, I had to begin the hunt for a new teddy coat. On top of the fact that I just needed a teddy coat because I missed it, I'd lost a lot of weight and now had the thermostat issue we wrote about in Chapter Four. I'm always cold, so I needed a really warm coat. I hunted, and hunted, but no teddy coat. Oh sure, many masqueraded as teddy coats (only partial teddy fur lining), and there were plenty of teddy coat wannabes, but alas, no teddy coat for Julie.

Then one day, there it was. Not my teddy coat, but a close relative. My teddy coat was tan, and this coat was black. I approached with cautious optimism, not knowing if I could handle another disappointment. I'd searched so long, so hard. I didn't dare hope that this could be the teddy coat I'd devoted my life to finding.

Reaching out, I touched the fur lining expecting to feel the scrape of cheap, imitation teddy fur. But to my surprise, I found the feel of the teddy fur I remembered. Could it be that this was merely a darker version of my cherished teddy coat? Indeed, it was! Oh, joy! My teddy coat had been found, and it was not a size 4x, but simply a misses size large.

Finding my teddy coat meant I would be warm, and it gave me high hopes of surviving the winter after all. My husband was relieved to know that I wouldn't freeze to death in the driveway before reaching my car. All was again right with the world.

But what of my first teddy coat, you ask? What was its fate? Well, at first it was reluctantly boxed up for sale, but I couldn't bear (no pun intended) to part with it, and I felt so guilty putting it away in that cold, lonely box. So, I staged a daring rescue while my husband was away, and it fulfilled a new role in my life: lap blanket. Yes, once again my teddy coat had found purpose and contentment, and I enjoyed its warm and soft embrace. Together we watch television, read books, and cuddled with the cats. My original teddy coat and I had been reunited. My teddy coats and I were going to live happily ever after.

Then a friend (also a Karen) had surgery. It was winter and she had no coat. I debated and debated. Finally, I made the decision to send my teddy coat to live with a nice lady on a farm. She needed a coat, and teddy coat needed a home and a purpose. I wish them all the happiness together that teddy coat and I found with each other.

Replacing your coat is not the end of the line, however. Did it occur to you that your head shrinks too? Yep. It shrinks. If you have nothing in your wardrobe but adjustable baseball caps, then you're probably going to luck out on this one. If, however, you like fitted caps, or have other hats in your accessory wardrobe, you will likely find that they'll end up too big, and they'll have to be replaced.

It doesn't stop with hats though. Let's examine other members of the accessory wardrobe family, shall we? Jewelry also becomes obsolete. Of course we're not suggesting that you ditch your wedding rings, toss your grandmother's locket, or dump the bracelet you received as an anniversary present. What we are telling you is that you may find that your jewelry is now out of scale to your new size. I know that because I was always a big person, and I always wore quite big jewelry so it looked like it "fit." By the time I lost about 80-90 lbs., I found that my jewelry was really just too big, and was overpowering both my outfits and me.

The obvious solution is to run right out and buy all new fine jewelry, right?! After all, diamonds go with everything you know.... But when you wake up from that dream, you figure out that you simply need to begin working on replacing things one piece at a time. Costume jewelry is good, but if you can afford it, buy yourself a nice piece of "real" jewelry as a reward every once in a while, because you deserve it.

Another tip from "Moi," the jewelry queen herself, is instead of rushing out and having your rings resized to your newly slim fingers, refrain from resizing for awhile. First of all, your fingers shrink quite a bit. I lost three rings sizes, so if I had my rings resized every time I shrank a ring size, it would have cost me, on average, about ten dollars per sizing, per ring. That really adds up if you're a jewelry maven like me! I would have had to mortgage my house to pay for my ring resizing!

What I did instead, was to go to a pawnshop that sells jewelry, and look for very thin, plain gold bands. I found ones that fit my new finger size, and now wear them in front of my other rings to hold them on. You really can't see them, they hold your rings on quite well, they can be used over and over again with different rings, and they cost about $6 per band (10k gold). It's much cheaper than paying for repeated ring resizing, and you don't lose all the gold that is taken out of your rings!

So, I've given you a good little tip on jewelry resizing, but I don't really have any good tips on inexpensively replacing your glasses. Your glasses may get too big for your slimmed down face, and that means your sunglasses as well. Sunglasses, if they aren't prescription, aren't too hard to replace. Heck, even the dollar stores carry sunglasses! But prescription glasses are another story, especially if you don't have optical coverage. We suggest keeping a close eye (no pun intended) on the specials offered at various optical centers, especially Sears® and Pearle Vision®, as they run some pretty amazing sales throughout the year.

And...speaking of things that go on your face, don't forget the expense that comes with buying new make-up for the ladies, and skin care products for both men and women. Once you begin to shrink, your face will change shape, and you may begin to see some lines where there were none before. You may also begin to see some droopy skin, or some hanging skin under your chin. This may be helped without the aid of plastic surgery, or Botox® injections simply by purchasing a quality moisturizer with sunscreen, and a skin firming product containing collagen, elastin, and/or Q10.

Many such products exist, but we suggest not heading for the cheapest thing on the market. Your looks are important to your self-esteem (men too), and you should buy a product that will give you the best benefit, not just one that will be easy on your wallet.

Don't buy cheap moisturizers either. We can't overemphasize the need to keep your skin moisturized from the outside, and hydrated from the inside. The drier your skin is, the more it will wrinkle, bag, and sag. Moist, firm skin looks younger and healthier. Even if you have oily skin, there are appropriate moisturizing products out there for you. Men, don't ignore me here! You need moisture too. Drink your water, and slap some moisturizer on your face and body. Your shrinking skin will thank you.

Not only does your skin need to be cared for while you shrink, but your hair does as well. We've already talked about the hair loss issue in Chapter Six, and we've clued you in to the fact that you should take the opportunity to update your look, whether or not you have hair loss issues. Many of us thought that we needed more hair to balance out our heads with our big bodies. I always referred to people with small heads and large bodies as illustrating the "peanut on a pumpkin" effect. Men do this too by growing their hair long, or wearing an outdated style that's just plain out of shape.

As you shrink, however, the proportion between your head and your body changes, and you may find that you don't need all that hair. We suggest going to any clothing store, and standing at least 15 ft. from a full-length mirror. This will let you appraise yourself as a whole person, rather than focusing simply on the bad or the good parts. Then look at the proportions of your hair to your head, and your head to your body. Take a friend who'll be brutally honest with you, and listen to what he or she has to say. Then make an appointment with a good stylist, cut that hair a bit, and update your look.

When you're done, don't sit in the chair 3 ft. from the mirror. Get up and stand 15 ft. away and honestly evaluate how your new cut looks in relation to your face, and in relation to the proportions of your body. Maybe it's the first cut, and maybe it won't be the last. Re-evaluate periodically as you shrink. In any event, you're bound to feel much lighter and incredibly better about yourself, if not a little more broke.

And… with the concept of being broke, comes the biggest offender of them all: replacing your general wardrobe. One of the best things that can happen to you when you lose weight is that you shrink and therefore move into smaller size clothing. One of the worst things that can happen to you when you lose weight is that you shrink and therefore move into smaller size clothing.

Most people when they lose weight only lose one or two sizes, and that means many things can be altered down. When weight loss surgery patients lose weight they generally lose a minimum of four sizes. I lost seven sizes going from a 28 to a 14. Karen lost ten sizes going from 34 to a 14. The average garment can only be altered a maximum of two sizes. I'll wait while you do the math.

Obviously, when you repeatedly shrink right through every thing you own, it's not realistic to keep replacing it over and over again. But it's also not realistic to keep wearing clothes that are literally hanging off you either. So what do you do? Well here are a few tips.

First, one of the obvious benefits of having surgery done through a multi-disciplinary practice is that they provide support groups. Aside from the intended purpose of the support groups, they allow you to meet other people who are approximately your size, and who have gone through the surgery before you or after you. What this facilitates is finding people with whom to "buddy-up" on a clothing co-op. As one shrinks out of something, another can shrink into it.

You don't spend very long in any one size, so the clothing certainly doesn't take a beating. In fact, as we've stated before, many of the items will pass to new owners without even having had the tags removed. It helps tremendously to know that clothing exists to get you to work and other events, and that you don't have to sell a kidney in order to pay for your clothing replacement needs.

As Karen and I went through this process, we buddied-up on almost everything. She knew that when I shrunk out of something, it was only a matter of weeks before she knew she'd shrink into it. (Remember her surgery was 6 weeks behind mine.) In fact, at one point Karen realized that I was buying all the replacement clothes for myself, while she was simply shrinking into mine. I couldn't find anyone to be on the giving end so I could be on the receiving end, as no other patients we met had jobs that required them to dress as formally for their jobs as we did. So, Karen started buying me some clothes because she knew that it was only a matter of time before they came to her, many having never been worn. At least that way we split the cost.

Now we didn't always have just one of any particular item waiting to go through the system. Occasionally we found something both of us wanted at the same time. Generally that desire was made stronger by the fact that it was on serious sale at the time as well. Case in point: the periwinkle blazer.

The first spring after our surgeries we both found a beautiful periwinkle blazer on sale for $29.99. We simply both had to have one as we both look great in that color (doesn't everybody though...?) So we both bought a blazer, and Karen knew that when I shrunk out of mine, I would be out of luck, and she'd be up one new blazer.

Well that time came within a few weeks, and I had to say good-bye to my new blazer. It wasn't quite as sad a parting as I'd had with my teddy coat, because I could visit it every once in a while. My blazer left me and moved in with Karen. Karen shrunk into that blazer and she enjoyed wearing it. I, however, was periwinkle blazer-less, and feeling a little moody about it.

So one day, on another of our famous "important-woman-business" shopping trips, I found another periwinkle blazer, but it was now on sale for $19.99. What luck! I immediately bought it knowing full well that Karen would be able to continue wearing periwinkle blazers far longer than I, and soon she would own this one too.

I stayed in that blazer for a little longer than the first, but eventually it joined its predecessor at Karen's house. Again I went into mourning for my blazer. A few weeks later, Karen had been out of town for a meeting and found yet another periwinkle blazer in a smaller size, and this time it was on clearance for $12.99! She bought it for me, and I was happy for the remainder of the summer. But that happiness was again short-lived. It seemed like only minutes before that blazer was moving out to join its kin at Karen's house. It seemed Karen was destined to remain perfectly clad in periwinkle.

I never saw another periwinkle blazer like that one again, but Karen ultimately ended up with full legal custody of four periwinkle blazers in descending sizes; none of which either one of us can wear anymore or have tailored down. We've since resolved not to engage in that type of behavior again. We've set the maximum legal limit for exact copies of clothing at two. Any more than that is just plain crazy.

In order not to appear crazy, and not to keep spending a ton of money on replacement clothes, here are a few more tips on how to get through this dilemma. First, when buying clothes, buy only on sale, or better yet "clearance," unless it's for a special occasion. Don't buy expensive clothes or investment pieces until you're almost done, or completely done shrinking. You'll just have to say good-bye to more expensive clothing, and more money lost. Also, don't poo-poo shopping at garage sales, resale stores, and consignment shops. Many good bargains are there for the taking.

Second, buy only separate pieces (not suits or matching outfits) and get very good at mixing and matching pieces. If you buy one piece of clothing to match only with another in order to make a specific outfit, you'll be bored, and your wardrobe will be severely limited. Also, if you shrink out of half of the outfit (and you will as parts of you will shrink at different rates than others), what will you do with the other half? Make sure to buy solid color, or minimal print pieces so that you can mix and match for maximum usage.

Third, when buying clothing, make sure that you buy clothes that have a lot of seams. Jackets should have back seams, and preferably princess seaming in the front and back. If you don't know what princess seaming is, ask a salesperson at a store. Remember that pieces can only be altered a maximum of two sizes. The more seams, and/or darts a piece has, the easier it is to have it altered if you really want to get maximum wear-time out of it. See Tips From the Tailor in the resources section.

Also, take the time to find a good tailor who charges reasonable rates. Many good tailors are out there, but some of them charge exorbitant rates. You could replace the item 2 or 3 times for what they want to cut it down one size. Do your shopping, and ask around. People with tailoring shops are not usually your best bet. Tailors or dressmakers who work from their homes generally charge less expensive rates.

Tailors can usually take care of more than one of the problems that arise, however, and that is as your clothes get bigger, they also get longer. If a skirt begins to get bigger, it gets longer too, so have the dressmaker take the skirt in, and shorten it at the same time.

Also, ladies you'll notice that as you begin to hit about size 18 or 16, many of the plus size clothes seem very long, especially blazers, t-shirts, and sweaters. If you think I'm kidding, put your clothes on and stand 15 ft. from a full-length mirror. Look at the proportions of your clothes. Now get your trusty friend (the one who'll be brutally honest), to pin up the hem of the skirt, or the bottom of the jacket or shirt a few inches. Get the sleeve lengths where they should be (approximately 1/2-3/4 of an inch above the thumb knuckle where it connects to the hand). Now look at the proportions on your body. You probably look smaller and taller. Clothes that are too long in proportion simply make you look heavier, and dowdier.

Another way to examine this is to have a friend take digital photos of you. This also helps with wrapping your head around what size you really are, and what you really look like at a particular point in time. The reason this works is because mirrors lie, and our minds lie. If you stand less than 6 ft. from a mirror, your mind will play tricks on you. Some days you'll think you look like a million bucks, and other days you'll think you look like you haven't lost a pound.

Similarly, the mind has a set configuration for recognizing itself, and it will often conform the images being viewed to that configuration. This is one of the basic reasons people look in the mirror and can't see the drastic changes (good or bad) that others see.

People who were thin for most of their lives, can't really see how much weight they've put on until they see a picture of themselves because it's not actual size, like it is in a mirror. In the same vein, those who've been heavy all their lives, have similar difficulties in adjusting their view of themselves as thinner people. It's hard to adjust this "gestalt." Pictures really help us figure out what image to have of ourselves now.

So you may be able to grasp the fact that you've lost weight, but don't get hung up on the numbers printed on the tag on your clothes. You must realize that women's clothes are not like men's. Men's clothes are generally based on actual measurements (17 in. neck, 34 in. waist, 32 in. inseam).

Women's clothing sizes are based on the "fit model" used to create the original patterns. In regular misses sizes, the female model used to fit the original pattern is generally one of those stick figures that walks down the runway in New York. The original pattern is generally a size 4 or 6, and will be dependent on that model's particular body shape, and the cut of the garment.

The manufacturers then usually take the pattern and simply size it up proportionately for each size after size 6. So, it's sort of like tracing 1 in. all the way around it to get the next size, and then tracing 1 in. all the way around that to get the following size, etc., etc.

Plus sizes generally work the same way except that they normally use a plus size model that is a size 12 or 14, and again the fit is dependent on how the model is proportioned. That's why some pants are bigger in the body and slimmer in the legs, and others are cut more fully through the hips and thighs. It depends on where the "fit model" carried her weight, and the cut of the garment.

If the fit model was in between a 12 and a 14, maybe the manufacturer just picked a number, we'll call it a 14, and then went up from there. That's why it may fit smaller than other size 14 clothes by other makers. If the manufacturer cut the garment and called it a 12, however, the garment will fit bigger than garments marked the same size. So what's the point of all this trivia? To let you know that you must shop in a range of three sizes. I can wear anything from a misses size 12 to a 18, or even a size 14w, on occasion if it really fits small.

I don't flip out any more about what the tag says. I go for fit and comfort (and more importantly sale price), more so than what size it says on the tag. Our clothes aren't standardized like men's because they aren't based on actual inch measurements. So stop beating yourself up about what the tag says. The general size that you "are" at any given moment is where you average out in clothes.

I average out at a misses size 14 all over now. As long as I'm not consistently moving up in clothing sizes, I'm okay. We all want to be able to shrink into the next smaller size, but don't get stuck on that. It is okay though to buy something (especially if it's on clearance) that is a bit too small, and hang it in your closet as "goal" clothing. You'll shrink into it soon enough.

In conclusion, I will tell you that losing a large amount of weight is very expensive. I will also tell you, however, that your food budget goes down considerably, and you won't be spending that $50 to $60 a week or more you were spending in the drive-thru or at restaurants. You won't be getting richer, but if you stop and look at it, you will have a little more money left over to help you with some of these expenses. Be creative, be frugal, and be happy you've lost the weight and are healthier, no matter what it might cost or how inconvenient it might be.

Pre-Op Emotional Issues

Well, we've told you about many of the other types of emotional issues you may experience if you have weight loss surgery, but we haven't really discussed the emotional upheaval you may experience during days and hours beforehand. During this time you begin to really grapple with the fact that you're finally going to give up some control of your eating, your weight, and your related medical conditions to other people. You may have thought you were okay with that, but in those hours before surgery it really begins to sink in that you're going to have to let these people help you, you're going to have to let them in and pay attention to what they say, and that this is a one way ride.

This process usually begins with the angst and anxiety that comes from knowing you are going to have to say good-bye to one of your closest, oldest, dearest, and most reliable friends for a while: food. You know that you have to gear up for the pre-operative weight loss program. For some that means a totally liquid protein protocol, and for others it may mean a high protein protocol that also involves protein supplement foods as well, but generally it does not involve pizza, burgers, fries, Ho-Hos, chips, and their friends.

There is a lot of grief and anxiety that accompanies this process, and if you don't watch it, you can actually make your situation a little worse. Our good friend and colleague, Dr. Scott Shikora from Tufts New England Medical Center calls it the "Last Supper Phenomenon." Be careful not to trick yourself into thinking that this is your last supper and that you will *never* be able to eat that food *ever* again. You will be able to eat the food again, and you're not saying good-bye forever — just a little while. Call it a vacation, a detox, or "going on a break." Just don't make it so final. That will help with some of the grief and with some of the weight that will pile on as you are preparing to try and take weight off of your liver and heart to prepare you for a more successful surgery and treatment process. Deal with the food realistically, and deal in facts not "food drama."

In addition to dealing with your food and controlling your food drama, you will also really begin to deal with the fact that you may finally be getting what you've always wanted: permanent relief from the nastiness that comes with being overweight. You will likely start to examine that in *ad nauseum* detail, mulling over whether this is really what you want or not. You think you've given it significant consideration thus far? You haven't even begun the mulling process yet until you hit those last hours before the O.R.

The last hours are when it becomes overwhelmingly real. Many patients begin to face the possibility, albeit a statistically insignificant possibility, that they could die from surgery. You know it is a possibility, and you also know that it's a remote possibility, but still it hits you squarely between the eyes and throws you for a loop.

The fear of the pain begins to creep in, and you remind yourself over and over again that there's medication for that. If you're going to have bypass, you begin to concentrate on the fact that your anatomy is going to be changed pretty much irreversibly, and you're no longer going to be in the condition your Maker made you. If you're going to have a Lap-Band®, you begin to fear having a device inside you permanently, and you begin to fear the needles and the fills, or what could go wrong with the device itself. You may just begin to fear the details of everything.

The fear of change really moves in and sets up housekeeping as well. You start to think about all the things that may become different, and strangely you don't necessarily see them as being positive anymore. You may find yourself clinging to the familiar because it's a known quantity. When the fear sets in you must keep reminding yourself, and have others remind you as well, "You can do anything afraid, that you can do unafraid." If that doesn't work, try "Always, always, always, always, always do what you are afraid to do." This is also a time to find your faith, whatever it may be, and hold on to that. It will help with the fear and emotional overload now and down the road, more than you know.

For some people the emotions are all over the map; happiness, sadness, fear, panic. For others it is manifested in sheer elation. This has never been more apparent to me than when I had my surgery and I was in the holding room right outside the O.R. In that room there are about twelve beds with people waiting to go in for various types of surgeries. It doesn't matter what type of surgery you're having, you may still go through this type of fear, analysis, emotional turmoil, and second-guessing.

When I was waiting to be brought to the O.R., I noticed other people who were waiting to have weight loss surgery done by Dr. Baker's partners. They appeared to be everything from happy and excited, to crying and scared, and one was almost morose. Personally, I was freaking out because despite the number of other surgeries I'd had in the previous two and a half years, I began to have flashbacks to my accident and the first night they took me into surgery. I wasn't prepared for that. I thought I had the fear of surgery licked. I thought I had it under control and it was a no-brainer. I was wrong.

I guess it kicked in for me because deep down I knew this surgery was going to be as life altering as the first one after my accident. That one determined whether I lived or died, walked or didn't walk. This one also determined, in a way, whether I really "lived" or not. I didn't expect the terror, the uncontrolled panic and hysteria, and the feeling that I wanted to leave as fast as I could, and didn't even care where I went. I wasn't prepared for any of that, and that scared me even more.

Intellectually, I knew that this surgery was a good thing, that it was the right thing, but emotions are pretty unpredictable little monsters, and they gave me a great big "gotcha." Others in the room were very confused, and kept asking nurses what kind of surgery I was having done. Other weight loss surgery patients, especially the ones that were happy and excited, were a bit perplexed, and I fear I kind of made them second guess their own happiness and commitment to going forward. Oooops! Sorry.

But as we keep telling you, each person is radically different from the next. We can't predict for you how you'll react, just know that you will and it's okay to do so. Karen, for example, was also a basket case. She was hit by a wave of emotion she and her family weren't prepared for either. She couldn't stop crying, she was terrified of the change coming in her life, and she was overwhelmed by the fear of the unknown.

Karen had such a death grip on her mom and me that I still have the scars on my fingers where she was squeezing my hand, and the diamonds on my wedding band cut my fingers open. I did finally manage to wrangle myself free and seek some medical attention for that (and an x-ray...), but I still feel bad about leaving her poor little mom to fend for herself. Sorry about that Mrs. Sparks.

Dr. Baker and his Physician Assistants, Matt and Randy, were entirely supportive and understanding, and helped both Karen and me during those last moments before going into surgery. They made sure that we got a little something to help calm us down before we went in. It was a good thing too, as after I got Karen to release the Vulcan Death Grip on my hand, she clamped onto the bed rail, and would have been responsible for replacing an expensive piece of medical equipment had she not started to relax just as the metal was about to snap!

Just as with my experience, there were several others waiting to go to surgery when Karen was in the pre-op holding area. This one particular woman was so excited she could hardly contain herself, and she just couldn't understand why Karen was upset and scared. She kept trying to talk to Karen and ask her questions. Karen was torn between screaming at this woman to just shut-up and leave her alone, and hiding under the covers. Fortunately they have those curtains you can draw around the bed as I feared it would have been the former rather than the latter, and it wouldn't have been any too polite or quiet.

So to draw this section to a close, we just want you to know that whatever range of emotions you feel, and whatever decides to jump up and down on you in those last hours before surgery, know that it is perfectly normal, and all will work out the way it is supposed to work out. Keep supportive, loving people close to you, let your medical team know exactly what you're feeling and let them help you, and take pity on those who offer to hold your hand. We're only here to help; paralysis and scarring isn't part of the bargain.

Surgical and Physical Issues

We're moving from pre-op to post-op now. The first thing we want to emphasize is that you must do what they ask you to do from the moment you wake up from surgery. They will ask you to get out of bed and walk around sometime within 12 hours after surgery. No, you will not want to get up and walk, but you have to anyway. It's for your own good.

Walking helps to get the blood flowing again, and prevents blood clots from forming. Walking also gets you breathing, helps to move the anesthetic out of your lungs and system, and helps to re-inflate your lungs so you won't have a pulmonary collapse. Walking is good, even if it doesn't feel good.

The next important piece of advice we can give you is to accurately and calmly assess your pain level (on a scale of 1-10, with 10 being the worst pain you've ever felt in your life), and report it to your nurse. Don't try and be a big brave soldier. You must break the pain cycle, and keep it broken. If they give you one of those little jeopardy buttons *(PCA – patient controlled analgesic device)* for the pain, then use it. You can't overdose on it. It's regulated, and you can press the thing all you want, but it will only give you a measured dose at set time intervals. So if it is set for every 10 minutes, you can push the button like there's no tomorrow, and it will only give you the correct dosage every 10 minutes.

Breaking the pain cycle is important. If you doze off, and you will, press it as soon as you wake up. You'll fall asleep and you'll think you've been asleep for hours, but you may find it's only been 8 minutes. Press the button anyway. It can't hurt, but it can help.

If you don't have a PCA, make sure to tell the nurse when you're becoming painful again. Don't try and tough it out. There's no point to that, unless you have some weird affinity for pain and suffering. If that's the case, you have bigger problems than being overweight. Just take the medication. You are not receiving enough to become addicted.

Dr. Baker says that even if you've had problems with pain medication addiction in the past, make sure that your doctor is aware of the issue, and it will be handled in an appropriate manner. Just because you've had a problem with addiction does not mean that you have to suffer through the pain with no help. Trust your medical team to know what to do to help you.

Also, when you go home, your doctor will most likely send you with some form of pain medication, probably in liquid form (for which you will be grateful). Follow the instructions and take the pain medication. Remember that we told you the pain is worst on days 2 through 5. For Lap-Band® patients, the medication should work for you as it would for any other person. For gastric bypass patients, however, be aware that medication tends to get into the bloodstream pretty fast after surgery, not unlike alcohol. So from the perspective of pain relief it works quite fast, but also know that other medications may kick in quite quickly too. Whether or not that is an issue is something you should discuss with your physician before surgery.

After surgery, the medical staff may also want you to breathe into the spirometer (the little device that you breathe in to make the balls move up and down). Although it may seem stupid, and it may seem hard to do, or cause some pain in your diaphragm, please don't ignore this little treatment. You don't have to do it forever, just for a couple of days. Take pity on your little lungs, and your whole body for that matter, and just be compliant. It's really quite necessary, and it is not designed just to annoy you, or just for the sake of being a pain in the neck. Waking you up to tell you to go to sleep, now that is designed to annoy you, and is just for the sake of being a pain in the neck!!!

So the moral of this story is: Do as you are told. Gee, just like mom said all those years ago. Again, they're not doing it for the good of their health, they're doing it for the good of yours. More wise words from my sister Cheryl that we've all internalized: "They are not the enemy."

Julie and Karen's Personal Theories About Stuff

Let me just say right off that this is a totally unscientific, untested, unfounded, unresearched portion of the book. These are 100% our personal observations, and they have no scientific merit whatsoever. That being said, we will also say that they have proven to work over and over again, so we do claim some form of validity and reliability in our totally non-scientific experiments.

The first theory has developed from an experiment I have been running for about the last 30 years of my life. Karen is new to the experiment, but she can report that she has been able to reproduce my results on a consistent basis. This theory is called the Skinny Mirror Theory.

For the last 30 or so years I have been testing just about any mirror I encounter to determine whether the mirror reflects an accurate image of me, or whether it reflects a slightly modified, somewhat "fun house" version of what I look like by making me appear taller and slimmer than I really am while not completely distorting the image.

Many such mirrors exist, and they should be noted as to their locations across the country. I've noticed that mid-priced to expensive clothing stores tend to invest in the placement of skinny mirrors throughout their facilities. I believe they understand the psychology behind the use of skinny mirrors in that customers tend to buy just about anything that makes them look thinner, no matter how hideous it may in fact be. Less expensive stores don't seem to care, they just hope you'll buy anything.

The danger in skinny mirrors is exactly as I've just stated: you may be prone to buying anything that makes you look thinner, no matter how hideous it might be. So, although having a skinny mirror in your home is a wonderful, life affirming thing, be mindful that the skinny mirrors in stores can have a hallucinogenic effect that may inhibit your judgment and impulse control.

To prevent skinny mirrors from inappropriately affecting your buying habits, be sure to stand at least 15 ft. from all full length mirrors in stores when evaluating a potential clothing purchase. This tends to negate the "overthinning" effect of the skinny mirror, and the attendant cascade of whatever brain chemicals are involved in the rabid buying behavior that goes on after that.

Skinny mirrors, however, make wonderful home companions. Once appropriate clothing has been purchased (by that we mean it is not hideous and has not been purchased while under the influence of a skinny mirror), the home skinny mirror will become a trusted friend that sends you on your way every day with a positive attitude and a spring in your step.

As a word of caution, "fat mirrors" also exist, and these are to be avoided at all costs. In the event a home skinny mirror cannot be located and procured, a regular accurate mirror will serve in its place until an appropriate replacement can be found. Under no circumstances should a fat mirror ever reside in your home whether by purchase or by gift. Fat mirrors are evil and should be destroyed on sight.

The next theory we've developed is called the Ketchup Theory. The Ketchup Theory is a fairly new theory for us, and like the rest of the theories that follow, were developed solely post-surgery. Although it involves ketchup, don't discount it off the bat if you are not a ketchup lover. It also involves other substances made with tomatoes, but the term "Ketchup, Tomato Soup, Tomato Sauce, Tomatoes, Salsa, Pizza Sauce Theory," was just a bit too long and unwieldy.

The Ketchup Theory deals with the effect that comes from eating foods accompanied by tomato-based products. We find, and we've asked others too, that foods tend to sit better and not fight back as much, if they are accompanied by a tomato-based product. As we said, there's no scientific proof for this, but we prefer to believe that it is because of the acid in the tomatoes.

As the new little pouch has virtually no acid makers in it at all (they're almost all in the remainder of the stomach), we think that the acid helps with breaking down the food a bit before it reaches the true stomach acid down in the small bowel. There may be no truth to this at all, but all we know is that whenever we eat food with a bit of ketchup, the food sits better.

I can eat a few french fries if I dip them in ketchup. If I eat more than two french fries without ketchup, they just don't sit well and I'm quite uncomfortable for a while. Now, the Ketchup Theory is not professing to allow you to eat a whole order of french fries. It will not do that for you, and you shouldn't be doing that anyway. If you do, you probably deserve the auto eject experience you're going to have.

What it does seem to do is allow you to eat a few fries so you feel like a regular person, without sending you into cramps or auto eject. Similarly, a bit of low-fat or fat-free spaghetti sauce on chicken gives it a nice flavor and helps it go down quite well. A 1/2 cup of tomato soup (with actual tomatoes), and a half of a wrap sandwich seems to work out quite well also. So don't run out and cover everything in the world in ketchup or tomato sauces. Remember that they have calories and other ingredients too, not the least of which is often a high sugar content from high fructose corn syrup. Tomatoes are high in lycopene and potassium, as well as vitamin K. If you're on blood thinners, be wary of how much tomato-based product you consume. If you're allergic to food acids like I am, then be careful in your consumption, and keep some anti-histamines handy.

The next theory is somewhat related to the Ketchup Theory, and is called the "Greasing the Skids Theory." By "greasing the skids" we mean making sure that you've had something to drink (preferably water) at least 10-15 minutes before you eat (as Carrie and Dr. Baker have told you), and if you haven't, then grease the skids by adding in some small form of light liquid as part of the meal itself. I'll explain.

As Carrie and Dr. Baker have said, you should drink some water 10-15 minutes before meals, and then about an hour after meals. The drinking before meals helps to control the need to tear into your food. But we've also found that if you don't have much liquid in the system, things might just get stuck in the pipes, so to speak.

If I get up in the morning and eat something without having had at least a half a bottle of water first, it just gets stuck, and then it hurts. I hate starting my day that way. Then I had the brilliant idea of just starting the day by eating a yogurt. After all, it is liquid, right? That didn't work well either. I made myself quite ill. I guess it's more solid than liquid or something.

From our experiences, it works best if you just drink some water and let it sit a couple of minutes before you eat. "But what if I can't drink 10-15 minutes before I eat? What if I'm not in a position to do that?" you ask. Well then the second half of the theory comes into play. We suggest, and we're not giving you a license to go crazy here, that you might have a bit of mustard on the side to dip meat into, or a 1/4-1/2 cup of soup *with* the meal, not before.

Maybe a little salsa (there's that Ketchup Theory again) could be put to use to make meat or other foods a bit more "wet." Do not, however, drown anything in sauces or condiments. Dipping is okay, drowning in it is not. You're just "greasing" the skids a little, not submerging them in liquid.

And speaking of liquid, that brings us to our final theory, the "Tea Theory." The Tea Theory is also very similar in nature to the Ketchup Theory in that it involves our suppositions regarding the tannic acid in tea. Now we're referring to tea as being either iced or hot, but not containing lemon. We have found, and almost every single person we've talked to has had the same response, that citric acid tends to be too strong and isn't tolerated well after gastric bypass. Some Lap-Banders seem to do well with citric acid products, while others do not. Maybe it has to do with the tightness of the band or something…I don't know. Citric acid is the type of acid found in citrus fruits like lemons, oranges, limes, and grapefruits.

Tea contains tannic acid, however, which appears to be somewhat on the strength of the acid in tomato-based products, and it seems to do the same thing. The difference is that you ingest it about an hour after eating, not while eating. The caution that comes with this theory, is to refrain from drinking it while eating, and from drinking too much of it. Not only does it contain caffeine which makes you hungrier because it is a gastric stimulant, but if consumed in large quantities, it does contain a significant amount of acid that can adversely affect your bones. Also, it will turn your teeth brown, so break out the whitening strips.

The tea does provide a nice little diversion from water now and again though, and decaffeinated tea is always an option. Tea seems to help with digestion, and in settling the stomach if you're feeling a little nauseous. If you like your tea sweet (for our friends in the South and from the British Isles), then may we humbly suggest that you *not* use regular sugar or artificial sweeteners. If it becomes a toss-up between artificial stuff or regular sugar, take the sugar every time.

Artificial sweeteners are incredibly bad for you. They actually break down in the body into formaldehyde (yes, the stuff that they embalm people with), and that formaldehyde does not break down further, but is actually stored in the brain. Many people suffer from terrible headaches and have found that when they stopped ingesting artificial sweeteners in any form (soda pop too) that their headaches virtually disappeared. My own sister and mother are two people for whom this has been true.

If you must sweeten things (and that's okay), we strongly suggest either brown sugar, honey, stevia, or Splenda® which is made from sugar. Please remember that all of these contain extra calories, and sugar turns to glucose, which when unused turns to stored fat in the body. You don't have to completely eliminate sugar, just be aware of how much and how often you ingest it.

Well, I guess that's about it for now. We really could have done a whole separate book on crazy little things like this, but we decided to let you find your own stuff to fill up your personal junk drawer. Along the way you'll discover your own unique oddities that work for you, and you'll be making notes for at least a year on these weird little experiences. As you do, just tuck them away in your mental junk drawer because just as in real life, no two junk drawers are the same, and they're each very specific to the home in which they reside.

So with that, this junk drawer is now full, and needs to be closed. The next time you need that odd but useful thing that doesn't seem to reside anywhere else, remember to check the junk drawer first.

SLAM!

Chapter Fifteen

SHRINK!
← SHRANK! ←
SHRUNK!

Randal S. Baker MD, FACS
Julie M. Janeway
Karen J. Sparks

As the title states, you've had surgery to *shrink*, you *shrank* down to a more healthy weight, and now you've pretty much *shrunk* to the size you want to maintain. Can you conjugate the verb "to shrink? I bet you can if you try...." (Apologies to Mr. Rogers. He probably won't be my neighbor now that I've made fun of him.) So, now that you've been through this process, what's left is maintaining your new weight and healthy lifestyle, and dealing with a few other little issues and questions that might crop up.

One of the most commonly raised patient questions goes something like this: "What about all that extra, flabby, hangy-down skin after you lose the weight? Isn't that a big problem?" I usually respond, "If in one to two years you have extra, flabby-type skin hanging around, it is an excellent problem to have!" I say this not to be dismissive or insensitive, but to point out that the apparent cosmetic dislike of excessive skin pales in significance to the medical problems related to the morbid obesity you had in the first place.

In other words, by the time you have baggy skin (if you have it at all — a lot of patients do not have excess skin issues), many, if not most of your serious weight related medical problems will be significantly improved, and maybe even gone. Unlike obesity, baggy skin does not lead to diabetes, high blood pressure, heart disease, arthritis, sleep apnea, stroke, and an increased risk of some cancers. Many long for the day when the only problem they have to deal with is some "hangy-down" skin! Having plastic surgery to remove excess skin is not, however, the automatic final step in the bariatric surgery process.

According to the American Society for Metabolic and Bariatric Surgery, in 2004 approximately 140,000 people had weight loss surgery in the United States alone, in 2005 it increased to 170,000, and the number is expected to hit a quarter million in 2007.[1] From 1998 to 2004 bariatric surgeries increased nine fold, and according to the American Society of Plastic Surgeons (ASPS), more than 66,000 post-bariatric plastic surgery procedures were performed in 2003 (remembering that many patients had more than one plastic surgery procedure performed).[2]

Body contouring plastic surgery has increased significantly in the last few years. According to the ASPS, the following proceduers have increased exponentially from 2000 to 2006:[3]

Buttock lifts	up 174%
Breast lifts	up 96%
Lower body lifts	up 4,887%
Thigh lifts	up 132%
Abdominoplasties	up 133%
Upper arm lifts	up 4,304%

Although it appears that bariatric surgery patients may be running to plastic surgery following massive weight loss, the ASPS reports that only about 15% of bariatric surgery patients actually seek plastic surgery for their redundant skin issues.[4] Body contouring after bariatric surgery has become a field of special interest to many plastic surgeons, and they are beginning to realize that bariatric patients have different needs and issues than non-bariatric body contouring patients. Body contouring and shaping plastic surgery is more difficult for the post-bariatric surgery patient because the skin has generally been permanently damaged by being so extremely stretched. As a result of this stretching, patients' skin will generally loosen with age faster than patients who have not been obese, which may result in a degradation of the surgical results.[5]

Another issue for post-bariatric surgery patients having plastic surgery is controlling post-operative nausea and vomiting resulting from anesthetic and other medications. Excessive vomiting may cause ulceration of the pouch or esophagus, and may damage the connections in the new gastric anatomy. This can be controlled well for all patients, but especially for weight loss surgery patients, by administering an intravenous dose of anti-nausea medications before or during surgery. Bariatric patients seeking plastic surgery after full weight loss should locate a plastic surgeon who is familiar with the special needs of weight loss surgery patients.

All this being said, there is a legitimate role for plastic surgery after significant weight loss. Major weight gain puts tremendous strain on the entire body, including the skin and fascia. The skin becomes stretched and usually shows strain patterns (translation: stretch marks) similar to those seen on the abdomens of women after pregnancy. For persons who lose large amounts of weight, the skin often does not regain its original shape. For these people, plastic surgery becomes an option.

In addition, the older you are, the less resiliency in your skin. Many people who lose weight in their 20s and 30s do not have nearly as much wrinkled and excess skin. Often when they lose all of their excess weight it becomes difficult to know that they were ever obese. As a general rule: the older you are, the greater the likelihood of more excessive skin after weight loss. But remember, excessive skin is not solely the domain of the "mature." It can affect people who are not yet even in their twenties depending on how stretched the skin became during the term of obesity.

For those patients who do end up with redundant skin issues, plastic surgery may be an option, but know that it is not usually covered by insurance as it is seen as a cosmetic and elective procedure. If you are experiencing rashes, welts, acne, yeast or other infections, skin breakdown, boils, or other dermatological issues in the redundant skin areas, see a physician. If you are interested in plastic surgery, the fact that you are repeatedly suffering from these types of issues may help get the surgery covered because it may become "medically necessary" to treat it surgically. Patients who also suffer from the skin interfering in their activities of daily life should report this to their doctors as well.

Some patients simply don't have insurance that will ever cover plastic surgery, and so they are basically stuck dealing with the unpleasant moisture, rubbing, rashes, etc. Whether you are waiting for bariatric or plastic surgery, or you are simply living with some of these nasty and irritating skin issues, consult your doctor or pharmacist about a wonderful treatment ointment and moisture barrier called Calmoseptine®. It does *not* require a prescription, and works exceptionally well on these types of problems. You don't have to stuff a half a box of kleenex in the skin folds anymore to try and keep the skin dry and keep it from chafing. Calmoseptine® is a great treatment option. You can also find them on the web at www.calmoseptineointment.com. So whether you are going to have plastic surgery or not, you can at least deal with excess skin issues plaguing you on a daily basis.

The most common surgical excess skin issue deals with the fat and skin on the lower abdomen. Significant weight loss can leave a large hanging "apron" of excess skin and fat below the stomach area which is called a *panniculus*. In some patients this can be what many women call a little "poochy tummy," and can look relatively normal. In other patients, however, it can hang down to the thigh and knee area obstructing walking, can pull or inordinately strain lower back and abdominal muscles, can cause yeast infections or become infected, causes hygiene issues, and can create terrible difficulties with proper clothing fit.

Probably the second biggest complaint is flabby skin that may appear in the upper arms and thighs. Again, not all patients encounter this problem. Men in particular, tend not to have issues with their arms or thighs. The reality is, however, that if you are going to have excess skin in these areas, no amount of toning or weight lifting is going to completely eliminate it.

Whether it's the arms, the thighs, or the abdomen, the fascia (connective tissue) region of the muscles also becomes stretched with weight gain. Unfortunately, fascia does not shrink significantly after weight loss surgery, or after having a baby either for that matter. Just like arms and thighs, it's a mistake to think that "toning" or exercise will help shrink the fascia on the belly. If you have loose skin anywhere, you have only two choices: deal with it and be grateful you're no longer obese and unhealthy, or have it removed.

So, what's involved in having it removed? Well, surgery is sometimes medically recommended if the large "fatty apron" has infections and open sores, or interferes with daily activities such as walking. As I pointed out earlier though, surgery for excess skin is entirely cosmetic, and most insurance companies only cover surgery if it is deemed "medically necessary."

Patients who desire plastic surgery often have to pay out-of-pocket, and plastic surgery is not cheap. There are options though, so if you've really got your heart set on having plastic surgery to deal with a problem, and you don't have insurance coverage, check out CareCredit. They finance medical procedures for people who don't have insurance coverage, including bariatric surgery by the way. You can learn more about them at www.carecredit.com. Perhaps taking a loan for plastic surgery might be a good trade-off for you.

It is also important to note that plastic surgery involves the trade of one cosmetic problem (loose skin) for another (scars). Most plastic surgeons will tell you that if you are unwilling to accept scars, you should not have plastic surgery as no surgeon can predict how the scars will heal on your body. Julie has told me many times that she would love to have some of the skin removed from her upper arms, but she is not willing to have to live with two more scars.

From past experience, Julie already knows that she scars badly, and to her, the excess skin is a small price to pay for the weight loss. Her arms are much smaller, she has no problem with clothing fit, and the skin is sound and causing no problems. Both she and I see no real need for plastic surgery on her arms. Does she have arms like Madonna? No. Does she need arms like Madonna? No. Is she healthy? YES.

For those determined to follow the plastic surgery path, however, there are a variety of surgeries available for the removal of excess skin and fat. The surgery that removes the excess panniculus, or skin and fat of the apron on the lower belly is called a *panniculectomy*. This surgery usually involves a large incision low on the abdomen where the excessive skin and fat are removed but the fascia is not touched. This is the type of surgery most likely to be covered, if at all, by your insurance company.

In contrast, an *abdominoplasty* includes removal of the excess skin and fat from the upper abdomen, along with tightening the fascia over the main muscle of the belly wall. Often times *liposuction* (suctioning of fat) is also done to contour the abdomen and waist line. This surgery gives a flatter appearance to the abdominal area and is often performed in conjunction with a panniculectomy (lower abdomen) in order to remove all the excess skin from the mid region of the torso.

These three surgeries together are sometimes referred to as a *mid-body lift*. Unfortunately, quite often this surgery is not covered by insurance, and patients are left to pay on their own. *Thigh lifts, arm lifts, facelifts,* and *total body lifts* can also be considered if necessary, but are almost always totally cosmetic and not covered by insurance.

A *medial thigh lift* is performed by making an incision along the inner thigh, and the location and length of the scar is based on the amount of skin that needs to be removed. Incisions can range from 4 inches, to the entire length of the thigh from the groin to just above the knee. Once the incision is made, the excess skin is removed, and the remaining skin is re-draped over the muscles.

If a thigh or leg lift is performed in conjunction with an abdominoplasty, and a *butt lift*, it is referred to as a *lower body lift*. A lower body lift may or may not include liposuction as well. A medial thigh lift addresses the excess skin on the inside of the thighs, while a lower body lift addresses the excess skin on the front, back, and outer thighs.

A *butt lift*, sometimes referred to as a *gluteplasty* or *glutepexy* (top of the buttocks), or *excisional back lipidectomy* (bottom of the lower back), is exactly what you would imagine it to be. It is the procedure that removes skin from the upper gluteal (buttock) and/or lower back region in order to lift and tighten all the skin below it. This procedure has an added benefit in that it tends to raise the skin on the back of the thighs a bit as well. The scar for a butt lift generally extends across the entire backside from hip to hip.

Moving up the body from hip to breast, another problem many women encounter is *masto ptosis*, or *breast droop* following significant weight loss. Breast droop is defined as the situation in which the nipple has actually drooped below the crease beneath the breast. In situations where the nipple remains above the crest, and only breast tissue sags below the crest, it is referred to as a pseudo-droop.

Breast augmentation surgery, or *breast implants* will improve pseudo-droop, but will not usually do anything for women who have drooping breasts. For this problem, a *breast lift* or *mastopexy* is the procedure that may be needed. In a breast lift a keyhole incision is made from the crest of the breast up and around the nipple. The nipple is moved up, and excess skin (and possibly fat) is removed. The breast incision is then closed, leaving an incision scar from the site of the new nipple placement down to the crest of the breast. An additional scar may appear across the crest of the breast depending on the size of the reduction that was performed, or if implants were placed. As a general rule, the more extensive the droop, the more extensive the scars.

If a patient develops excess skin in the upper arms, the only way to improve this problem is through an *arm lift*, or *brachioplasty*. The brachioplasty is done in a very similar fashion to the medial thigh lift. The major disadvantage of an arm lift is that the scars will extend down the length of the inside of the upper arm, from armpit to elbow. If you wear long sleeves to cover the excess skin on your arms, will you be forced to wear long sleeves to cover the scars on your arms? If so, then why put yourself through a surgical procedure, as all surgeries have the potential for complications and other issues? The advantages and disadvantages must always be weighed in determining whether or not to have plastic surgery. It can be very beneficial and affirming, but can also lead to the creation of other problems you could just as well do without.

Another issue many weight loss patients would rather do without is the problem of sagging skin on their faces or neck. Other excess skin issues can be covered by clothing, but sagging facial or neck skin is a real problem in that it can't really be covered, and it makes patients feel older and less attractive. Feeling better about yourself, your health, and your appearance are basic reasons for losing weight to begin with, so results that contradict that are often unacceptable to patients who have worked so hard to change their bodies.

A *face lift* or *rhytidectomy* will lift sagging cheeks, eliminate those pesky jowls, and contour the jawline. It can also remove excess fat under the chin or lift sagging skin on the neck. What it will not do, is eliminate wrinkles, sun damage, acne scars, and other skin issues. For those types of skin problems other procedures such as *derm-*

abrasion, chemical peels, and *laser resurfacing* may be available, and you should consult with a dermatologist or plastic surgeon. Sagging eyelids or foreheads can require different surgeries as well.

Face lift scars generally start above your ear, move down in front of your ear, and go behind the earlobe into the hairline. Another incision is made under the chin. Most scars fade quite well, and can be hidden with makeup. After 3 months or so, the scars are usually undetectable, although no surgeon can make that guarantee. Face lifts are one of the least invasive reconstructive procedures for bariatric patients, compared to procedures such as lower body lifts, and total body lifts that can place in the body 600 or more incision stitches during one operation.

Many of the plastic surgeries that are done on patients after weight loss surgery also involve *liposuction.* Liposuction is done two ways: *tumescent* and *ultrasonic.* Tumescent, or *true tumescent* liposuction is the type of fat suctioning surgery that has been performed in the United States since the 1970s. This form of liposuction involves filling the fat with tumescent fluid (saline with adrenaline and lidocaine) to make the fat stiffer, and reduce bleeding and discomfort.

Once the fat has been stiffened by the tumescent liquid, it is then suctioned out by the insertion of long thin rods called *cannulas.* The tiny incisions involved are often hidden in skin creases, and are generally no bigger than the incisions made for laparoscopic bariatric surgery.

Ultrasonic liposuction on the other hand, involves the infusion of tumescent fluid to stiffen the fat, but rather than suctioning the stiffened fat out in its globular form, the surgeon uses an ultrasonic rod (energy waves similar to sound, but higher frequencies) to liquify the fat before it is removed. The rod is inserted through tiny incisions as well. As it passes by the fat it liquefies it, and it is then suctioned out in a fluid form.

Plastic surgery professionals are split over the issue of which technique is better. Although both techniques have a very low incidence of blood loss to begin with, there is slightly less blood loss with ultrasonic. Discomfort seems to be about equal for both. The best advice we can give you is to consult with your plastic surgeon on which technique is right for you. Plastic surgeons will usually recommend the technique with which they are most familiar and that is always a plus for the patient, unless you are willing to volunteer to be the patient on which they learn a new technique.

For weight loss surgery patients in general, it is best to wait at least one and a half years (18 months) post-bariatric procedure before considering any type of plastic surgery. Patients fare far better when they wait for their weight to stabilize, because their bodies are healthier going into surgery. Patients who wait for plastic surgery experience fewer infections, respiratory complications, and wound reopenings. Those who forge ahead with premature surgery will often desire to have the surgery repeated because of further laxity of the skin as a result of further weight loss.

Generally plastic surgery is not medically necessary, and there is no real rush to get into it. Many patients do not choose to pursue this type of surgery, and that option is fine as well. The goal is to learn to live as realistic and normal a life as possible, with as few surgical interventions as possible.

With that said, I believe a word about realistic expectations is needed at this juncture. Plastic surgery will help some with overall appearance and self-acceptance but don't expect the "extreme makeover" hype as seen in many television shows. You are not likely going to look like Barbie Beauty after surgery if you didn't resemble her before. And guess what? You don't need to! You are fine being you.

The most important thing is that you are no longer suffering from obesity, have improved or resolved its serious related medical conditions, and you are now much more healthy and vital than you were before. It has been my experience that some patients are just not happy with themselves in general, and keep looking toward plastic surgery (and even bariatric surgery) to make a fairy tale ending to a not-so fairy tale life. These expectations are often hollow and lead to disappointment.

Like any other surgery, plastic surgery has risks: some significant, and some not so significant. These must be realistically discussed with your surgeon prior to any attempt at "reconstruction" or "body contouring." Just keep in mind that the excess skin dilemma (assuming there are no serious skin issues) is a not-so-bad circumstance to find oneself in after claiming a total success and victory over morbid obesity.

Ladies, if you have to wait for plastic surgery, elect not to have it, or are otherwise prevented from having it, remember that there are good support garments out there that can help with carrying around torso skin, hiding or disguising it better, and assist with clothing fit. There are lots of catalogs, stores, and boutiques that cater to these sorts of products, but Julie and Karen recommend that you check out Lipo In A Box®. This company makes support, shapewear, and other garments, and specializes in weight loss surgery patients. Connie Elder, owner of Lipo In A Box® is a friend of Julie and Karen's and her products have been seen and featured in O Magazine, Glamour, QVC, as well as on The View and the Today Show. So check them out too at www.lipoinabox.com.

In addition to supporting the skin and feeling good on the outside, it's important to keep doing what's right for you on the inside. Maintenance is key to long-term success with plastic surgery as well as bariatric surgery. Unhealthy eating and little exercise will challenge and reverse some of the best plastic surgery results. As noted repeatedly in this book, a total lifestyle change will be necessary to achieve the best result possible, with or without plastic surgery.

Keeping up the habits you developed to get the weight off, and continually developing new and better ones is what the maintenance portion is all about. If you think it's just going to stay off, you're wrong. You'll have to work at it like everybody else, for the rest of your life.

Keep your life in perspective and appreciate it every day, even when the days are tough for whatever reason. Remind yourself that balance is a new life credo. Balance all things: food, exercise, self-concept, work, attitude, ego, etc. Don't go overboard on any one thing. This metamorphosis was designed to give you a good start on a good life, now it's up to you to maintain it. It was not designed to move you off in any one direction so far as to become completely unrecognizable in any aspect from the person who started the journey.

Periodically take photographs of yourself, and really look at them. Make sure that you're not just seeing what you want to see in the mirror, or what your mind wants to see as being you. Make sure you aren't putting the weight back on. Make sure that you aren't turning yourself into someone you're not, like trying to reclaim lost youth by sporting clothing your 13 year old daughter wears!

Being your age, whatever that may be, is okay. Celebrate the fact that you have lived, and given your previous weight circumstances, that you have survived those years. Be glad for the knowledge, wisdom, insight, experiences, and love you have felt through those years. Be happy with what you have accomplished, and don't fixate on what you have missed. There's nothing more pathetic than someone in their thirties (or later), male or female, trying to act and dress like they are still in their early twenties (or worse yet, teens!).

It's okay to feel young. It's okay to act as a vital, alive person. But remember to be who you are and make the most out of what is happening now, not waste it trying to relive lost years or opportunities. Put the past in the past. Embrace the here-and-now, and look excitedly toward the future. You deserve it!

Chapter Sixteen

THE FINAL BATTLE: — DEFEAT — OF THE CLONES

Randal S. Baker MD, FACS

You've made it to the end of this book, and that means we've pretty thoroughly explored weight loss surgery, one particular method of dealing with obesity. Surgery is the most effective means available today for dealing with the disease and its related maladies. But what about in the future? How will obesity be treated, or possibly eliminated in the future? Will we really have to live for another 50 or 100 years putting up with all those obnoxious miracle-diet commercials that are simply clones of each other? Will the miracle-diet clones take over the airwaves of the future? Good Heavens, we hope not!

More than likely the future will *not* be populated with a growing profusion of miracle-diet clones claiming to cure obesity and "whatever else ails ya!" I have no doubt, however, that these clones will continue to exist in some form or another as the age old tradition of "snake oil" sales seems to defy time, space, and social progress. Sadly, the clones will co-exist for a little while at least, while advances in varying technologies aimed at defeating obesity (and hopefully defeating the miracle-diet clones as well!) continue to evolve.

The future will likely see several diverse approaches to treating and/or eliminating the obesity epidemic. As the cause is essentially a combination of genetic predispositions and environment, scientists will have to combat the issue on both fronts. At present the surgical battle-plan offers a way to "fool" the genetic predispositions, and force some environmental changes. Less food makes one feel full, overeating leads to nausea and vomiting, and eating the wrong foods can lead to dumping (auto eject). The weapon is an effective one, but isn't available to all combatants in the battle.

Currently, surgery is only recommended for patients in the *morbidly obese* camp (BMI greater than 40), because the risk/benefit ratio is not as medically justifiable for people in the *overweight* and *obese* categories (BMI between 25 and 39). Remember that approximately 65% of the U.S. population is *overweight* and *obese*, and that number is increasing dramatically, but the surgical option is not generally available to them in their battle with the bulge.

I believe that improvements will continue to make surgery safer, as well as to possibly open up the field for the use of less-invasive surgical techniques (laparoscopic RYGB or Lap-Band®) for patients even in the obese category. The use of less invasive "micro-surgical" techniques on patients in all obesity related categories may even become commonplace in the future battle to win the war on weight.

We may also see the development of surgical and non-surgical products designed to provide fullness and encourage weight loss. Recently, a device called an *implantable gastric stimulator* was being tested in the United States. This device, more commonly referred to by researchers as a *gastric pacemaker*, is about the size of a matchbox. It is surgically implanted under the skin of the abdomen, and a connecting wire is implanted in the wall of the stomach. The device aims at emitting electrical pulses to the stomach muscles to create a feeling of fullness. It is hoped that this feeling of fullness will then cause the patient to eat less.

The pacemaker's electrical emissions create a feeling of fullness by slowing down the process of peristalsis, and making the patient feel full with less in the stomach. The mechanism is not unlike the decreased empting of the stomach that occurs with the stomach flu. Signing up for permanent "stomach flu" may not be most people's idea of a good way to lose weight. In addition, results have been sporadic, and complications like gastric perforation, lead dislodgement, pain, nausea, and vomiting are not infrequent. The amount of weight lost with pacing is significantly less than with present bariatric surgeries. Ultimately, the question remains whether the technology will be helpful for those in the obese category, for whom surgery is presently not an option.

The gastric pacemaker has received approvals in several European countries and Canada, and has recently completed clinical trials in the United States. Studies in other countries have shown that patients typically lose only around 20% of their excess weight, but such a loss will still have a positive effect on their health. Results of a multicenter, randomized, controlled, double-blind study in the U.S. showed no significant difference in weight loss with the pacing stimulated vs. nonstimulated patient participants.

The final study of the American experience was published in 2005 by the researchers from Tufts New England Medical Center in Boston. Patients in the study showed no more weight loss than the control group after 7 months, and after 29 months (over 2 years) excess weight loss approached 20%. After adjusting the criteria for patient participation in the study a second group showed excess weight loss of 23% after 16 months. Additionally, many patients suffered electrical lead dislodgements which had to be corrected surgically.[1] An additional study showed that it was also ineffective as a back-up procedure for adjustable gastric band patients who had the band removed due to band migration (slippage) or erosion.[2]

So, the results were basically that it didn't cause death (although patients could die from the general complications of having surgery itself), and it wasn't a complete bust. Most people, however, can, and have lost 20% or more of their excess weight over 29 or more months just with diet, exercise, and behavior modification. The study was not long enough to determine long-term weight loss maintenance complications, or effects on the body.

In a variation on a theme, Enteromedics™ has developed a new theoretical treatment for obesity called VBLOC, or Vagal Blocking for Obesity Control. VBLOC involves an implantable electrical device that sends very high frequency, low power signals through leads to block vagal nerve transmission. The vagal nerves regulate much of the activity of the stomach and pancreas, and are also believed by some researchers to play a role in the signaling of satiety and hunger. Enteromedics™ believes that it will help regulate multiple functions in the ingestion and digestion of calories, without distorting normal anatomy.[3] The obviously missing component here is that calories in and calories out are generally not really a significant part of the equation anymore once one becomes obese. (See Dr. Buffington's Prologue again for a refresher). VBLOC is not currently available, and is in human trials in countries outside the U.S. But, kudos go out to them for continuing to look for a better alternative. Time will tell if VBLOC will work.

And finally, in the vein of implantable devices, the Bioenteric Intragastric Balloon (the BIB) is currently undergoing human trials both in the U.S. and abroad. The BIB is implanted in the body via an endoscope that passes through the mouth, down the esophagus, and into the stomach (not through surgical incisions). It is intended to restrict food intake in obese patients. Although less invasive and cheaper than gastric bypass or adjustable gastric banding, it can only be left in place for a maximum of 6 months.[4]

Preliminary studies from Singapore, Greece, Italy, China, Israel, Brazil, The Netherlands, France, and the U.S. report that the BIB is not a long-term solution for the treatment of obesity in any form.[5] These studies state that the major complications and complaints with the BIB include: general gastric intolerance, nausea, gastric discomfort, vomiting, aspiration on vomit resulting in death, gastric ulcers, erosions, balloon rupture, gastroesophageal reflux, balloon meteorism (upward rise), bowel obstruction, esophageal perforation, and gastric perforation.[6]

Further, the studies concluded that any weight loss was reasonably preserved at the end of the six month implantation period, but by one year, when all the patients had been without BIBs for at least 6 months, the average weight loss for the group compared to pre-BIB weight was only about 1.5 kg or just over 3 pounds. Weight loss was greater in male obese patients with a BMI greater than 40.[7] The best indication for use of the BIB was for morbidly obese patients with BMIs over 40, and for super-obese patients (BMI greater than 50) in preparation for bariatric surgery. Eligible patients should be encouraged to undergo bariatric surgery rather than rely on the BIB to achieve long-term reliable weight loss.[8]

In the researchers' experience, treatment with BIB is useful from an educational point of view, and can be used to select patients for bariatric surgery only within a multi-disciplinary team. BIB placement can be considered an effective first stage treatment of high-risk, super-obese patients in need of surgical intervention.[9] Although not without risk, it is generally a simple procedure leading to satisfactory weight loss, improvement in co-morbidities, and reduction of the post-operative mortality and complication rates associated with surgery.[10] In potential super-obese candidates for laparoscopic Roux-en-Y gastric bypass, pre-operative placement of an intragastric balloon can reduce the excess weight by 10% within 3 months. Extending this period failed to improve these results further.[11]

Patients undergoing a laparoscopic gastric sleeve (LGS), however, as a first stage procedure showed a faster and greater weight loss than those using a BIB after 6 months. Moreover, LGS is a safe procedure, and results indicate that both average weight loss and percentage of excess weight loss were better in the LGS group. The BMI decreased substantially more in the LGS group as well. Although the BIB procedure shows efficacy in reducing weight, the gastric sleeve group does so faster and to a greater amount, thus suggesting that this may be a superior procedure as a first stage for super-obesity.[12]

In a variation on the BIB theme, BaroNova Therapeutics Inc., has a gastric retention technologies group that has created a polymer pill that expands to take up space in the stomach for 1 week after ingestion. The theory here is that the pill would degrade and pass through the gastrointestinal system. The pill would be intended for ingestion at regular intervals and adjusted accordingly based on response.[13] No human trials have yet been performed, but the concept does lead one to a number of questions, including how the pill would pass, how well it would work if it was continually shrinking, and what it is made of. Things that make you say "Hhmmmm......."

No matter what they eventually come up with, if it ultimately works, all of these potential devices, applications, and procedures should be offered through comprehensive, multi-disciplinary centers that can care for all of the weight related changes (medication, dietary, behavioral, emotional, and exercise), which ensue with obesity and weight loss. None of the surgical or non-surgical options will work in isolation, so the nutrition, behavioral/emotional, and exercise issues must be addressed as well.

As the invasive nature of the procedures and the attendant potential complications decrease, we may see more surgical application not only for people who are significantly less than *morbidly obese*, but also for children and adolescents as well. The obesity epidemic in children and adolescents is already at an all-time high. This demographic is where we really need to aim our efforts in order to halt the overwhelming advance toward obesity, and cut it off at its root source.

With regard to the awareness of childhood obesity, the future is beginning now. Various countries around the world have begun to look seriously at the weight and health of their nations' children, and to assess the potential long-range ramifications on the economy and social structure of their nations as a result of the epidemic.

Indeed, many U.S. states have Bills that are pending, or been recently passed that are aimed at addressing the childhood obesity problem. From cracking down on the poor nutritional content of school lunch programs, to increased, mandatory daily physical education requirements, states are looking long and hard at the weighty matter of heavy kids.

The other main way to affect this epidemic is by a major change on the environmental side of the equation. Television, computers, and video games have resulted in less physical activity in children, fewer calories burned, and more pounds being carried. A new generation of games and toys, however, could possibly begin to reverse this trend.

In fact, Julie was telling me about another physician friend of hers, Dr. Edmond Ducommun, who has been working with a neuropsychologist colleague on a device that would be implanted in children's shoes, much like the device that makes the little light in their athletic shoes light up when they walk. The device won't make their shoes glow, but it will keep track of how many steps they take.

The device then relays the message to a storage unit that is worn on the wrist and doubles as a watch. The "watch" tallies the steps and converts the total number of steps involved into credits that are used for time spent on the computer, television, gaming station, or DVD player. The watch transmits the accumulated credits to receivers attached to these components, thereby limiting little Johnny's use of them, and encouraging him to run around and play more so he can play his video game again later.

Now, I know what you're thinking, and I thought it too: "How are you going to keep the kid from just sitting there banging the shoe repeatedly while he's watching the television in order to rack up more credits?" Well, apparently they've thought of that, and have built in some safeguard that involves some major formula referencing weight, pressure, impact, torque, velocity, mass, and a bunch of other physics-type things that involve way too much math.

I also asked what would happen if Johnny didn't have enough credits to watch T.V., and came into the room while Susie was watching it on her credits. Would the T.V. turn off to prevent Johnny from getting a free ride? They claim to have thought of that as well and have some system in place that will prevent one device from canceling out another. It will purportedly work on the same system used to prevent one keyless entry remote from opening all cars of a similar make parked in the area, or preventing all the garage doors in the subdivision from going up or down at the same time when you press your door opener remote. I guess if Susie is watching and Johnny sits down to watch too, the safeguard for that is still parental supervision.

This product has already been proto-typed, is patent-pending, and is now in the design enhancement process. It's just one of many new products being created to get kids back outside and moving like they should be. It can be put into almost anything: a basketball, on a bike, on a free weight, on a tennis racquet, or on a baseball bat. If you want to measure the movement force of something, it can be incorporated. The possibilities are almost endless. Maybe it will be the big "must-have" item for parents for the 2010 Holiday season.

For now, we just need to encourage kids to be active and play outside more often (weather and other conditions permitting). My kids recently received a laser tag game with which they stampede throughout the house (more than usual), chasing each other with lasers and helmets. The house and furniture have taken a beating, but the kids are getting good exercise and having fun in the process.

For those of you in Florida or Arizona wondering why my kids are cavorting inside the house, just remember we have two basic seasons in Michigan: winter (the longest), and road construction (the harshest). At present, it's winter, but we've seen orange barrels beginning to sprout, so construction must be just around the corner!

If we are to properly treat the obesity epidemic in the future, an overall emphasis on more activity will be essential to help restructure the present obesity encouraging environmental conditions. In fact, by the year 2030, daily life might just sound a little like this:

> "Where's Jason?" Devin asked. "He's playing his 'Exploring Mars' game in the virtual reality room," Rebecca replied. "He's been at it since he came home from school. He has about 15 more minutes until he reaches his exercise requirement credits for today, but I suspect that he'll be in there until we call him for dinner. He loves that new game, but he keeps whining that the Martian landscape is too steep, and he gets tired of climbing before he can close in on the lost treasure."
>
> Devin thought a minute and said, "I don't know what he's whining about, when we were kids we had to drive ten miles, up hill, both ways, in the blinding snow, and biting cold, with no heated seats, just to get to a friend's house so we could sit in the basement, eat cheese puffs, and play video games! These kids just don't know how easy they have it with balanced meals and snacks, interactive 3-D games, and climate controlled environments. We were forced to sit on the basement floor for a million hours a year playing stupid, unrealistic games. They can play games in what-ever climate and conditions they want, they aren't forced to ruin their backs and posture like we were, and their snacks not only taste good, but are good for them too! Kids today take everything for granted!"

If this is the future, then some things will never change! In addition to empha-sis on increased exercise, better nutrition, and surgical interventions, pharmaceutical breakthroughs may also be seen, but these will likely be expensive and plagued with side effects. Most of you are all too familiar with the nasty effects of the anti-obesity drugs that are currently approved for use in the United States. The new "wonder drug" diet clone that is on the horizon is Rimonabant, also known as Acomplia® or Zimulti®. Rimonabant is the first in a new class of therapeutic agents called Cannabinoid-1 Receptor Blockers (CB1). Rimonabant is approved in Europe and other countries, and is used in the treatment of obesity and related conditions. Put simply, it is sup-posed to suppress appetite signals from the brain and fatty tissue that promotes eat-ing, and regulate body weight and adipose tissue function. It has an "anti-munchie" effect that works by turning off brain receptors that stimulate appetite.[14]

The Rimonabant in Obesity (RIO) trials have shown that Rimonabant induces weight loss of more than 5% in about 30-40% of patients, and greater than 10% of the patients in the clinical trials were generally overweight and obese, but not morbid-ly obese. Thus, the loss of 5% of an overweight patient's body weight has significantly more positive effect on the patient's health than would a 5% reduction in the excess body weight of a morbidly obese individual.[15]

Side effects in clinical trials for obesity treatment included vomiting, nausea, depression, and dizziness. Improvements in waist circumference, lowered triglycerides, and lowered blood pressure were also noted. Sanofi-Aventis, the makers of Rimonabant also claim that Rimonabant may reduce the risk of heart disease by boosting levels of HDL, or "good" cholesterol.[16]

Rimonabant recently received an almost unanimous FDA investigation committee recommendation that it *not* be approved by the FDA for use in the United States. What this means for the long-range outlook of this drug is unknown. It is the first in the endocannabinoid class of drugs, and future developments in this class of drugs may be adversely affected as well. Currently, researchers are investigating other hormones and chemical pathways in the body and their effects on weight regulation, appetite, fat storage, and a variety of other systemic effects.[17]

Recently, I heard a report about the newly discovered hormone, *ghrelin*. It has been found that ghrelin levels are different in thin people and obese people.[18] In fact, researchers have discovered that after weight loss ghrelin levels change drastically, so now the race is on to find a drug to deal with this hormone.[19] During one of the studies of a potential drug to inhibit ghrelin production, they discovered that ghrelin is actually also involved in memory.[20] The rats did lose weight but they didn't know it, and they couldn't remember where they lived, who each other were, or how to get back to the cage! So there you go.

All medications have side effects and/or adverse effects. Many of these side effects do not become apparent until wide spread usage is engaged. (Take Celebrex® and Phen-fen® as examples.) Although the pharmaceutical industry will probably want to assail me with literature to the contrary, I think the major effective obesity breakthroughs will not be in this area. The "in your face" quick fix miracle-diet clones will not likely be significantly thwarted by any pharmaceutical advances either. They'll simply pick up on some of the "junk science" like Hoodia and Ephedra, and spin it into another clone offering a miracle cure for your weight problems.

Another area of potential, if not eventual success, is related to gene therapy. According to geneticists, more than one gene is responsible for obesity. It is thought that there are many gene sequences that predispose humans toward obesity.[21] To be able to "fix" these genetic sequences would be a huge breakthrough, but we're probably not going to see that for some time. A lot of miracle-diet clones will prevail before this research area comes through with a decent arsenal of weapons ready to do battle in the weight wars, and defeat the miracle-diet clones.

Gene therapy will represent a breakthrough for multiple medical maladies not just obesity, but unfortunately it is a long way off.[22] Perhaps, gene therapy might affect the future somewhat like this:

> *Lucas passed through the antiviral decontaminator and paused briefly as the detection unit identified another mutated avian virus that somehow got on his clothes. After decontamination he entered the kitchen and called out "Laura, I'm home. How did the doctor's visit go?" Laura came into the kitchen and said, "It went great. The*

baby is doing well, but the genetic sequence screen identified dysfunctional leptin and alpha-ghrelin related genes, which will predispose little Mary Beth or Noah for obesity. It also found some other pro-pancreatic cancer sequence thingy, and the genetic sequence for heart disease. On the walk home I stopped and set up an appointment for a G.O.N.E procedure (genetic outpatient neomalgene eradicator) to correct the problems." "That's good. At least they didn't find anything significant," Lucas replied.

The year 2030 may not even be far enough in the future for us to see the use of genetic correction therapy, so until then the current methods of preventing obesity through good nutrition and exercise will have to suffice.

Speaking of nutrition, however, I expect that the future will see an increased emphasis being placed on eating a more balanced diet, and reducing the amount of saturated fat, trans fat, sugar, grease, and processed foods we consume. We're already seeing a trend toward better nutrition, even in the fast food industry. We're seeing wrap sandwiches that eliminate much of the breads used in regular sandwiches, more salads are being offered with dressings that have lower fat content, more whole grains are showing up in foods, and fruit is even appearing in many fast food restaurants for both children and adults to help balance our diets.

Ensuring a good balanced diet requires work, and the work is made more complex by the fast paced lives we live. We rarely have our meals together as families anymore, and trying to control all nutrition sources, especially in our children's lives is difficult. Until we develop a program for the computers in our "smart homes" to keep track of our caloric intake and exercise, we need to have some significant "work arounds" to help us stay fit and healthy.

We and our children need to learn how to go into a restaurant and not come out having been "bigger sized." Draconian "diets" do not work as no one can stand the monotony of the featured foods, or the deprivation of foods that taste good for long periods of time. And, as we've concluded, miracle-diet clones are nothing but "snake oil" in a new package.

A basic balanced approach with an emphasis on proper types of food and overall calories ingested will be necessary for long-term success. We need to learn and apply that knowledge now, and teach it consistently and regularly to our children so we can keep them from having to worry about dealing with weight problems. For our children, going to school and memorizing the food pyramid while eating snack cakes and chips at lunch and not having the most important food groups from the pyramid in the school and home is a recipe for defeat. Defeat in this instance, is equivalent to fat and weight gain.

Emphasis on creating good tasting food choices from the base of the food pyramid should be stressed. Today many of the important food groups are mostly available as tasteless cardboard consistency gruel. Most healthy whole grain cereals taste like gravel with sand thrown in. And most of these "healthy" cereals have boxes with boring nutrition facts and insipid graphics that probably taste better than the contents. If I have to eat gravel, at least let me look at exciting puzzles and cartoons to keep my mind off the taste and texture! Grape Nuts® could learn a thing or two from Fruit Loops®, and vice versa.

In addition to good tasting healthy foods, and amusing packaging to help us eat better, perhaps the future will bring us technologies to track our nutritional consumption as well. It may be a unit linked to the computers that will automate our homes, or maybe it will be hand-held like a PDA, I don't know. Maybe the future will be a little like this:

> *Haleigh yelled, "Honey, I'm home! What's for dinner? I'm starving!" Jordan laughed as he took Courtney's school bag off the couch and put it at the bottom of the stairs, "When aren't you starving? I've been busy all day with a conference call to Tokyo, so I set the Cookmaster to 'auto chef'" said Jordan. "It says it planned a special tuna and rice dish to completely balance this week's food pyramid program. Courtney and I even get some dessert tonight because we haven't used all our simple carbohydrate quotas for the week. Courtney can actually have seconds on dessert because the school lunch program has an even more restrictive carb quota than we do, but I'm not telling her that!" Haleigh groaned; tuna casserole again. "Do I get dessert?" she asked. "No, because you keep eating fast food for lunch, and you're way over your carb quota for the week. If you'd let the Cookmaster prepare your lunch and take it with you to work, maybe you could eat dessert when you got home," said Jordan. "The next time you're at the drive-thru maybe you should 'small size' your order from the healthwise menu, and eat less junk food on your breaks," Jordan added. Haleigh, nodded her head in agreement, and said, "I'll start on that tomorrow, but for tonight I'm eating Courtney's extra dessert. What she doesn't know won't hurt her!"*

Not only is personal responsibility for proper nutrition and exercise essential, but an overall emphasis by entire communities is necessary as well. Effective education and real programs with results are needed, not just symbolic "feel good" seminars. Recently, I attended such a meeting where a well-meaning and well-intentioned group presented its "child first" weight control program.

The program focused mainly on the emotional side of the issue. I support treating this part of the problem entirely, as self-loathing is a defeatist behavior, and poor self-esteem feeds the cycle of eating and self-loathing. But, it's only one component of the entire issue, and a comprehensive multi-disciplinary approach is essential to long-term success.

A peronalized action plan for weight management, modification of inappropriate eating behaviors, and monitored compliance with nutrition and exercise components were not being addressed at all. As a result of this approach, the kids were, unfortunately, still gaining unhealthy weight, but at least they felt better about themselves while doing so. I know it sounds like I am skewering some sacred cows or being anti-politically correct, but these feel good symbolic gestures are NOT working!

We need substance over symbolism to repulse obesity and those obnoxious miracle-diet clones. We need real action and real treatment, not just some well-intentioned band-aid being placed over a gaping chest wound! Obesity is a disease, and is best treated through prevention before symptoms occur. In this case, prevention isn't worth a pound of cure, it's worth a mountain range of cure!

In the mean time, as society's weight problems continue to increase, we really need to focus our collective attention on both obesity cure and prevention. We need a laser-fine focus that will begin to dramatically change the future of obesity as a disease and epidemic, and finally win the war on weight. Only then will all the quick fix miracle-diet clones really be vanquished, as true and lasting healthy lifestyles emerge. Alas, I fear it won't come soon enough. Until then... I still have some of my famous lemon extract for sale....

Chapter Seventeen

⟋ ADDITIONAL RESOURCES ⟍

Julie M. Janeway
Karen J. Sparks

THE BARIATRIC PATIENT'S PLAN TO SUCCEED!

- Eat when you are hungry. Pay attention to when you feel *satisfied* — STOP eating!
- Do not drink with meals, or for about an hour after eating.
- Take your Building Blocks® vitamins and calcium every day!
- Get your protein in first! Get a *minimum* of 60-70g of protein in every day from your actual food, and then supplement it with Bariatrix' SmartForme prtoein bars, shakes, or other *quality* protein sources if necessary.
- Minimize, but do *not* eliminate, complex carbs like bread, rice, potatoes, and pasta. Eat balanced meals and get some of each of the food groups. Watch your food portions!
- Watch your sugar intake (things that end in "ose" — glucose, fructose, sucrose). Watch for hidden sugars like sugar alcohols (things that end in "tol" — malitol, sorbitol, xylitol).
- Make healthy food choices, and plan your food ahead as much as you can. *Value yourself* enough to do this.
- Chew everything well, and slow down your eating.
- Drink 64 oz. of non-caffeinated, non-carbonated, non-sugared liquid a day — preferably water.
- Get some movement in every day, even if it's just vacuuming or walking out to get the mail.
- If you start a structured movement program, pick one that you can stick with, and one that isn't too much for you to handle. Start slow but consistent, and move up slowly. You have a lifetime to get to that hour of working out per day!
- Determine your food, situation, and emotional triggers, and make a plan to deal with them.
- Set *realistic* goals, stop beating yourself up, and focus on the positive. Celebrate your Little Victories!
- Surround yourself with supportive people. Go to your SUPPORT GROUP meetings and events! It's SUPPORT *not* therapy!
- Follow-up with your medical team for the rest of your life! They got you this far, they'll keep you on track for the rest of the journey.

Every great success is a series of Little Victories!™

QUESTIONS FOR MY PRIMARY CARE DOCTOR

- How would I benefit from weight loss surgery?

- What other options are open to me?

- What are my best options now?

- Do you feel I am healthy enough for surgery if that is the option I choose?

- What are the next steps I should take?

- Can you refer me to a bariatric surgeon in a multi-disciplinary practice?

- Is there an American Society for Metabolic and Bariatric Surgery (ASMBS), Surgical Review Corporation (SRC) or American College of Surgeons (ACS) certified Center of Excellence (COE) nearby?

QUESTIONS FOR MY SURGEON

- Is this practice a Center of Excellence? If not, are you applying for, or moving toward Center of Excellence certification?

- What types of weight loss surgery procedures have you performed?

- What surgeries do you offer at your practice and which surgeon performs them?

- How many of each type of weight loss procedure have you performed?

- If I choose the adjustable gastric band, how often do I have to return for band fills?

- Who performs the band fills?

- For a band, what is your philosophy regarding how tight the band should be directly following surgery?

- For a band, what is your philosophy on the use or discontinuation of the band once my weight loss goal has been achieved?

- What professional organizations do you belong to that relate to weight loss surgery?

- Can this surgery be performed using minimally invasive techniques such as laparoscopy?

- Can I be considered a candidate for surgery even though I have one or more associated health conditions (co-morbidities) related to my weight problem?

- If I've had an ulcer, will that make a difference whether or not I can have weight loss surgery?

- Does your practice have age limitations for patients choosing a surgical option?

- Does your practice have weight or BMI limitations for patients choosing a surgical option?

- Does your practice accept Medicare/Medicaid? (If appropriate to your situation.)

- If my insurance requires me to engage in a medically managed weight loss program for a specified period of time before they will give approval for surgery, does your practice offer such a program?

- Why might I need to have a gastrointestinal (GI) evaluation?

- Do I have to lose weight before having surgery? Why? How much?

- Will I be asked to stop smoking?

- Which weight loss procedure is best for me? Why? What are the risks and potential complications involved?

- What pre-operative tests or evaluations will you perform? Why?

- Is this a multi-disciplinary practice?

- What is the immediate follow-up care plan for your practice? Long-term follow-up?

- If I am from out of the practice's geographic area, how will my follow-up be managed?

- What role does my primary care doctor play in this process?

- What role do my other treating physicians (if any) play in this process?

- How long will I be in surgery?

- What is the anticipated length of my hospital stay?

- Will I need a naso-gastric tube? If so, why?

- Will any drains have to be left in after surgery?

- Is a blood transfusion/infusion required? If so, why?

- What precautions do you undertake to prevent deep vein thrombosis (DVT) or pulmonary embolism?

- What is an incisional hernia, and what is the probability of having one after surgery?

- For gastric bypass, what type of staple line reinforcement do you use? (Insist on staple line reinforcement).

- How will my pain be managed?

- How long will I be off solid foods?

- What type of protein supplement will I be on? What does it taste like? What are the nutritional aspects of it? Will you consider using Bariatrix' SmartForme products?

- Do you use a vitamin formulated specifically for bariatric surgery patients like Building Blocks® bariatric vitamins? (Do not accept a practice that uses over-the-counter general vitamins that you see advertised on T.V. Require vitamins especially for bariatric surgery patients.)

- Will this procedure modify the dosages or use of any of my current medications?

- Will I be able to take oral contraceptives after surgery?

- Is sexual activity restricted?

- How long will it be before I can return to pre-surgery levels of activity?

- How soon will I be able to drive?

- Are you affiliated with a qualified and experienced bariatric reconstructive plastic surgeon to who I can be referred if I should need such services following weight loss?

- Do you have any information about weight loss surgery costs and payment options?

- What is the typical excess weight loss and improvement of associated health conditions for your other patients?

- Do you have patients who are willing to share their experiences, both positive and negative?

- What information can you give me to help family and friends better understand this surgery?

- Does your practice provide support groups run by appropriately trained support group leaders?

- Does your practice provide counseling services?

- What are your expectations of me as a patient if I decide on a surgical treatment?

- After receiving an insurance approval how long will it take before I am booked for surgery?

Every great success is a series of Little Victories!™

EXPLORING MY INNER SHADOWS

This is a great exercise to help you to understand some of your emotional eating patterns. Follow the directions below and take it with you when you see the behaviorist on your assessment visit.

INSTRUCTIONS: Put a **circle** around the number that best describes the degree to which you **experience this quality in your life.** For example: "How much love do I experience in my life?" Put a **square** around the number to indicate the degree to which you **use food to compensate for any deficiency in this quality.** For example: "When I feel unloved, how much do I turn toward food?"

	Least									Most
Love	1	2	3	4	5	6	7	8	9	10
Joy	1	2	3	4	5	6	7	8	9	10
Peace	1	2	3	4	5	6	7	8	9	10
Patience	1	2	3	4	5	6	7	8	9	10
Kindness	1	2	3	4	5	6	7	8	9	10
Self-Control	1	2	3	4	5	6	7	8	9	10
Forgiveness	1	2	3	4	5	6	7	8	9	10
Guilt	1	2	3	4	5	6	7	8	9	10
Confidence	1	2	3	4	5	6	7	8	9	10
Purpose	1	2	3	4	5	6	7	8	9	10
Significance	1	2	3	4	5	6	7	8	9	10

The more your **circles are to the right, (except for guilt)** and the more your **squares are to the left, the better.**

NOW ASK YOURSELF:

• Where are your circles?

• What made you circle that particular number?

• Where are the squares?

• What made you put a square around that particular number?

• For any of the qualities, did you put a square around a number higher than the number you circled? Why? How can you change that in your life?

• Are you seeing any patterns emerging as to how you use food in emotional situations?

• How is this affecting your image of yourself?

• How is this affecting the respect and value you give yourself?

If you want to win your war with weight, talk with a behaviorist about resolving these eating patterns. Good luck!

Developed by Scott H. Glass, MS, MA, LLP ©*2005. Little Victories Medical/Legal Consulting & Training*™ *Little Victories Support University*™. *All Rights Reserved.*

MEDICAL WARNING SIGNS

If any of the following occur, **immediately** seek medical attention.

If you are a bariatric surgical patient: immediately contact your bariatric surgeon's office and/or go to an emergency room and give them the name and phone number for your bariatric surgeon.

- Blood in urine or stool

- Severe pain and/or a heat to the touch in the back of the calf

- Can't get food down or won't stay down for more than 36 hours

- Can't keep liquid down

- Wound sites open, re-open, or won't heal

- Piercing pain in right side

- Significant bruising

- Recurring pain in the abdomen

- Low grade fever lasting longer than 12 hours (not flu related – 100.8 degrees or higher); or higher grade fever lasting longer than 1 hour (102 degrees or higher)

- Heart arrhythmias or palpitations

- Chest pain, pain radiating down left arm, or up into jaw

- Shortness of breath

- Unusual constipation or diarrhea

- Nausea lasting longer than 6 hours

- Vomiting lasting longer than a half hour continuously, or 3 hours intermittently

- Recurring fainting, dizziness, lightheadedness, or tingling or numbness in hands and/or feet

- Hives, rashes, symptoms of allergic reactions

- Torso Scramps (see definition in Chapter Four)

- Internal torso pain (gut pain or discomfort)

- Blurry vision or recurring vision changes

Reviewed by Stephen R. Hendrick, MD, FACS
Bariatric Surgeon – Henry Ford Health Systems, Wyandotte Campus

MEDICATIONS THAT CAN CAUSE WEIGHT GAIN

• Antipsychotics, especially olansepine

• Antidepressants: tricyclics, selective serotonin reuptake inhibitors, monoamine oxidase inhibitors, mirtazepine, lithium

• Corticosteroids

• Oral contraceptives and progestagenic compounds

• Beta blockers

• Oral hypoglycemic agents: glitazones (peripheral rather than visceral gain), sulphonylureas

• Insulin

• Anticonvulsants: phenytoin, sodium valproate

• Antihistamines: many antihistamines, although weight gain is greater with older agents

• Pizotifen, used as a prophylactic migraine treatment

• Some hypertension (blood pressure) control medications

• Some cancer treatment medications

• Some thyroid medications

Check with your doctor or pharmacist if you have questions about any medication's potential for causing weight gain.

Nutrient & Deficiency Functions/Symptoms (Functional Intracellular Analysis™)

Source: SpectraCell Laboratories 2007

NUTRIENT	DEFICIENCY	WHAT IT DOES	WHERE IT'S FOUND	SYMPTOMS AND PROBLEMS
B1 Thiamine	VERY COMMON	Carb conversion, breaks down fats & protein, digestion, nervous system, skin, hair, eyes, mouth, liver, immune system	Pork, organ meats, whole grain and enhanced cereals, brown rice, wheat germ, bran, brewer's yeast, blackstrap molasses	Heart, age-related cognitive decline, Alzheimer's, fatigue
B2 Riboflavin	VERY COMMON	Metabolism, carb conversion, breaks down fat & protein, digestion, nervous system, skin, hair, eyes, mouth, liver, antioxidant	Brewer's yeast, almonds, organ meats, whole grains, wheat germ, mushrooms, soy, dairy, eggs, green vegetables	Anemia, decreased free radical protection, cataracts, poor thyroid function, B6 deficiency, fatigue, elevated homocysteine (leads to heart issues)
B3 Niacin Niacinamide	LESS COMMON	Energy, digestion, nervous system, skin, hair, eyes, liver, eliminates toxins, sex/stress hormones, improves circulation	Beets, brewer's yeast, meat, poultry, organ meats, fish, seeds and nuts	Cracking, scaling skin, digestive problems, confusion, anxiety, fatigue
B6 Pyridoxine	COMMON	Enzyme protein metabolism, red blood cell (RBC) production, reduces homocysteine, nerve & muscle cells, DNA and RNA, B12 absorption, immune function	Poultry, tuna, salmon, shrimp, beef liver, lentils, soybeans, seeds, nuts, avocados, bananas, carrots, brown rice, bran, wheat germ, whole grain flour	Depression, sleep and skin problems, elevated homocysteine, increase heart disease risk
B12 Cyanocobalamin	VERY COMMON	Healthy nerve cells DNA/RNA, red blood cell production, iron function	Fish, meat, poultry, eggs, milk, and milk products	Anemia, fatigue, constipation, loss of appetite/weight, numbness and tingling in the hands & feet, depression, dementia, poor memory, oral soreness
BIOTIN Vitamin H	LESS COMMON	Carbs, fat, and amino acid metabolism (the building blocks of protein)	Salmon, meats, vegetables, grains, legumes, lentils, egg yolks, milk, sweet potatoes, seeds, nuts, wheat germ	Depression, nervous system, premature graying, hair, skin

		Function	Sources	Deficiency
FOLATE Folic Acid	VERY COMMON	Mental health, infant DNA/RNA, adolescence & pregnancy, with B12 to regulate RBC production, iron function, reduce homocysteine	Supplementation, fortified grains, tomato juice, green vegetables, black-eyed peas, lentils, beans, spinach, leafy greens, asparagus	Anemia, immune function, fatigue, insomnia, hair, high homocysteine, heart disease
PANTO-THENATE	LESS COMMON	RBC production, sex and stress-related hormones, immune function, healthy digestion, helps use other vitamins	Meat, vegetables, whole grains, legumes, lentils, egg yolks, milk, sweet potatoes, seeds, nuts, wheat germ, salmon	Stress tolerance, wound healing, skin problems, fatigue
VITAMIN A Retinol	LESS COMMON	Eyes, immune function, skin, essential cell growth and development	Milk, eggs, liver, fortified cereals, orange or green vegetables and fruits	Night blindness, immune function, zinc deficiency, fat malabsorption
VITAMIN D D3 Cholecalciferol	VERY COMMON	Calcium and phosphorus levels, calcium absorption, bone mineralization	Sunlight, milk, egg yolk, liver, fish, fortified breakfast cereals	Osteoporosis, calcium absorption, thyroid issues
VITAMIN E Alpha Tocopheryl	VERY COMMON	Antioxidant, regulates oxidation reactions, stabilizes cell membrane, immune function, protects against cardiovascular disease, cataracts, macular degeneration	Wheat germ, liver, eggs, nuts, seeds, cold-pressed vegetable oils, dark leafy greens, sweet potatoes, avocados, asparagus, sunflower seeds, cooked spinach, safflower oil	Skin, hair, rupturing of red blood cells, anemia, bruising, PMS, hot flashes, eczema, psoriasis, cataracts, wound healing, muscle weakness, sterility
CALCIUM Calcium Citrate (for bariatric surgery patients)	VERY COMMON	Bones, teeth, helps heart, nerves, muscles, body systems work properly, needs other nutrients to function	Dairy, wheat/soy flour, molasses, brewer's yeast, Brazil nuts, broccoli, cabbage, dark leafy greens, hazelnuts, oysters, sardines, canned salmon	Osteoporosis, osteomalacia, osteoarthritis, muscle cramps, irritability, acute anxiety, colon cancer risk

NUTRIENT	DEFICIENCY	WHAT IT DOES	WHERE IT'S FOUND	SYMPTOMS AND PROBLEMS
CHROMIUM	COMMON	Assists insulin function, increased fertility, carbohydrate/fat metabolism, essential for fetal growth/development	Supplementation, brewers yeast, whole grains, seafood, green beans, broccoli, prunes, nuts, potatoes, meat, raisins	Metabolic syndrome, insulin resistance, decreased fertility
MAGNESIUM	VERY COMMON	300 biochemical reactions, muscle/nerve function, insulation regulation, heart rhythm, immune system, strong bones, regulates calcium, copper, zinc, potassium, vitamin D	Green vegetables, beans & peas, nuts and seeds, whole unprocessed grains, avocados, acorn squash, kiwi	Appetite, nausea, vomiting, fatigue, numbness, tingling, cramps, seizures, personality changes, heart rhythm, heart spasms, erratic blood sugar levels
SELENIUM	COMMON	Antioxidant, works with vitamin E, immune function, prostaglandin production	Brewer's yeast, wheat germ, liver, butter, cold water fish, shellfish, garlic, whole grains, sunflower seeds, Brazil nuts	Destruction to heart/pancreas, sore muscles, fragility of red blood cells, immune system
ZINC	MOST COMMON	Supports enzymes, immune system, wound healing, taste/smell, DNA synthesis, normal growth & development during pregnancy, childhood, adolescence, testosterone regulation	Oysters, lean red meat, poultry, beans, nuts, seafood, whole grains, fortified breakfast cereals, dairy, chickpeas	Growth retardation, hair loss, diarrhea, impotence, eye & skin lesions, loss of appetite, taste, wound healing, mental lethargy, depressed immune system
COQ10 Coenzyme Q-10	COMMON	Powerful antioxidant, stops oxidation of LDL cholesterol, energy production, important to heart, liver, and kidneys	Oily fish, organ meats, and whole grains	Congestive heart failure, high blood pressure, angina, mitral valve prolapse, fatigue, gingivitis, immune system stroke, cardiac arrhythmias

CARNITINE	LESS COMMON	Energy, heart function, oxidize amino acids for energy, metabolize ketones	Red meat, dairy, fish, poultry, tempeh (fermented soybeans), wheat, asparagus, avocados, peanut butter	Elevated cholesterol, liver function, muscle weakness, reduced energy, impaired glucose control
N-ACETYL CYSTEINE (NAC) & GLUTA-THIONE	COMMON	Glutathione production, lowers homocysteine, lipoprotein(a), heal lungs, inflammation, decrease muscle fatigue, liver detoxification, immune function	Meats, ricotta, cottage cheese, yogurt, wheat germ granola, and oat flakes	Free radical overload, elevated homocysteine, cancer risk, cataracts, macular degeneration, immune function, toxin elimination
ALPHA LIPOIC ACID	COMMON	Energy, blood flow to nerves, glutathione levels in brain, insulin sensitivity, effectiveness of vitamins C, E, antioxidants	Supplementation, spinach, broccoli, beef, brewer's yeast, some organ meats	Diabetic neuropathy, reduced muscle mass, atherosclerosis, Alzheimer's, failure to thrive, brain atrophy, high lactic acid
POTASSIUM	COMMON	Blood pressure, heart and kidney function, muscle contraction, digestion	Supplementation, citrus and other fruits, bananas, potatoes, broccoli, vegetables, low-fat dairy products, whole grains, fish, lean meats	Blood pressure issues, blood sugar issues, kidney problems, muscle cramps, poor digestion, metabolism issues

MEDICATION AND NUTRIENT INTERACTION CHART

MEDICATION	NUTRIENTS	MECHANISM
Antacids	Iron Phosphates	Malabsorption Binding
Tetracyclines	Iron (antacids) Calcium	Chelation Calcium binding in bones
Cholestyramine	Triglycerides, Calcium, Fat Soluble Vitamins	Malabsorption, bile-acid sequestration
5-Fluorouracil	Protein	Malabsorption, reduced peptidases
Metformin	Vitamin B12	Malabsorption; mucosal damage
Colchicine	Vitamin B12	Malabsorption
Para-aminosalicylic acid	Folate, Potassium	Reduced levels and synthesis
Ethanol	Folate Magnesium Zinc Vitamin B6	Uncertain Possible malabsorption; increase in stool Increased urinary loss Reduced conversion to pyridoxal phosphate
Methyldopa	Vitamin B6	Metabolic antagonism
Isoniazid	Vitamin B6, Tryptophan	Competition for active enzyme site
Penicillamine	Vitamin B6	Increased urinary loss
Diphenylhydantoin	Folate	Uncertain
Primidone	Folate, Iron	Cell formation; megaloblastic anemia
Methotrexate	Folate	Direct antagonism; competition for active enzyme site
Pyrimethamine	Folate, Iron	Cell formation; megaloblastic anemia, leucopenia
Triaminopteride	Folate	Direct antagonism
Trimethoprim	Folate	Blood dyscrasias
Coumadin	Vitamin K	Decreased synthesis
Barbiturates	Vitamin K	Induction of warfarin inactivation
Oxyphenbutazone	Vitamin K	Enhancement of warfarin action (displacement of albumin binding)
Oral contraceptives	Vitamin B6 Tryptophan Folate	Altered metabolism Increased protein binding Reduction in red cell levels

PRECAUTIONS WHEN USING ALCOHOL
AFTER BARIATRIC SURGERY

Dr. Cynthia K. Buffington
Florida Hospital – Celebration Health Bariatric Center

A 36 year old female gastric bypass patient left a party after having only two alcoholic beverages, drove her car into oncoming traffic, causing the death of a 12 year old child.* Her blood alcohol level was above the legal limit for the operation of a motor vehicle, and was far higher than would have been expected from the two alcoholic beverages she claimed to have consumed. Was the patient telling the truth about the amount of alcohol she drank at the party, or did her surgery affect the way her body absorbed or metabolized the alcohol?

A recent study reported in the British Journal of Clinical Pharmacology found that the gastric bypass procedure significantly affects alcohol absorption and its inebriating influence. According to the study, a group of gastric bypass patients, three years post-surgery, and their non-surgical control group consumed an alcoholic drink containing 20% alcohol (95% ethanol), and blood alcohol levels were examined over a period of time. The data showed that blood alcohol levels of the gastric bypass patients were far higher and required much less time to peak than those of the non-surgical controls.

The more rapid absorption of alcohol and heightened blood alcohol levels would cause the bariatric patient to have a more pronounced feeling of inebriation during and shortly after drinking. And, such effects could have serious ramifications with regard to driving an automobile or performing other skilled tasks such as operating heavy machinery, piloting a plane, or any other task that may influence the safety of the individual or others.

Why would alcohol absorption be higher for someone who has had gastric bypass (or any other surgical procedure that reduces the size of the stomach and bypasses the upper portion of the gut)? With the gastric bypass procedure, 95% of the stomach and the upper gut (duodenum and a portion of the jejunum) are bypassed. Alcohol passes directly from the stomach pouch, usually without restriction, into the second portion of the gut, known as the jejunum. This portion of the gut has a large surface area and readily and rapidly absorbs the alcohol.

In addition to anatomical changes in the GI tract that influence alcohol absorption, the gastric bypass patient (or patient having had any bariatric procedure), may also be more sensitive to the intoxicating effects of alcohol because of the reduced caloric intake caused by the surgery. A number of studies have found that alcohol absorption is far higher if fasting, or when consumed on an empty stomach than if provided with a meal or consumed soon thereafter.

During the first several months following gastric bypass or any other bariatric surgical procedure, total daily calorie intake is quite low. Drinking alcohol, even small amounts, at this time, would increase significantly an individual's risk for intoxication.

In the rapid weight loss period following bariatric surgery, alcohol consumption could have far more serious consequences than just inebriation — namely brain damage, coma, and death. How is this possible?

Muscle, heart, liver, and other tissues use fat and sugar (glucose) for fuel. The brain, however, requires sugar (glucose) to function. To avoid low sugar, the body stores sugar in the form of glycogen. However, glycogen stores can be depleted in a short period of time with prolonged work or exercise, starvation, or a diet low in carbohydrates. When this happens, the body has two back-up mechanisms that help to provide the brain and nervous system the sugar required to function.

One of the mechanisms whereby sugar is produced is a process called gluconeogenesis, a chemical pathway that converts certain components of protein, lactic acid, and other substances into sugar. Fat cannot be converted into sugar. The production of sugar by gluconeogenesis, however, is run by energy produced by the incomplete breakdown of fat into ketone bodies via a process known as ketosis.

Ketone bodies can be used by all tissues, including the brain, for fuel. And, ketones can also be converted into sugar via gluconeogenesis. In this way, the brain and nervous system can function normally, even during times of low calorie intake, such as during the rapid weight loss period following bariatric surgery.

The production of ketones is what causes the sweet or distinct smell in the urine and on the breaths of bariatric patients during the rapid weight loss period after surgery. And, during this time, it is extremely important that alcohol NOT be consumed. Why?

Alcohol inhibits gluconeogenesis and ketosis. This means the brain and nerves are depleted of the fuel needed to function. The consequences of such fuel depletion initially are disorientation, confusion, semi-consciousness, coma, and ultimately death.

Drinking alcohol in the early postoperative period may have other adverse effects on health. Frequent vomiting, low calorie intake, not taking multivitamins, and malabsorption may cause a number of vitamin and mineral deficits, including thiamine. Alcohol further reduces the absorption of thiamine, causing severe deficits and a condition known as Beriberi. Beriberi, in turn, may cause congestive heart failure, nerve damage, muscle cramping and pain, crippling, brain damage, a loss of memory and inability to learn, confusion, disorientation, coma, and death.

Drinking alcohol after surgery may also reduce maximal weight loss success. Alcohol has no nutrient benefits and contains high numbers of calories that may cause weight gain or prevent weight loss. One 12 oz. can of beer, for instance, contains 150 calories; 3.5 oz. of wine contains 70 calories; 1.5 oz. of gin, rum, vodka or whiskey contains between 97 and 124 calories; and 1.5 oz. of liquor contains 160 calories.

Based on all the information provided above, should the bariatric patient abstain from alcohol totally? The bariatric patient should absolutely NOT drink alcohol during the rapid weight loss period and definitely not if consuming no or low carbohydrates, not taking appropriate bariatric vitamin and mineral supplements, vomiting frequently, or not able to keep appropriate food down. With time, however, there is no reason an individual should not be able to enjoy an occasional drink, provided they are aware that it only takes a small amount of alcohol to produce an inebriating effect. With such knowledge, appropriate precautions should be taken, such as waiting a sufficient length of time after drinking to drive or perform other skilled tasks.

The age of the individuals involved in the accident described and some details have been changed so that those involved may remain anonymous.

TIPS FROM THE TAILOR

Diane Trimble
Lansing, Michigan

Julie and Karen here again. Diane is the tailor we use, and she's phenomenal. She's got decades of experience and she's been kind enough to share her experience with all of you.

If you need a tailor (and you will if you have surgery...), Diane suggests:

Checking with local fabric stores for their lists of area seamstresses and tailors. Many qualified people run their tailoring or dressmaking businesses from their homes and don't advertise outside of business cards and word of mouth. These tailors are quite good, and usually much less expensive than tailoring shops. Ask to see their work, and ask for references.

Many drycleaners offer alteration services. Find out the scope of the services offered, as well as the prices. You may find that the alteration services offered by the drycleaner are best used for things like mending small tears, replacing buttons, and replacing shoulder pads, etc. Actual garment reconstruction is probably best left to tailors who have the time and facilities to properly fit and measure your garment on you rather than simply taking a written description. As for buying clothes for the shrinking person, Diane suggests:

MEN: Do not buy pre-pleated pants. They may fit well when you are heavy, but as you shrink you will create problems with bagginess in the front, and tailoring that down becomes very difficult and can be expensive.

MEN and WOMEN: When buying blazers or suit jackets, make sure to buy them with center back seams if at all possible. This will allow not only for reducing the size of the garment through the torso, but also for some lift in the shoulders to decrease the breadth there as well.

WOMEN: Buy jackets and blazers with bust darting or princess seams as well.

WOMEN: Buy skirts with many seams, few pleats, and no waistband if possible. This makes tailoring much easier and cheaper.

MEN and WOMEN: Buy single breasted blazers. Tailoring double breasted blazers down is much more difficult and expensive. Incidentally, double breasted blazers tend to make people look wider anyway, and are much more difficult to fit in the first place.

MEN and WOMEN: Take care to notice the hem length on pants, skirts, and dresses as you shrink. What used to be the right length may now look sloppy or dowdy and it defeats the purpose of weight loss. Keep an eye out for that.

MEN and WOMEN: Similarly, keep an eye out for sleeve/cuff length as you shrink too.

MEN: Did you know that it is often much cheaper to have your Big and Tall Men's ties shortened than to buy new ties? Ask your tailor for a price.

MEN and WOMEN: Depending on how fast you need your garment altered, it's better to actually have your tailor make the garment just a bit more snug than you would actually wear it, because by the time you get it back and put it on, you will probably have shrunk again, and at least you won't have completely wasted your money.

MEN and WOMEN: When bringing clothes to have them altered, bring the shoes you normally wear with the garment. Even if you are simply intending to have a garment taken in, bring the shoes because the hem length might change.

WOMEN: When having garments re-fitted, remember to wear the foundation garments you would normally wear with the garment. So if you normally wear a specific kind of bra (one that fits properly!), or you wear control top pantyhose, then wear them to the fitting. It will make a big difference in how things come out.

MEN and WOMEN: When being measured or pinned for alterations, remember to stand straight up, hands at your sides, and look straight ahead. If you look down to watch the tailor mark your pants or skirt, when you get the garment back it can be as much as an inch to an inch and half too short, and will probably be uneven.

EVERYONE: Don't bring all your clothes to have them altered at once. Remember: you have to have something to wear while other garments are being altered.

EVERYONE: Remember that clothes can generally only be taken down a maximum of two sizes before they lose their shape and proportions. Don't expect miracles from the tailor. They can only work with what's already been cut and sewn. They're not magicians!

Every great success is a series of Little Victories!™

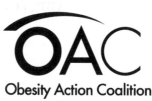

Obesity Action Coalition

The Mission of the Obesity Action Coalition (OAC) is to elevate and empower those affected by obesity through education, advocacy, and support.

The OAC aims to educate patients, family members, and the public about obesity and morbid obesity. In addition, the OAC will increase obesity education, work to improve access to medical treatments for obese patients, advocate for safe and effective treatments, and strive to eliminate the negative stigma associated with all types of obesity.

By building a coalition of members ranging from patients and their family members to healthcare professionals, the OAC and its members will focus national attention on obesity; organize all those concerned as advocates for action, advances, and change; and visibly affect and impact the healthcare community and the public. The OAC is recognized by the Internal Revenue Service as a 501(c)(3) public charity.

Join the OAC for one year - FREE!!*
Call 1-800-717-3117
Use complimentary membership code TRS-2

Your membership strengthens the voice of all those dealing with obesity and ensures that education remains at the forefront of the fight against the disease. Various membership levels are available. Membership in the OAC is on an annual basis and is accompanied with numerous benefits.

As a member you will receive:

· Official charter membership card/certificate
· OAC News – the OAC's quarterly educational and advocacy newsletter
· Subscription to Obesity Action Alert – a monthly electronic newsletter distributed on the first of each month
· Representation through advocacy in addition to information on state and national advocacy issues concerning patients

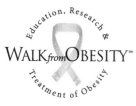

The ASBS Foundation and the OAC proudly bring you the Walk from Obesity, the nation's largest gathering of individuals affected by obesity. In cities all across the country, obesity sufferers and survivors alike will join forces and walk to raise money for research, education, prevention, and treatment of obesity. To date, the Walk from Obesity has raised more than $1.6 million to support research and educational programs on behalf of those affected by obesity.

Proud Supporters of the OAC and the Walk from Obesity.

LV Press

Free membership excludes Institutional and Chairman's Council memberships.

LIST OF ORGANIZATIONAL RESOURCES

The organizations, agencies, and web sites presented here were selected based on the value of the information presented on obesity, being overweight, weight loss treatments or resources, and related conditions. The appearance in this chapter of any organization, agency, or web site, (or any products, programs, or services they may advertise or offer), does not constitute an endorsement by the publisher, Michigan Weight Loss Specialists, or any of the main or contributing authors or sponsors of this book. While the information in these resources and web sites may be useful to those contemplating a weight loss program, anyone wishing to do so should consult a skilled bariatric physician or surgeon.

* Indicates site has a physician locator service

Michigan Weight Loss Specialists
4100 Lake Drive, SE, Suite B01
Grand Rapids, MI 49546
(616) 974-4400
1-877-877-MMPC Toll Free
www.mmpc.com (click on Bariatrics)

American Diabetes Association
1701 North Beauregard Street
Alexandria, VA 22311
(800) DIABETES (800-342-2383)
www.diabetes.org

The American Diabetes Association is the nation's leading nonprofit health organization providing diabetes research, information, and advocacy. The mission of the organization is to prevent and cure diabetes, and to improve the lives of all people affected by diabetes.

American Dietetic Association
120 S Riverside Plaza, Suite 2000
Chicago, IL 60606-6995
(312) 877-1600
www.eatright.com

The American Dietetic Association promotes optimal nutrition, health, and well-being for all persons, as well as advocating for its membership comprised mainly of registered dietitians and nutritionists.

American Heart Association
7272 Greenville Avenue
Dallas, TX 75231
(800) AHA-USA1 (800-242-8721)
www.americanheart.org

The American Heart Association is a national voluntary health agency whose mission is to reduce disability and death from cardiovascular diseases and stroke.

American Medical Association (AMA)
515 North State Street
Chicago, IL 60610
(800) 621-8335
www.ama-assn.org

Founded more than 150 years ago, AMA's strategic agenda remains rooted in its historic commitment to standards, ethics, excellence in medical education and practice, and advocacy on behalf of the medical profession and the patients it serves.

American Society for Aesthetic Plastic Surgery (ASAPS) *
36 W 44th Street, Suite 630
New York, NY 10036
(212) 921-0500
www.surgery.org

Founded in 1967, ASAPS is the leading professional organization of plastic surgeons certified by the American Board of Plastic Surgery who specialize in cosmetic plastic surgery.

American Society for Bariatric Physicians (ASBP) *
2821 S Parker Road, Suite 625
Aurora, CO 80014
(303) 770-2526
www.asbp.org

The American Society of Bariatric Physicians is an international association of allied health care professionals with special interest and experience in the comprehensive treatment of overweight, obesity, and related disorders. Their purpose is to establish and maintain practice guidelines, and provide education to their members, the health care industry, and the public.

American Society for Bariatric Surgery (ASBS)
Now: American Society for Metabolic and Bariatric Surgery (ASMBS) *
1100 SW 75th Drive, Suite 201
Gainesville, FL 32607
(352) 331-4900
www.asbs.org

Founded in 1983, ASMBS is the largest society in the world for this medical specialty. Many of the specialty's foremost American surgeons comprise this society's leadership, and have established an excellent organization with educational and support programs for surgeons and allied health professionals.

Bariatrix Nutrition
PO Box 65069
Burlington, VT 05406
800-468-3438
www.bariatrix.com

In addition to their innovative weight management and nutritional supplement products, Bariatrix provides consumers with a wealth of nutrition and weight management information. The info page is regularly updated with selected articles, helpful links, sample diets, and recipes. We also recommend signing up on the homepage for their e-Bulletin which provides featured products, info, feedback and more!

Building Blocks® Essential Bariatric Vitamin Supplements
4800 NE 20th Terrace, Suite 303
Fort Lauderdale, FL 33308
877-419-1568
www.bbvitamins.com

Essential bariatric vitamins and mineral supplements. Building Blocks® is committed to improving the health and well-being of the bariatric patient by providing an effective and easy-to-follow daily supplement protocol for both bypass and gastric band patients. These supplements provide maximum absorption and bioavailability in multiple forms to meet the needs of the pre-operative through post-operative timeframe - liquid to chewable to capsule. The Stepping Stone protocol helps eliminate the confusion patients often have regarding what vitamins to take for their nutritional needs.

CBS Health Watch
www.cbsnews.com/sections/health/main204.shtml

Medscape takes consumer health information to a new level with CBS Health Watch, which offers an array of high-quality information and interactive tools to help consumers and their families manage their daily personal health.

Calmoseptine®
16602 Burke Lane
Huntington Beach, CA 92647-4536
(800) 800-3405
www.calmoseptineointment.com

Calmoseptine® is a multi-purpose moisture barrier ointment formulated to temporarily relieve discomfort and itching. Originally created in the 1930's as a diaper rash ointment, it is now widely used by hospitals and other medical care facilities as a treatment for a variety of skin irritation conditions, including the conditions suffered by bariatric patients with excess skin. Calmoseptine® is available at any pharmacy in North America without a prescription. It is a very effective, easy to apply, helpful resource for patients with excess skin irritation issues.

Canadian Obesity Network
www.obesitynetwork.ca

The Canadian Obesity Network (CON) focuses the expertise and dedication of more than 1,000 member researchers, clinicians, allied health care providers and other professionals with an interest in obesity in a unified effort to reduce the mental, physical, and economic burden of obesity on Canadians. Membership application is available to everyone.

CareCredit
GE Card services
PO Box 960061
Orlando, FL 32896-0061
www.carecredit.com

CareCredit helps patients pay for costly healthcare procedures that insurance doesn't cover. They offer convenient monthly payment options, no up-front costs, no prepayment penalties and no annual fees. They also offer extended payment plans with low, fixed interest rates if you need more time to pay for your procedure. CareCredit offers a long list of credible healthcare organization endorsements. They are a GE Money Company, so you know you they are reliable and credible. More than six million cardholders have used CareCredit to get the healthcare services they wanted or needed over the past 20 years.

Centers for Disease Control and Prevention (CDC)

1600 Clifton Road
Atlanta, GA 30333
(404) 639-3534 (800) 311-3435
www.cdc.gov

The Centers for Disease Control and Prevention (CDC) is recognized as the leading federal agency for protecting the health and safety of people — at home and abroad — by providing credible information to enhance health decisions, and promoting health through strong partnerships. The CDC serves as the national focus for developing and applying disease prevention and control, environmental health, and health promotion and education activities designed to improve the health of the people of the United States.

Ethicon Endo-Surgery, Inc.
BariatricEdge

4545 Creek Road
Cincinnati, OH 45242
1-800-USE-ENDO
www.bariatricedge.com

Ethicon Endo-Surgery is a Johnson & Johnson company dedicated to helping patients find and understand credible information about weight loss surgery options and procedures.

International Bariatric Surgery Registry (IBSR)

Dept. of Surgery, University of Iowa Hospitals & Clinics
200 Hawkins Drive, 1504 JCP
Iowa City, IA 52242-1086
(800) 777-8442
healthcare.uiowa.edu/surgery/ibsr

The purpose of the IBSR is to promote optimum care of patients undergoing surgical treatments for severe obesity, and to give medical providers standardized clinical data collection and analysis.

Lap-Band® System

www.lapband.com

The LAP-BAND® System is an adjustable gastric band designed to help you lose excess body weight, improve weight related health conditions and enhance quality of life. This site explains the best information available concerning the Lap-Band®. Patient focused, easy to use.

Lipo in a Box®
Connie Elder International, LLC
PO Box 290219
Nashville, TN 37229-0219
(615) 885-1800
www.lipoinabox.com

The goal of Lipo in a Box® is to continue developing products for women that help them look and feel better. Connie Elder realized there was a need for a foundation garment product that offered control, shaping, and all-day comfort. It occurred to her that the technology found in medical-related compression garments might also work for shapewear. Connie notes, "This is NOT Grandma's girdle; it can be a solution to your figure problems or even complement your surgical procedure as an aftercare garment." Employing the same science used in compression garments, Lipo in a Box® shapewear is snug where you want support and comfortable where you need comfort.

National Eating Disorders Association
Eating Disorders Awareness and Prevention, Inc.
603 Stewart Street, Suite 803
Seattle, WA 98101
(206) 382-3587
www.edap.org

EDAP is the nation's largest nonprofit organization devoted to the awareness and treatment of eating disorders.

National Heart, Lung, and Blood Institute (National Institutes of Health)
NHLBI Information Center
PO Box 30105
Bethesda, MD 20824-0105
(301) 592-8573
www.nhlbi.nih.gov

The National Heart, Lung, and Blood Institute (NHLBI) provides leadership for a national program in diseases of the heart, blood vessels, lung, blood, blood resources, and sleep disorders. The Institute plans, conducts, fosters, and supports an integrated and coordinated program of basic research, clinical investigations and trials, observational studies, demonstrations, and educational projects.

The National Institutes of Health (NIH)
9000 Rockville Pike
Bethesda, MD 20892
(301) 496-4000
www.nih.gov

Founded in 1887, the National Institutes of Health is one of the world's foremost medical research centers. It is comprised of 25 separate institutes and centers, all part of the U.S. Department of Health and Human Services.

North American Association for the Study of Obesity *
8630 Fenton Street, Suite 918
Silver Spring, MD 20910
(301) 563-6526
www.naaso.org

The North American Association for the Study of Obesity is an interdisciplinary scientific society dedicated to the study of obesity. They are committed to encouraging research on the causes and treatment of obesity, and to keeping the medical community and public informed of new advances.

Sleepnet.com *
www.sleepnet.com

This is an educational web site that provides visitors with information on sleep disorders, terms and definitions, tips for better sleep, as well as useful links to other well rated informational web sites.

The Surgeon General's Call to Action to Prevent and Decrease Overweight and Obesity 2001
www.surgeongeneral.gov/topics/obesity

WebMD
webmd.com/solutions/sc/weight-loss-surgery
my.webmd.com/health_and_wellness/food_nutrition/lose_weight/default.htm

WebMD provides connectivity and a full suite of services to the healthcare industry that improve administrative efficiencies and clinical effectiveness enabling high-quality patient care.

Weight-Control Information Network (National Institute of Diabetes and Digestive and Kidney Disorders at the National Institutes of Health)
1 WIN Way
Bethesda, MD 20892-3665
(202) 828-1025 1-877-946-4627
www.niddk.nih.gov

The Weight-Control Information Network (WIN) is a national information service of the National Institute of Diabetes and Digestive and Kidney Disease (NIDDK), National Institutes of Health (NIH). WIN was established in 2004 to provide health professionals and consumers with science-based information on obesity, weight control, and motivation.

Obesity Action Coalition
4511 North Himes Avenue, Suite 250
Tampa, FL 33614
www.obesityaction.org

The Obesity Action Coalition is a non-profit patient organization dedicated to educating and advocating on behalf o the millions of Americans affected by obesity. By strictly representing the interests and concerns of obese patients, the OAC is a unique organization with a patient-focused approach to obesity. Membership application available to everyone.

Smallsteps.gov
www.smallsteps.gov

119 ideas for movement and exercise. Sponsored by the U.S. Department of Health and Human Services.

Smart Nutrition Company (SmartForme)
40 Allen Road
PO Box 65069
Burlington, VT 05406
877-895-3511
www.smartforme.com

Bariatric diet and Bariatric nutrition products developed for bariatric surgery patients, SmartForme is a convenient source for high-protein nutrition. The bariatric product line is an impressive array of tasty, functional foods that are widely used to supplement the dietary phases surrounding bariatric weight loss surgery. SmartForme products use only the highest quality ingredients from around the world, and they focus on meeting the wants and needs of bariatric patients through development of products suggested by, and tested by bariatric patients!

The Rudd Center for Food Policy and Obesity – Yale University
Rudd Center for Food Policy & Obesity
309 Edwards Street
Yale University
New Haven, CT 06520-8369
(203) 432-6700
www.yaleruddcenter.org

The mission of the Rudd Center is to improve the world's diet, prevent obesity, and reduce weight stigma through creative connections between science and public policy, targeted research, frank dialogue among key constituents, and a commitment to real change. The Rudd Center assesses, critiques, and strives to improve practices and policies related to nutrition and obesity so as to inform and empower the public, promote objective, science-based approaches to policy, and maximize the impact on public health.

Make it a rule of life never to regret

and never to look back.

Regret is an appalling waste of energy;

you can't build on it;

it is only good for wallowing in.

KATHERINE MANSFIELD

Chapter Eighteen

⟶ GLOSSARY OF TERMS ⟵

Abdominal cavity – The abdomen or abdominal cavity contains all of the digestive organs.

Abdominoplasty – A surgical procedure used to make the abdomen more firm by removing loose skin, excess fat, and tightening the fascia.

Absorption – Process by which digested food is absorbed by the lower part of the small intestine into the bloodstream.

Addiction – Compulsive, uncontrolled dependence on a substance, habit, or practice to such a degree that cessation causes severe emotional, mental, or physiologic reactions.

Adhesions – The process of adhering or uniting of two surfaces or parts, especially the union of the opposing surfaces of a wound. Inflammatory bands that connect opposing serous surfaces.

Adipose – Fatty; pertaining to fat.

Agoraphobia – An anxiety disorder characterized by fear of being in an open, crowded, or public space such as a field, tunnel, bridge, congested street, or busy department store where escape is perceived as difficult or help not available in case of sudden incapacitation.

Allergies – Hypersensitive reactions to common, often intrinsically harmless substances, most of which are environmental or chemical.

Altzheimer's disease – Progressive mental deterioration characterized by confusion, memory failure, disorientation, restlessness, speech disturbances, and inability to carry out purposeful movement.

Amino acids – An organic chemical compound composed of one or more basic amino groups and one or more acidic carboxyl groups. Twenty of more than 100 amino acids that occur in nature are the building blocks of proteins.

Analgesic – Any of a class of drugs designed to reduce pain in the body.

Anastomosis – Surgical connection between two structures.

Anemia – Decrease in hemoglobin in the blood to below normal levels. It can be caused by decrease in red cell production, an increase in red cell destruction, or a loss of blood. It is related to low iron levels.

Anesthesia – Loss of sensation resulting from pharmacologic depression of nerve function or from neurological dysfunction.

Anti-depressants – Pertaining to a substance or measure that prevents or relieves depression.

Antihistamine – Any substance capable of reducing the physiologic and pharmacologic effects of histamine release in the body in response to allergic inflammatory reactions.

Arm lift – See brachioplasty.

ASBS – American Society for Bariatric Surgery; now American Society for Metabolic and Bariatric Surgery (ASBMS).

Bariatric – Pertaining to weight or weight reduction.

Biliopancreatic diversion – A restrictive and Malabsorptive surgical obesity procedure; an improvement on the jejuno-ileal bypass. Used more in Europe than the United States.

Bioenteric intragastric balloon (BIB) (intragastric balloon) – Device implanted in the body via an endoscope that passes through the mouth, down the esophagus, and into the stomach (not through surgical incisions). It is intended to restrict food intake in obese patients. Not yet approved in the United States.

Bleeder – Blood vessel that bleeds, especially one that is cut during a surgical procedure.

Blood counts – A determination of the number of red and white blood cells per cubic millimeter of blood. (Complete blood counts.)

Blood pressure – The pressure exerted by the circulating volume of blood on the walls of the arteries and veins and on the chambers of the heart.

Blood transfusion – Transfer of blood or blood components of an individual (donor) to another individual (receptor).

BMI – Body Mass Index-Method of calculating degree of excess weight. Based on weight and body surface area.

Body contouring – A cosmetic surgery to remove excess skin from the abdomen, breasts, arms, and thighs after significant weight loss.

Bowel leakage – Leakage of bowel contents following the cutting and closure of the bowel during surgery; the leakage of an anastomosis of the bowel.

Bowel obstruction – Blocking or clogging of any portion of the bowel.

Brachioplasty – "Brachio" meaning arm, and "plasty" meaning molding, formation, or surgical repair of a specified body part.

Breast augmentation – See mammoplasty.

Breast cancer – A malignant disease of the breast tissue. The incidence increases with age from the third to the fifth decade and reaches a second peak at age 65. Risk factors include obesity, certain genetic abnormalities, a family history of breast cancer, late menopause, diabetes, and hypertension.

Breast droop – See masto ptosis.

Breast implant – The surgical placement of prosthetic material in a breast either to increase the breast's size, or for reconstruction.

Breast lift – See mastopexy.

Butt lift – See glutepexy or gluteplasty.

Calcium – An alkaline earth metal element. The fifth most abundant element in the human body and is mainly present in the bone.

CT – Abbreviation for computed tomography. A radiographic technique that produces an image of a detailed cross section of tissue. It is a painless, noninvasive, test that requires no preparation.

Carafate® – A gastric protective used to treat and prevent ulcers.

Candidiasis – An infection caused by a species of yeast-like fungi called Candida. Diaper rash, vaginitis, and thrush are common topical manifestations of candidiasis.

Capillaries – Blood vessels.

Carbohydrate – Any of a group of organic compounds the most important of which are the saccharides, starch, cellulose, and glycogen. Carbohydrates constitute the main source of energy for all body functions, particularly brain functions, and are necessary for the metabolism of other nutrients.

Cardiac dysfunction – Pertains to a heart that is unable to function normally; may also pertain to abnormality in function of the esophageal opening of the cardiac portion of the stomach.

Cardiovascular – Pertaining to heart and blood vessels.

Charles Horton Cooley – Sociologist (1864-1929). Symbolic Interactionist; taught at the University of Michigan; coined the term "looking glass self" to describe the process by which our sense of self develops.

Chemical peel – A therapy to eliminate wrinkles, blemishes, pigment spots, and sun-damaged areas of the skin using a chemical solution to peel away the top skin layers to reveal smoother skin with tighter cells. Also called chemical exfoliation.

Circadian rhythms – A pattern based on a 24 hour cycle, especially the repetition of certain physiologic phenomena, such as sleeping and eating.

Clinically severe obesity – Body Mass Index of 40 or more, which is roughly equivalent to 100 pounds or more over ideal body weight. Also known as Morbid Obesity.

Clotrimazole – A broad-spectrum anti-fungal agent of the imidazole group used in topical applications to treat fungal and yeast infections.

Cognitive dissonance – A state of tension resulting from a discrepancy in a person's emotional and intellectual frame of reference for interpreting and coping with his or her environment. It usually occurs when new information contradicts existing assumptions or knowledge.

Colon – Large intestine beginning at the end of the small intestine and ending at the rectum.

Colon cancer – Cancer of the portion of the large intestine extending from the cecum to the rectum.

Co-morbidity – Illness (i.e., arthritis, hypertension) or disabling conditions associated with clinically severe obesity or obesity-related health conditions.

Complete Blood Count (CBC) – A determination of the number of red and white blood cells per cubic millimeter of blood. Hemoglobin or hematocrit levels (reflecting general iron stores) are also routinely reported as part of this test.

Congestive heart failure (CHF) – Heart failure in which the heart is unable to maintain an adequate circulation of blood in the bodily tissues or to pump out the venous blood returned to it by the veins.

Contraindications – Any symptom or circumstance indicating the inappropriateness of an otherwise advisable treatment (i.e., alcoholism; drug dependency; severe depression; sociopathic (antisocial) personality disorder).

Controlled-release – Released or activated at predetermined intervals or gradually over a period of time.

Coronary artery disease (CAD) – The abnormal condition that may affect the heart's arteries and produce various pathologic effects, especially the reduced flow of oxygen and nutrients to the myocardium.

Criteria – Defines potential candidate for surgery treatment.

Cytotec – Brand name for the generic drug Misoprostol. An anti-ulcer medication generally prescribed for use in preventing ulcers associated with the use of NSAIDs, or for treating duodenal ulcers.

Deep vein thrombosis (DVT) – A disorder involving a blood clot in one of the deep veins of the body, most commonly the iliac or femoral veins of the leg.

Degenerative joint disease – Inflammation of the joint which causes degenerative changes.

Dehydration – Excessive loss of water from body tissues.

Demerol – Brand name for generic meperidine hydrochloride. A narcotic analgesic (pain killer). Prescribed for moderate to severe pain.

Depression – A mood disturbance characterized by feelings of sadness, despair, or discouragement resulting from and normally proportionate to some personal loss or tragedy. Also, an abnormal emotional state characterized by exaggerated feelings of sadness, melancholy, dejection, worthlessness, emptiness, and hopelessness that are inappropriate and out of proportion to reality.

Dermabrasion – A treatment for the removal of superficial scars of the skin by the use of revolving wire brushes or sandpaper. An aerosol spray is used to freeze the skin for this procedure. Often used to reduce scars from severe acne.

Diabetes – A clinical condition characterized by the excessive excretion of urine. Generally, abbreviation for diabetes mellitus which is a complex disorder of carbohydrate, fat, and protein metabolism that is primarily a result of a deficiency or complete lack of insulin secretion by the beta cells of the pancreas, or resistance to insulin. See also, type 1 diabetes, type 2 diabetes.

Diarrhea – The state in which an individual experiences a change in the normal bowel habits characterized by the frequent passage of loose, fluid, unformed stools.

Diflucan – A trademark for a broad-spectrum anti-fungal agent. Brand name for generic drug fluconazole.

Digestion – Process by which food is broken down by the stomach and upper small intestine into absorbable forms.

Dilation – Process of enlarging a passage or anastomosis.

Dilatation – See dilation.

Dilaudid – Trademark for dilaudid hydrochloride, an opium based analgesic (pain killer). Also known as hydromorphone hydrochloride.

Disease – A condition of abnormal vital function involving any structure, part, or system of an organism. A specific illness or disorder characterized by a recognizable set of signs and symptoms, attributable to heredity, infection, diet, or environment. A process injurious to health and/or longevity.

Distention – The state of being swollen.

Diuretic – A drug or other substance tending to promote the formation and excretion of urine.

Dominant culture – The portion of the entire culture that dictates the prevailing power, privileges, and social status, and occupies the best positions in these categories.

Dramaturgy – Also dramaturgical analysis. Theory developed by sociologist E. Goffman to explain social interaction between individuals; social life is analyzed in terms of drama or the stage.

Dumping syndrome – Uncomfortable feeling of nausea, lightheadedness, upset stomach, diarrhea, associated with ingestion of sweets, high-calorie liquids, high fat foods or dairy products.

Duodenum – First twelve inches of small intestine immediately below stomach. Bile and pancreatic fluids flow into the duodenum through ducts from the liver and pancreas respectively. This is where much of the iron and calcium is absorbed.

Dysentery – An inflammation of the intestine, especially the colon that may be caused by chemical irritants, bacteria, protozoa, or parasites. Characterized by frequent and/or bloody stools and abdominal pain.

Edema – Swelling.

EKG – Abbreviation for electrocardiograph; a device used for recording the electrical activity myocardium to detect transmission of the cardiac impulse through the conductive tissues of the muscle. EKG allows diagnosis of specific cardiac abnormalities.

Endometrial cancer – Cancer of the mucous membrane lining of the uterus. It is the most prevalent gynecologic cancer most often occurring in the fifth and sixth decades of life. Risk factors associated with endometrial cancer include medical history of infertility, late menopause, uterine polyps, diabetes, hypertension, and obesity.

Endoscopy – The visualization of the interior of organs and cavities of the body with an endoscope.

Enteric coated – A coating put on a pill or capsule so that it doesn't dissolve until it reaches the small intestine.

Enzymes – A complex produced by living cells that causes chemical reactions in organic matter. Most enzymes are produced in tiny quantities and facilitate reactions that take place within the cells. Digestive enzymes, however, are produced in relatively large quantities and act outside of the cells in the digestive tube.

Erving Goffman – Sociologist (1922-1982); Symbolic Interactionist. Developed the social interaction theory called dramaturgy.

Esophagus – The esophagus is a long muscular tube, which moves food from the mouth to the stomach.

Essential fatty acids – Essential in the diet for proper growth, maintenance, and functioning of the body playing important roles in metabolism. The best dietary sources are natural vegetable oils, such as soy and corn oils; margarines blended with vegetable oils; wheat germ; edible seeds, such as pumpkin, sesame, and sunflower; and fish oils (Omega-3, fish and vegetable oils: Omega-6 vegetable and seed oils).

Excisional back lipidectomy – "Excise" meaning to remove completely, "back" referring to the rear portion of the torso, and "lipidectomy" referring to fat removal by surgical means.

Extended-release – Released or activated gradually over a period of time.

Face lift – See rhytidectomy.

Fascia – The fibrous connection membrane of the body that may be separated from other specifically organized structures, such as the tendons and ligaments, and that supports, covers, and separates the muscles.

Fat oxidation – The breaking down of fat into energy.

Fat soluble – Preferring or needing to reside in fat tissue.

First-pass effect – A process whereby drugs are initially absorbed through the intestinal system, move into the blood stream, and pass through the liver before they are redistributed back into the intestinal system for absorption by the body and are ready to perform the intended function.

Fluconazole – Generic name for Diflucan, a broad-spectrum anti-fungal agent.

Foley catheter – A rubber catheter (tube) with a balloon tip to be filled with a sterile liquid after it has been placed in the bladder. This kind of catheter is used when continuous drainage of the bladder is desired such as in surgery.

Folic acid – A yellow crystalline water-soluble vitamin essential for cell growth and reproduction.

Fundus – The base or the deepest part of an organ; the portion farthest from the mouth of the organ.

Gallbladder – A pear-shaped excretory sac lodged in the surface of the right lobe of the liver. It stores and concentrates bile which it receives from the liver. During digestion of fats the gallbladder contracts ejecting bile through the bile ducts into the duodenum.

Gallbladder disease – An abnormal vital function of the gallbladder characterized by a recognizable set of signs and symptoms.

Gallstone – Also known as biliary calculus. A stone formed in the biliary tract consisting of cholesterol or bile pigments and calcium salts. If stones cannot pass spontaneously into the duodenum they can be removed surgically.

Gastric – Pertaining to stomach.

Gastric bypass – Any of a number of surgical procedures that reconstruct the route of the gastric system.

Gastroesophageal reflux disease – A back flow of contents of the stomach into the esophagus that is often the result of incompetence of the lower esophogeal muscle. Gastric juices are acid and therefore produce burning pain in the esophagus.

Gastrointestinal protectant – Medications that either produce prostaglandins or inhibit acid production to protect the stomach or gastrointestinal linings from irritants or ulcer causing agents.

Gastrointestinal tract – Pertaining to stomach or intestine.

Gastrojejunostomy anastomosis – Upper connection of the Gastric Bypass operation.

Gastroplasty – A surgery performed to reshape or repair any stomach defect or deformity.

Gene therapy – The insertion of genes into an individual's cells and tissues to treat a disease, and hereditary diseases in particular.

Genetic – Pertains to transmitted hereditary characteristics.

Gestalt – A single physical, psychologic, or symbolic configuration, pattern, or experience that consists of a number of elements and has an effect as a whole different from that of the sum of its parts.

Ghrelin – A hormone produced in the lining of the stomach that stimulates appetite.

Glucose – A simple sugar found in foods, especially fruits, and a major source of energy present in the blood and animal body fluids.

Gluteplasty – "Gluteus" meaning any of the three muscles that form the buttocks, and "plasty" meaning to reshape of reform. See also butt lift.

Glutepexy – "Gluteus" meaning any of the three muscles that form the buttocks, and "pexy" meaning to affix or re-affix. See also butt lift.

Gout – A disease associated with an inborn error or uric acid metabolism that increases production or interferes with excretion of uric acid. Excess uric acid is converted to sodium urate crystals that pass through the blood and become deposited in joints and other tissues. The big toe is often a common site for the collection of urate crystals.

Gut – Intestine, digestive tract.

Hair follicle – A tiny tube of epidermal cells originating in the dermis and containing the root of a hair shaft.

HDL cholesterol – Abbreviation for high-density lipoprotein. HDL is a plasma protein made mainly in the liver and is involved in transporting cholesterol to the liver to be disposed. HDL is the good cholesterol.

Heparin – A naturally occurring substance that acts in the body as an anticlotting factor to prevent intervascular clotting.

Hernia – A weakness in the abdominal wall resulting in a detectable bulge.

Herniation – Process in which a hernia is formed.

Hormones – A complex chemical substance produced in one part or organ of the body that initiates or regulates the activity of an organ or a group of cells in another part.

Hydrogenation – The addition of hydrogen and removal of oxygen from a substance.

Hyperlipidemia (high cholesterol) – An excessive level of blood fats.

Hyperosmolality – Presence of highly concentrated substances capable of producing dumping syndrome.

Hypertension – High blood pressure.

Hypotension – Low blood pressure.

Hypothalamic-pituitary-adrenal axis – The combined system of neuroendocrine units that regulate the adrenal gland's hormonal activities in a negative feedback network.

Hypothyroidism – An underfunctioning thyroid gland.

Hypoventilation syndrome – An abnormal condition of the respiratory system in which the volume of air that enters the lungs and takes part in the gas exchange is not adequate for the body's needs.

Identity – Relating to who we are as individuals and people; defines which groups to which we belong. Can be based on either physical appearance or on collection of experiences, but most commonly believed to be based on both.

IFSO – International Federation for the Surgery of Obesity.

Ileum – The last ten feet of small intestine; responsible for the absorption of fat-soluble vitamins A, D, E, and K and other nutrients.

Ileus – Obstruction of the bowel caused by the immobility of the bowel.

Immune system – A system of tissues and organs that protects the body against pathogenic organisms and other foreign bodies.

Implantable gastric stimulator (gastric pacemaker) – A device surgically implanted under the skin of the abdomen with a connecting wire implanted in the wall of the stomach. The device emits electrical pulses to the stomach muscles to create a feeling of fullness that will cause the patient to eat less and lose weight. Not yet approved in the United States.

Infantile projectile vomiting – Process of vomiting that involves severe outthrust of contents, often seen in small infants.

Infection – The invasion of the body by micro-organisms that reproduce and multiply causing disease by local cellular injury, secretion of a toxin, or antigen-antibody reaction in the host.

Inflammatory disease – A disease state in the body caused by irritated and swollen cells or tissues.

Insulin – A naturally occurring polypeptide hormone secreted by the beta cells in the pancreas in response to increased levels of glucose in the blood as well as the parasympathetic nervous system.

Intravenous – Pertaining to the inside of a vein.

Iron supplements – Supplements often given in pill or liquid form to augment the iron level in the body's blood.

I.V. – Abbreviation for the term intravenous.

Jejunum – The middle ten feet of small intestine extending from the duodenum to the ileum; the part responsible for digestion.

Jejuno-ileal bypass – A surgical procedure bypassing the jejunum and ileum. No longer performed in the United States.

Keratin – A fibrous sulphur containing protein that is the primary component of the skin, hair, nails, and enamel of the teeth.

Kilogram – Measure of weight equal to 2.2 pounds.

Lactose intolerant – A sensitivity disorder resulting in the inability to digest lactose (milk sugar) from dairy products because of inadequate production of, or defect in the enzyme lactase.

Lap-Band® – Brand name for a particular adjustable gastric band.

Laparoscopy – Method of visualizing and surgically treating intra-abdominal problems with long fiber-optic instruments.

Large intestine – Lower portion of the intestinal tract. In the large intestine, excess fluids are absorbed and a firm stool is formed. The colon may absorb protein, when necessary.

Laser resurfacing – A dermatological procedure that involves the use of lasers to even the surface and contour of the skin.

LDL cholesterol – Abbreviation for low-density lipoprotein. LDL is a plasma protein provided by the liver, and delivers lipids and cholesterol to the body tissues. LDL is the bad cholesterol.

Leptin – A protein hormone produced by fat cells that regulates blood sugar and affects regulation of body weight and metabolism, and stimulates satiety.

Level One Trauma Care – A level of care classification based on type of care given, the number of people being served, and the people providing the care. A level one trauma care center provides trauma medical care for the most urgent and critical patients, serves an entire geographic region, has specialized equipment and facilities for the care of these patients, and the medical personnel are specifically trained in this type of medical practice.

Liposuction – A technique for removing adipose (fat) tissue with a suction pump device. It is used primarily to remove or reduce localized areas of fat around the abdomen, breast, legs, face, and upper arms where the skin is contractile enough to redrape in a normal fashion.

Looking-Glass Self – Term coined by sociologist Charles Horton Cooley to describe the process by which one develops a sense of self in response to perceived behaviors and reactions of others.

Lortab® – Liquid Vicodin® elixir for post-surgical pain management containing morphine derivatives.

Lower body lift – The combination of a medial thigh lift, abdominoplasty, and gluteplasty or glutepexy are commonly referred to as a lower body lift. May also include excisional back lipidectomy and/or liposuction.

Lung collapse – Disinflation of one or both of the lung organs.

Macronutrients – Nutrients required in the greatest amounts for the normal physiologic processes of the body; carbohydrate, protein, fat, and water.

Magnesium – A silver white mineral element.

Mammoplasty – Reshaping of the breasts through plastic surgery, performed to reduce or lift sagging breasts, to enlarge small breasts, or to reconstruct a breast after tumor removal.

Mastopexy – Repositioning or lifting of the breasts through plastic surgery.

Masto ptosis – An abnormal condition in which one or both of the nipples of the breasts droop near or below the breast crease beneath the breast.

Medial thigh lift – A surgical procedure pertaining to the center portion of the thigh intended to remove excess skin and lift the remaining skin and underlying tissue.

Menstrual irregularities – Abnormal functioning of the menstrual cycle that may include shortened or prolonged menstrual cycles, abnormally heavy or light menses, pain with menstruation, and other symptoms.

Metabolism – The aggregate of all chemical processes that take place in living organisms resulting in growth, generation of energy, elimination of wastes, and other body functions as they relate to the distribution of nutrients in the blood after digestion.

Metabolites – A substance produced by metabolic action or necessary for a metabolic process. An essential metabolite is one required for a vital metabolic process.

Metaphysical – Of or relating to the transcendent or a reality beyond what is perceptible to the senses.

Micronutrients – Any dietary element essential only in minute amounts for the normal physiologic processes of the body, including vitamins and minerals or chemical elements such as zinc or iodine.

Minoxidil – Generic drug name for any of a series of antihypertensives or hair growth stimulants. See Rogaine.

Misoprostol – Generic name for brand name drug cytotec. Anti-ulcer medication.

Monounsaturated fat – Unsaturated fats having only one double or triple bond of carbon atoms in the hydrocarbon chain. Found in foods such as fowl, pecans, cashews, almonds, peanuts and olive oil. Considered a good fat.

Morbid obesity – Body Mass Index of 40 or more, which is roughly equivalent to 100 pounds or more over ideal body weight.

Morbid – Pertaining to disease, illness, increased risk of death.

Morphine – A white crystalline alkaloid derived from the opium poppy. Used as an analgesic (pain killer).

Mortality – Pertaining to death.

Multi-disciplinary approach – Team approach to evaluation and treatment of clinically severe obesity; includes surgical, internal medicine, nutrition, behavioral, and exercise physiology assessment and treatment.

Nasogastric tube – Any tube passed into the stomach through the nose.

Nausea – A condition characterized by an unpleasant, wave-like sensation in the back of the throat, gastric system, or abdomen that may or may not result in vomiting.

Negative conditioning – A form of behavior modification in which the presentment of something immediately after occurrence of a particular behavior, will decrease the rate of recurrence of the behavior.

Nervous breakdown – An attack of a mental or emotional disorder of sufficient severity as to be incapacitating and/or requiring hospitalization.

Neurochemicals – Concerned with, and having effects on the biochemicals of the nervous system.

NIH – National Institutes of Health.

Nitrosamines – Potentially cancer causing compounds produced by reactions of nitrites with amines or amides normally present in the body.

NSAID – Non-steroidal anti-inflammatory drug.

Nutritional supplementation – Assisting with or providing a balanced dietary intake of foods and nutrients either through food substances or vitamin and mineral substances.

Nystatin – Generic name for a vaginal anti-infective, or a general anti-fungal agent.

Obesity – Pertaining to excessive weight or adipose tissue.

Obstructions – Narrowing of an anastomosis or segment of gastrointestinal tract which slows normal passage of food or waste materials.

Osmosis – The movement of a pure solvent such as water through a differentially permeable membrane from a solution that has a lower solute concentration to one that has a higher solute concentration. The membrane is impermeable to the solute, but permeable to the solvent.

Osmotic pump – A miniature medication infusion pump for continuous and controlled dosing delivery.

Osteoarthritis – A form of arthritis in which one or many joints undergo degenerative changes. Arthritis is an inflammatory condition of the joints characterized by pain, swelling, heat, redness, and limitation of movement.

Overweight – More than normal in body weight after adjustment for height, body build, and age or 10-20% above the person's "desirable" body weight.

Panniculus – A sheet or layer of tissue; the superficial fascia which contains an abundance of fat deposits on various parts of the body; a collection of fat and skin that protrudes on the abdomen or lower belly.

Panniculectomy – The plastic surgery procedures that removes the excess panniculus, or skin and fat of the apron on the lower belly.

Panic attack – An episode of acute anxiety that occurs unpredictably with feelings of intense apprehension or terror, accompanied by dizziness, sweating, trembling, and chest pain or palpitations. The attack may last several minutes and may occur again in certain situations.

Peristalsis – The coordinated, rhythmic serial contraction of smooth muscle that forces food through the digestive tract, bile through the bile duct, and urine through the ureters.

PCA – Patient controlled analgesia. A drug delivery system that dispenses a preset intravascular dose of a narcotic pain medication when the patient pushes a switch on an electric cord. The patient administers a dose of narcotic when the need for pain relief arises. A lockout interval automatically inactivates the system if the patient tries to increase the amount of narcotic with the preset period.

Pediatric – Of or pertaining to infants, children, or minors.

Peptides – A molecular chain compound composed of two or more amino acids joined by peptide bonds.

Pharmacology – The study of the preparation, properties, uses and actions of drugs.

pH level – Abbreviation for potential hydrogen, a scale representative of the relative acidity (or alkilinity) of a solution, in which a value of 7.0 is neutral, below 7.0 is acid, and above 7.0 is alkaline.

Pica – A craving to eat nonfood substances such as dirt, clay, chalk, glue, ice, starch, paper, or hair. This appetite disorder may occur with some nutritional deficiency states (particularly iron deficiency), with pregnancy, and in some forms of mental illness.

Plastic surgery – The alteration, replacement, or restoration of visible parts of the body, performed to correct a structural or cosmetic defect. The medical term "plastic" refers to something that is conformable, or capable of being molded.

Pneumonia – An acute inflammation of the lungs, often caused by inhaled bacteria, viruses, or fungi.

Polyunsaturated fat – Unsaturated fats having more than one double or triple bond of carbon atoms in the hydrocarbon chain. Found in foods such as fish, corn, walnuts, sunflower seeds, soybeans, and safflower oil.

Port – A device that serves as an entrance or conduit for the insertion of medical devices or instruments, or for the delivery of medication or nutrients.

Post-traumatic stress disorder (PTSD) – A disorder characterized by an acute emotional response to a traumatic event or situation involving severe environmental stress, such as a natural disaster, airplane crash, serious automobile accident, military combat, or physical torture.

Potassium – An alkali metal element in the body that helps to regulate neuromuscular excitability and muscle contraction.

Prostaglandins – A natural substance produced in the body that provides protection for the stomach and pouch linings.

Proton pump inhibitors (PPIs) – An agent that inhibits gastric acid secretion. Protects against ulcer production by preventing acid production. Also known as a gastric acid pump inhibitor.

Pseudo-droop – A form of masto ptosis in which the nipple of the breast does not droop below the crease of the breast.

Pseudotumor-cerebri headaches – A condition characterized by increased intracranial pressure, headache, blurring of the optic disc margins, and vomiting. Headaches that mimmic the signs of a tumor when no tumor is present.

Psychotherapy – Evaluation and treatment of mentally related disorders.

Pulmonary – Pertains to the lungs.

Pulmonary embolism (PE) – The blockage of a pulmonary artery by fat, air, tumor tissue, or blood clot that usually arises from a peripheral vein (most frequently one of the deep veins of the legs).

Pulse-oximetry monitor – A device that measures the amount of saturated hemoglobin in the tissue capillaries.

Pylorus – The pylorus is a small round muscle located at the outlet of the stomach and the entrance to the duodenum (the first section of the small intestine). It closes the stomach outlet while food is being digested into a smaller, more easily absorbed form. When food is properly digested, the pylorus opens and allows the contents of the stomach into the duodenum.

Rapid gastric emptying – See dumping syndrome.

Respiratory dysfunction – Pertains to a lung or lungs that are unable to function normally.

Rhytidectomy – A plastic surgery procedure in which wrinkles and other signs of aging are eliminated. See also face lift.

Rogaine – See minoxidil.

Role exit – Leaving a particular role or set of behaviors, responsibilities, and experiences behind in order to temporarily or permanently abandon the role, or to replace the role with another.

Roles – Particular sets of behaviors, responsibilities, experiences, and manners of acting, being, or reacting. Can include specific wardrobes or props that are included to facilitate the role (a uniform, a briefcase).

Roux-en-Y Gastric Bypass – A surgical method of reconnecting the stomach and upper small intestines in roughly in a Y shape, for the purposes of creating a restrictive and malabsorptive weight loss treatment.

Saline solution – A solution containing sodium chloride.

Satiety – The state of being satisfied as in the feeling of being full after eating.

Saturated fat – A fatty acid in which all of the carbon atoms in the hydrocarbon chain are joined by single bonds. They exist mostly as components of fats or other lipids of animal origin. Foods rich in saturated fat include beef, lamb, pork, veal, whole milk-products, butter, most cheeses, and some plant products such as cocoa butter, coconut oil, and palm oil.

Sclerotherapy – The use of sclerosing (tissue hardening) chemicals to treat conditions such as hemorrhoids, esophageal ulcers, or to reduce the size of a dilated anastomosis.

Sedation – An induced state of quiet, calmness, or sleep, as by means of a sedative or hypnotic medication.

Sedentary – Requiring a minimal amount of physical effort; a condition of inaction; sitting.

Self-concept – The composite of ideas, feelings, and attitudes that a person has about his or her own identity, worth, capabilities, and limitations. Includes self-perception, self-esteem, and adopted roles as components, but also includes one's idea of the self as person; how the roles are played (role performance), and what one brings to this planet and this existence that makes them the unique individual they are.

Self-esteem – The regard one holds one's self in. The value one places on one's self. The personal judgment of self-worth.

Self-perception – Also, self-image. The total concept, idea, or mental image one has of one's self and of one's role in society; the person one believes one's self to be. How one sees or perceives one's self physically, mentally, emotionally, intellectually, spiritually, and socially.

Serotonin – A naturally occurring derivative of tryptophan found in blood platelets and in the cells of the brain and intestine. In the intestines it stimulates the muscles to contract, and in the central nervous system, it acts as an important neurotransmitter. Carbohydrates are important to the production of serotonin.

Severe obesity – Also known as morbid obesity.

Sleep apnea – A sleep disorder characterized by periods in which respiration is absent. The person is momentarily unable to contract respiratory muscles or to maintain airflow through the nose and mouth.

Small intestine – The small intestine is about 15 to 20 feet long (4.5 to 6 meters) and is where the majority of the absorption of the nutrients from food takes place. The small intestine is made up of three sections: the duodenum, the jejunum, and the ileum.

Spasm – Twitching or involuntary contraction of a specified sort.

Staples – Surgically sterile devices for connecting tissue; usually permanent and made of stainless steel or titanium.

Stenosis – An abnormal condition characterized by the constriction or narrowing of an opening or passageway in a body structure.

Steristrips – Small, sterile adhesive bandage strips used after surgery to close small incision sites.

Steroids – Drugs used to relieve swelling and inflammation.

Stomach – The stomach, situated at the top of the abdomen, normally holds just over 3 pints (about 1500 ml) of food from a single meal. Here the food is mixed with an acid that is produced to assist in digestion. In the stomach, acid and other digestive juices are added to the ingested food to facilitate breakdown of complex proteins, fats, and carbohydrates into small, more absorbable units.

Stress urinary incontinence – The state in which an individual experiences a loss of urine of less than 50 ml occurring with increased abdominal pressure, such as experienced during coughing, sneezing, laughing, and lifting.

Strictures – Narrowing of anastomosis or section of intestine; often related to inflammation, external pressure, or scarring.

Stroke – Also known as cerebrovascular accident (CVA). An abnormal condition of the brain characterized by bleeding in the brain that may permanently damage tissue resulting in a variety of deficits.

Serum ferritin – A reliable test for the assessment of iron stores in the blood. Blood serum iron levels may show a deficiency before hemoglobin levels show a deficiency in a CBC.

Subculture – The values and related behaviors of a group that distinguishes its members from the larger culture; a world within a world.

Sudden Cardiac Death (SCD) – Death that occurs unexpectedly and from 1 to 24 hours after the onset of symptoms, with or without known pre-existing conditions.

Suppository – An easily melted medicated mass for insertion into the rectum, urethra, or vagina. Drug administration by rectal suppository is especially useful in cases of vomiting and certain digestive disorders.

Sustained-release – Gradual release of an active agent over a period of time, allowing for a sustained effect.

Therapy – Treatment.

Thrush – Candidiasis of the tissues of the mouth characterized by the appearance of creamy white patches of mucus on an inflamed tongue or gums.

Timed-release – Gradual release over a prolonged period of time.

Torso – The body excluding the head, neck, and limbs.

TPN (total parenteral nutrition) – The administration of a nutritionally adequate hypertonic solution through an indwelling catheter. The procedure is used in situations including prolonged coma, severe uncontrolled malabsorption, extensive burns, and other conditions in which feeding by mouth cannot provide adequate amounts of nutrition.

Trans fat – Fatty acids found in margarines and shortenings or as artifacts after hydrogenation.

Transfusion – The introduction into the blood stream of whole blood or blood components such as plasma, platelets, or packed red cells. Also, blood infusion.

Transit contact time – The time a medication spends in the intestinal tract determines how much is actually absorbed.

Triage – Establishing priorities of patient care for urgent treatment while allocating scarce resources.

Triglyceride – A simple fat compound consisting of three molecules of fatty acid and glycerol. They make up most animal and vegetable fats and are the principal lipids in the blood where they circulate within lipoproteins.

Tumescent – A solution that causes a certain type of swelling, edema, or stiffness.

Type 1 diabetes – Also known as Type 1 Diabetes Mellitus. A disorder of glucose and insulin metabolism in which patients are insulin dependent, and the condition may be caused by an autoimmune process. Contributing factors to the development of diabetes are heredity, obesity, sedentary lifestyle, high-fat low-fibre diets, hypertension, and aging.

Type 2 diabetes – Also known as Type 2 Diabetes Mellitus. A disorder of glucose and insulin metabolism in which patients are not insulin dependent, although they may use insulin for correction of symptomatic hyperglycemia (high blood sugar). Approximately 60%-90% of these patients are obese, and the condition is often improved by weight loss.

Ultrasonic – Pertaining to ultrasound waves.

Ultrasound – Sound waves at the very high frequency over 20kHz (vibrations per second).

Upper body lift – A combination of an arm lift and a breast lift, and may include the upper back.

Vagal Blocking for Obesity Control (VBLOC) – An experimental implantable electrical device that sends very high frequency, low power signals through leads to block vagal nerve transmission. The vagal nerves regulate much of the activity of the stomach and pancreas, and are also believed by some researchers to play a role in the signaling of satiety and hunger. Not yet approved in the United States.

Valve – A valve at the entrance to the stomach from the esophagus allows the food to enter while keeping the acid-laden food from "refluxing" back into the esophagus, causing damage and pain. Another valve separates the small and large intestines to keep bacteria-laden colon contents from coming back into the small intestine.

Vertical Banded Gastroplasty – A surgical procedure in which the stomach is subdivided and a vertical band is placed to form a restrictive component to aid in weight loss.

Vomiting – The forcible voluntary or involuntary emptying of the stomach contents through the mouth.

Chapter Nineteen

⟨ REFERENCE CITATIONS ⟩

PROLOGUE

Increased Capacity for Fat Storage and Reduced Capacity for Fat Utilization

1. Large V, Peroni O, Letexier D, Ray H, Beylot M. Metabolism of lipids in human white adipocytes. *Diabetes Metab* 2004; 30:294-309.

2. Sorisky A. From preadipocyte to adipoycte: Differentiation-direct signal of insulin from the cell surface to the nucleus. *Crit Rev Clin Lab Sci* 1999; 36:1-34.

3. Zhou YT, Wang ZW, Higa M, Newgard CB, Unger RH. Reversing adipocyte differentiation: implications for treatment of obesity. *Proc Natl Acad Sci* 1999; 96:2391-5.

4. Blaak EE. Basic disturbances in skeletal muscle fatty acid metabolism in obesity and type 2 diabetes mellitus. *Proc Nutr Soc* 2004; 63:323-30.

5. Hickner RC, Privette J, McIver K, Barakat H. Fatty acid oxidation in African American and Caucasian women during physical activity. *J Appl Physiol* 2001; 90:2319-24.

6. Kelley DE. Skeletal muscle triglycerides: an aspect of regional adiposity and insulin resistance. *Ann NY Acad Sci* 2002; 135-45.

7. Ritov VB, Menshikova EV, He J, Ferrell RE, Goodpaster BH, Kelley DE. Deficiency of subsarcolemmal mitochondria in obesity and type 2 diabetes. *Diabetes* 2004; 54:8-14.

8. Kelley DE. Influence of weight loss and physical activity interventions upon muscle lipid content in relation to insulin resistance. *Curr Diab Rep* 2004; 4:165-8.

Chronic Stress Response

9. Bjorntorp P. Do stress reactions cause abdominal adiposity and comorbidities? *Obes Rev* 2001; 2:73-86.

10. Rosmond R, Bjorntorp P. Quality of life, overweight, and body fat distribution in middle-aged men. *Behav Med* 2000; 26:90-4.

11. Ottosson M, Lonnroth P, Bjorntorp P, Eden S. Effects of cortisol and growth hormone on lipolysis in human adipose tissue. *J Clin Endocrinol Metab* 2000; 85:799-803.

12. http://www.ncbi.nlm.nih.gov; Goldstone AP. The hypothalamus, hormones, and hunger: alterations in human obesity and illness. *Prog Brain Res* 2006; 153:57-73.

13. Overgaard D, Gamborg M, Gyntelberg F, Heitmann BL. Psychological workload and weight gain among women with and without familial obesity. *Obesity* 2006; 14:458-63.

14. Valsamakis G, Anwar A, Tomlinson JW, Shackleton GH, McTeman PG, Chetty R, Wood PJ, Banerjee AK, Holder G, Barnett AH, Stewart PM, Kumar S. 11beta-hydroxysteroid dehydrogenase type 1 activity in lean and obese males with type 2 diabetes mellitus. *J Clin Endocrinol Metab* 2004; 89:4755-61.

Appetite Regulators

15. http://www.ncbi.nlm.nih.gov; Arora S, Anubhuti. Role of neuropeptides in appetite regulation and obesity - a review. *Neuropeptides* 2006; 40:375-401.

16. http://www.ncbi.nlm.nih.gov; Adan RA, Tiesjema B, Hillebrand JJ, la Fleur SE, Kas MJ, de Krom M. The MC4 receptor and control of appetite. *Br J Pharmacol* 2006; 149:815-27.

17. http://www.ncbi.nlm.nih.gov; Bloom SR. Regulation of food intake by gastrointestinal hormones. *Curr Opin Gastroenterol* 2006; 22:626-31.

18. http://www.ncbi.nlm.nih.gov; Talley NJ. Gut-brain neuropeptides in the regulation of ingestive behaviors and obesity. *Am J Gastroenterol* 2006; Oct: 6.

19. http://www.ncbi.nlm.nih.gov; Cummings DE. Ghrelin and the short- and long-term regulation of appetite and body weight. *Physiol Behav* 2006; 89:71-84.

20. http://www.ncbi.nlm.nih.gov; Garattini S, Bizzi A, Caccia S, Mennini T, Samanin R. Progress in assessing the role of serotonin in the control of food intake. *Clin Neuropharmacol* 1988; 11:S8-32.

21. Konturek SJ, Konturek JW, Pawlik T, Brzozowski T. Brain-gut axis and its role in the control of food intake. *J Physiol Pharmacol* 2004; 55:137-54.

22. http://www.ncbi.nlm.nih.gov; Bloom SR. Gut peptides in the regulation of food intake and energy homeostasis. *Endocr Rev* 2006; 27:719-27.

Hormones and Obesity

23. Peeke PM, Chrousos GP. Hypercortisolism and obesity. *Ann NY Acad Sci* 1995; 771:665-76.

24. Bjorntorp P. Endocrine abnormalities of obesity. *Metabolism* 1995; 44:21-3.

25. De Pergola G, Giagulli VA, Garruti G, Cospite MR, Giogino F, Cignarelli M, Giorgino R. Low dehydroepiandrosterone circulating levels in premenopausal obese women with very high body mass index. *Metabolism* 1991; 40:187-90.

26. Holdstock C, Engstrom BE, Ohrvall M, Lind L, Sundbom M, Karlsson FA. Effect of bariatric surgery on adipose tissue regulatory peptides and growth hormone secretion. *Asia Pac J Clin Nutr* 2004; 13 (Suppl): S41.

27. Mayes JS, Watson GH. Direct effects of sex steroid hormones on adipose tissues and obesity. *Obes Rev* 2004; 5:197-216.

28. Diamanti-Kandarakis E, Bergiele A. The influence of obesity on hyperandrogenism and infertility in the female. *Obes Rev* 2001; 2:231-8.

29. Nam SY, Lobie PE. The mechanism of effect of growth hormone on preadipocyte and adipocyte function. *Obes Rev* 2000; 1:73-86.

Products of Fat

30. Ahren B, Havel PJ, Pacini G, Cianflone K. Acylation stimulating protein stimulates insulin secretion. *Int J Obes* 2003; 27:1037-43.

31. Gullicksen PS, Della-Fera MA, Baile CA. Leptin-induced adipose apoptosis: Implications for body weight regulation. *Apoptosis* 2003; 8:327-35.

32. Vendrell J, Broch M, Vilarrasa N, Molina A, Gomez JM, Gutierrez C, Simon I, Soler J, Richart C. Resistin, adiponectin, ghrelin, leptin, and proinflammatory cytokines: relationships in obesity. *Obes Res* 2004; 12:962-71.

33. Bullo M, Salas-Salvado J, Garcia-Lorda P. Adiponectin expression and adipose tissue lipolytic activity in lean and obese women. *Obes Surg* 2005; 15:382-6.

34. Cottam DR, Mattar SG, Barinas-Mitchell E, Eid G, Kuller L, Kelley DE, Schauer PR. The chronic inflammatory hypothesis for the morbidity associated with morbid obesity: implications and effects of weight loss. *Obes Surg* 2004; 14:589-600.

35. Lee YH, Pratley RE. The evolving role of inflammation in obesity and the metabolic syndrome. *Curr Diab Rep* 2005; 5:70-75.

36. http://www.ncbi.nlm.nih.gov; Enriori PJ, Evans AE, Sinnayah P, Cowley MA. Leptin resistance and obesity. *Obesity (Silver Spring)* 2006; 14:254S-258S.

37. Havel PJ. Control of energy homeostasis and insulin action by adipocyte hormones: leptin, acylation stimulating protein, and adiponectin. *Curr Opin Lipidol* 2002; 13:51-9.

38. Faraj M, Havel PJ, Phelis S, Blank D, et al. Plasma acylation-stimulating protein, adiponectin, leptin, and ghrelin before and after weight loss induced by gastric bypass surgery in morbidly obese subjects. *J Clin Endocrinol Metab* 2003; 88:1594-602.

Medications that Cause Weight Gain

39. Sharma AM, Pischon T, Hardt S, Kunz I, Luft FC. Hypothesis: Beta-adrenergic receptor blockers and weight gain: A systemic analysis. *Hypertension* 2001; 37:250-4.

40. Blickle JF. Thiazolidiendiones: clinical data and perspectives. *Diabetes Metab* 2001; 27:279-85.

41. http://www.ncbi.nlm.nih.gov; Faulkner G, Cohn TA. Pharmacologic and nonpharmacologic strategies for weight gain and metabolic disturbance in patients treated with antipsychotic medications. *Can J Psychiatry* 2006; 51:502-11.

42. Fava M. Weight gain and antidepressants. *J Clin Psychiatry* 2000; 61:37-41.

43. Carver C. Insulin treatment and the problem of weight gain. *Diabetes Educ* 2006; 32:910-7.

44. Newcomer JW, Haupt DW. The metabolic effects of antipsychotic medications. *Can J Psychiatry* 2006; 480-91.

45. Biton V. Weight change and antiepileptic drugs. *Neurologist* 2006; 12:163-7; Wofford MR, King DS, Harrell TK. Drug-induced metabolic syndrome. *J Clin Hypertens* 2006; 8:114-9.

Chapter Two — Enlightenment

1. Staple line buttressing material developed by R. Baker, J. Foote and W.L. Gore and Associates, Seamguard®.

2. Baker, R., Foote, J., Kemmeter, P., Brady, R., Vroegop, T., Serveld, M. (2004). The science of stapling and leaks. *Obesity Surgery*, 14(10). 1290-8.

Chapter Three — The New and Improved, Amazing, All Natural Lemon Diet

1. Buchwald, H. (2007) Is morbid obesity a surgical disease? *General Surgery News, Obesity Care Suppl;* June; 6:9-15; www.ifso2007.com; Sturm, R., Ringel, J., Andreyeva, T. (2004). Increasing obesity rates and disability trends. *Health Affairs,* 23 (2). 199-205; United States, Centers for Disease Control, National Center for Health Statistics. Overweight prevalence. (2002). Washington DC: US Government Printing Office; Buchwald, H., Avidor, Y., Braunwald, E., et al. (2004). Bariatric surgery: a systematic review and meta-analysis. *Journal of the American Medical Association*, 292(14). 1724-37; Liping, L., Meydani, M. (2003). Angiogenesis inhibitors may regulate adiposity. *Nutrition Reviews,* 61(11). 384-387; Rosner, S. (2002). Obesity: the disease of the twenty-first century. *International Journal of Obesity Related Metabolic Disorders*, 26. S2-S4; http://www.ASBS.org/html/rationale/rationale.html (Rationale for the Surgical Treatment of Obesity).

2. Buchwald, H. (2007) Is morbid obesity a surgical disease? *General Surgery News, Obesity Care Suppl;* June; 9-15.

3. http://www.familystudies.org/alcoholism&genetics.htm (a site of the University of California — San Francisco, Department of Neurology, Gallo Clinic and Research Center — Human Genetics Project); Shuckit, M. (1999). New findings on the genetics of alcoholism. *Journal of the American Medical Association,* 281 (20). 1875-1876; Bouchard, C. (1994). The Genetics of Obesity. Boca Raton: CRC Press. 245.

4. United States. Alcohol Alert: National Institute on Alcohol Abuse and Alcoholism. (1992). No. 18, PH 357. Washington DC: U.S. Government Printing Office.

5. Cardon, L., Carmelli, D., Fabsitz, R., Reed, T. (1994). Genetic and environmental correlations between obesity and body fat distribution in adult male twins. *Human Biology* 663. 465-479; Price RA, Gottesman II. Body fat in identical twins reared apart: roles for genes and environment. (1991) *Behavior Genetics* Jan; 21(1): 1-7.

6. Jensen, G., Rogers, J. (1998). Obesity in older persons. *American Dietetic Association Journal,* (98). 1308-131.

7. United States. Surgeon General's call to action to prevent and decrease overweight and obesity. (2001). Washington DC: U.S. Government Printing Office; Olshansky JF, Passero DJ, Hershow RC, et al (2005). A potential decline in life expectancy in the United States in the 21st Century. *N Engl J Med* 352: 1135-7.

8. Anderson DA, Wadden TA. (2004) Bariatric surgery patients' views of their physicians' weight related attitudes and practices. *Obesity Research* Oct; 12(10): 1587-95; Schwartz, M., Chambliss, H., Brownell, K, Blair, S., Billington, C. (2003). Weight bias among health professionals specializing in obesity. *Obesity Research,* 11. 1033-1039; Teachman, B., Brownell, K. (2001). Implicit anti-fat bias among health professionals: is anyone immune? *International Journal of Obesity Related Metabolic Disorders,* 25. 1525-1531; Loomis, G., Connolly, K., Clinch, C., Djuric, D. (2001) Attitudes and practices of military family physicians regarding obesity. *Military Medicine,* 166. 121-125.

9. Wang SS, Brownell KD, Wadden TA. (2004) The influence of the stigma of obesity on overweight individuals. *International Journal of Obesity Related Metabolic Disorders* Oct; 28(10): 1333-7; Puhl, R., Brownell, K. (2001). Bias, discrimination, and obesity. *Obesity Research,* 9(12). 788-805.

10. Garner, D., Wooley, S. (1991) Confronting the failure of behavioral and dietary treatments for obesity. *Clinical Psychology Review,* 11(6). 729-780; Harris MB, Walters LC, Waschull S. (1991) Altering attitudes and knowledge about obesity. *Journal of Social Psychology* Dec; 131(6): 881-4.

11. Goldbeter A. (2006) A model for the dynamics of human weight cycling. *Journal of Biosciences* Mar; 31(1): 129-36; Jandacek RJ, Anderson N, Liu M, et al. (2005) Effects of yo-yo diet, caloric restriction, and olestra on tissue distribution of hexachlorobenzene. *American Journal of Physiology, Gastrointestinal and Liver Physiology* Feb; 288(2): G292-9; No authors listed (1999) Yo-yo dieting promotes gallstones. *Health News* April 15(5): 5; http://www.med.umich.edu/opm/newspage/2003/yoyodiet.htm. (Study links yo-yo dieting to poor post-menopause heart health.)

12. http://www.nih.gov/nihrecord/01_18_2005/story09.htm. Ghosh, A. (2005). Focus on women: seminar explores obesity research, stigma.

13. Major GC, Doucet E, Trayhurn P, Astrup A, Trembaly A. (2007) Clinical significance of adaptive thermogenesis. *International Journal of Obesity* Feb; 31(2): 204-12; Miller WC. (1999) How effective are traditional dietary and exercise interventions for weight loss? *Medicine and Science in Sports and Exercise* Aug; 31(8): 1129-34; Perri, M., Fuller, P. (1995). Success and failure in the treatment of obesity: where do we go from here? *Med Exerc Nutr Health,* 4. 255-272; National Task Force on the Prevention and Treatment of Obesity: very low calorie diets. *(1993). Journal of the American Medical Association,* 270. 967-974; Safer, D. (1991). Diet, behavior modification and exercise: a review of obesity treatments from a long-term perspective. *South Med J,* 84(12). 1470-4; Weintraub, M., et al. (1992). Long-term weight control study IV weeks (156-190): The second double-blind phase. *Clin Pharmacol Ther,* 51. 608-614; Powers, P., Dietel, M. ed. (1989). Conservative treatments for morbid obesity, in surgery for the morbidly obese patient. Lea & Feibiger: Philadelphia. 27-37; United States. National Institutes of Health. Clinical guidelines

on the identification, evaluation, and treatment of overweight and obesity in adults: The evidence report. (1998). Bethesda, MD: US Department of Health and Human Services; Jain, A. (2004). What works for obesity? A summary of the research behind obesity interventions. BMJ Publishing Group: London, England.

14. *Id.*

15. Shoelson SE, Herrero L, Naaz A. (2007) Obesity, inflammation, and insulin resistance. *Gastroenterology* May; 132(6): 2169-80; Ogden CL, Yanovski SZ, Carroll MD, Flegal KM. (2007) The epidemiology of obesity. *Gastroenterology* May; 132(6): 2087-102; Hell, E., Miller, K., Moorehead, M., et al. (2000). Evaluation of health status and quality of life after bariatric surgery: comparison of standard roux-en-y gastric bypass, vertical banded gastroplasty, and laparoscopic adjustable silicone gastric banding. *Obesity Surgery*, 10. 214-19; United States. National Institutes of Health. Consensus Statement 84. Bethesda, MD: US Department of Health and Human Services.

16. Finkelstein, E., Fiebelkorn, I., Wang, G. (2004). State-level estimates of annual medical expenditures attributable to obesity. *Obesity Research,* Jan. 18-24; Craig, B., Tseng, D. (2002). The cost-effectiveness of bariatric surgery. *American Journal of Internal Medicine,* 113. 491-8; Allison, D., Zannolli, R., Vienkat, K. (1999). The direct healthcare costs of obesity in the United States. *American Journal of Public Health,* 89. 1194-1199.

17. Lakdawalla, D., Bhattacharya, J., Dana, P. (2004). Are the young becoming more disabled? *Health Affairs,* 23. 168-176; Sturm, R., Ringel, J., Andreyeva, T. (2004). Increasing obesity rates and disability trends. *Health Affairs,* 23(2) 199-205.

18. Weber, M., Muller, M., Bucher, T., et al. (2004). Laparoscopic gastric bypass is superior to laparoscopic gastric banding for treatment of morbid obesity. *Annals of Surgery,* 240(6). 975-983; Hell, E., Miller, K., Moorehead, M., et al. (2000). Evaluation of health status and quality of life after bariatric surgery: comparison of standard roux-en-y gastric bypass, vertical banded gastroplasty, and laparoscopic adjustable silicone gastric banding. *Obesity Surgery,* 10. 214-19; Pories, W., Swanson, M., MacDonald, K., et al. (1995). Who would have thought it? An operation proves to be the most effective therapy for adult onset diabetes mellitus. *Annals of Surgery,* 222(3). 339-50; Chapman, A., Kiroff, G., Game, P., et al. (2004). Laparoscopic adjustable gastric banding in the treatment of obesity: a systematic literature review. *Surgery,* 135(3). 326-51.

19. Mason EE, Renquist KE, Huang YH, Jamal M, Samuel I. (2007) Causes of 30-day bariatric surgery mortality: emphasis on bypass obstruction. *Obesity Surgery* Jan; 17(1): 9-14; Flum DR, Salem L, Elrod JA, et al. (2005) Early mortality among Medicare beneficiaries undergoing bariatric surgical procedures. *Journal of the American Medical Association* Oct 19; 294(15): 1903-8; Chapman, A., Kiroff, G., Game, P., et al. (2004). Laparoscopic adjustable gastric banding in the treatment of obesity: a systematic literature review. *Surgery,* 135(3). 326-51.

20. Mason EE, Renquist KE, Huang YH, Jamal M, Samuel I. (2007) Causes of 30-day bariatric surgery mortality: emphasis on bypass obstruction. *Obesity Surgery* Jan; 17(1): 9-14; Sapala, J., Wood, M., Schuhknecht, M., Sapala, M. (2003). Fatal pulmonary embolism after bariatric operations for morbid obesity: a 24-year retrospective analysis. *Obesity Surgery,* 13(6). 819-25.

21. Luukkonen, P., Kalima, T., Kivilaakso, E. (1990). Decreased risk of gastric stump carcinoma after partial gastrectomy supplemented with bile diversion. *Hepatogastroenterology,* 37(4). 392-394; Lacaine, F., Houry, S., Huguier, M. (1992). Stomach cancer after partial gastrectomy for benign ulcer disease: a critical analysis of epidemiological reports. *Hepatogastroenterology,* 39(1). 4-8; Tersmette, A., Giardiello, F., Tytgat, G., Offerhaus, G. (1995). Carcinogenesis after remote peptic ulcer surgery: the long-term prognosis of partial gastrectomy. *Scandinavian Journal of Gastroenterology Supplement,* 212. 96-99.

22. Hamoui N, Anthone GJ, Kaufman HS, Crooks PF. (2006) Sleeve gastrectomy in the high risk patient. *Obesity Surgery* Nov; 16(11): 1445-9; Mognol P, Chosidow D, Marmuse JP. (2006) Laparoscopic sleeve gastrectomy (LSG): review of a new bariatric procedure and initial results. *Surgical Technology International* 15:47-52; Ou Yang SO, Loi K, Jorgenson J, Talbot M. (2007) HP25 Laparoscopic sleeve gastrectomy for morbidly obese patients. *ANZ Journal of Surgery* May; 77 suppl 1:A45; Langer FB, Bohdjalian A, Felberbauer FX, et al. (2006) Does gastric dilation limit the success of sleeve gastrectomy as a sole operation for morbid obesity? *Obesity Surgery* Feb; 16(2): 166-71.

23. Ou Yang SO, Loi K, Jorgenson J, Talbot M. (2007) HP25 Laparoscopic sleeve gastrectomy for morbidly obese patients. *ANZ Journal of Surgery* May; 77 suppl 1:A45; Freszza EE. (2007) Laparoscopic vertical sleeve gastrectomy for morbid obesity: the future procedure of choice? *Surgery Today* 37(4):275-81; Hamoui N, Anthone GJ, Kaufman HS, Crooks PF. (2006) Sleeve gastrectomy in the high risk patient. *Obesity Surgery* Nov; 16(11): 1445-9.

24. *Id.*

25. Dixon AF, Dixon JB, O'Brien PE. (2005) Laparoscopic adjustable gastric banding induces satiety: a randomized blind crossover study. *Journal of Clinical Endocrinology & Metabolism* 90(2): 813-819.

26. Chapman, A., Kiroff, G., Game, P., et al. (2004). Laparoscopic adjustable gastric banding in the treatment of obesity: a systematic literature review. *Surgery,*135(3). 326-51.

27. The Art of Adjustments with the Lap-Band®System. Allergan. Santa Barbara, CA.

28. *Id.*

29. Dargent J. Esophageal dilation after laparoscopic adjustable gastric banding: definition and strategy. (2005) *Obesity Surgery* June/July; 15(6):843-8.

30. Ponce J, Paynter S, Fromm R. (2005) Laparoscopic adjustable gastric banding: 1,014 consecutive cases. *Journal of the American College of Surgeons* Oct 201(4): 529-35.

31. Allen JW. (2007) Laparoscopic gastric band complications. *The Medical Clinics of North America.* May; 9(13): 485-97; Ponce J, Paynter S, Fromm R. (2005) Laparoscopic adjustable gastric banding: 1,014 consecutive cases. *Journal of the American College of Surgeons* Oct 201(4): 529-35.

32. Allen JW. (2007) Laparoscopic gastric band complications. *The Medical Clinics of North America* May; 9(13): 485-97; Ponce J, Fromm R, Paynter S. (2006) Outcomes after laparoscopic adjustable gastric band for slippage or pouch dilation. *Surgery for Obesity and Related Diseases* Nov-Dec; 2(5): 627-31.

33. Lopez PP, Patel NA, Koche LS. (2007) Outpatient complications encountered following Roux-en-Y gastric bypass. *The Medical Clinics of North America,* May; 91(3): 471-83; Nguyen NT, Wilson SE. (2007) Complications of antiobesity surgery. *Nature Clinical Practice – Gastroenterology and Hepatology* Mar; 4(3): 138-47; Tanenberg, R., Pories, W. (2002). Surgery for obesity. *Diabetes Forecast.* 55(4). 81-86; Chapman, A., Kiroff, G., Game, P., et al. (2004). Laparoscopic adjustable gastric banding in the treatment of obesity: a systematic literature review. *Surgery,* 135(3). 326-51; Sapala, J., Wood, M., Schuhknecht, M., Sapala, M. (2003). Fatal pulmonary embolism after bariatric operations for morbid obesity: a 24-year retrospective analysis. *Obesity Surgery,* 13(6). 819-25; Melinek, J., Livingston, E., Cortina, G., Fishbein, M. (2002). Autopsy findings following gastric bypass surgery for morbid obesity. *Archives of Pathology & Laboratory Medicine,* 126(9). 1091-5; http://www.memorial-health.net — (Possible complications from gastric bypass surgery.); Spaw, A., Husted, J. (2005). Bleeding after laparoscopic gastric bypass: case report and literature review. *Surgery for Obesity and Related Diseases,* 1(2). 99-103.

34. Doro C, Dimick J, Wainess R, et al. (2006) Hospital volume and inpatient mortality outcomes of total hip arthroplasty in the United States. *Journal of Arthroplasty* Sept; 21(6 suppl 2): 10-16; Tarity TD, Herz AL, Parvizi J, Rothman RH. (2006) Ninety-day mortality after hip arthroplasty: a comparison between unilateral and simultaneous bilateral procedures. *Journal of Arthroplasty* Sept; 21(6 suppl 2): 60-64; Ganhi R, Petruccelli D, Devereaux PJ, Adili A, et al. (2006) Incidence and timing of myocardial infarction after total joint arthroplasty. *Journal of Arthroplasty* Sept; 21(6): 874-7; Blom A, Patterson G, Whitehouse S, Taylor A, Bannister G. (2006) Early death following primary total hip arthroplasty: 1,727 procedures with mechanical thrombo-prophylaxis. *Acta Orthopaedica* June; 77(3): 347-50; Dobbs RE, Parvizi J, Lewallen DG. (2005) Perioperative morbidity and 30-day mortality after intertrochanteric hip fractures treated by internal fixation or arthroplasty. *Journal of Arthroplasty* Dec; 20(8): 963-6; Ritter, M., Harty, L., Davis, K., Meding, J., Berend, M. (2003). Simultaneous bilateral, staged bilateral, and unilateral total knee arthroplasty: a survival analysis. *Journal of Bone and Joint Surgery,* 85-A(8). 1532-7; Sheppeard, H., Cleak, D., Ward, D., O'Connor, B. (1980). A review of mortality and morbidity in elderly patients following Charnley total hip replacement. *Archives of Orthopaedic and Traumatic Surgery,* 97(4). 243-8; Chapman, A., Kiroff, G., Game, P., et al. (2004). Laparoscopic adjustable gastric banding in the treatment of obesity: a systematic literature review. *Surgery,* 135(3). 326-51.

35. Flum, D., Dellinger, E. (2004). Impact of gastric bypass operation on survival: a population based analysis. *Journal American College of Surgery,* 199. 543-551; http://www.njbariatricspc.com/tips/risk.asp.

36. Buchwald, H., Avidor, Y., Braunwald, E., et al. (2004). Bariatric surgery: a systematic review and meta-analysis. *Journal of the American Medical Association,* 292(14). 1724-37.

37. *Id.*

38. Pories, W., Swanson, M., MacDonald, K., et al. (1995). Who would have thought it? An operation proves to be the most effective therapy for adult onset diabetes mellitus. *Annals of Surgery,* 222(3). 339-50.

39. Spivak, H., Hewitt, M., Onn, A., Half, E. (2005). Weight loss and improvement of obesity-related illness in 500 U.S. patients following laparoscopic adjustable gastric banding procedure. *American Journal of Surgery, 189(1).* 27-32; Frigg, A., Peterli, R., Peters, T., Ackermann, C., Tondelli, P. (2004). Reduction in co-morbidities 4 years after laparoscopic adjustable gastric banding. *Obesity Surgery,* 14(2). 216-23.

40. Folope V, Coeffier M, Dechelotte P. (2007) Nutritional deficiencies associated with bariatric surgery. *Gastroenterologie Clinique et Biologique* April; 31(4): 369-77; Singh S, Kumar A. (2007) Wernicke encephalopathy after obesity surgery: a systematic review. *Neurology* Mar 13; 68(11): 807-11; Carrodequas L. Kaidar-Person O, Szomstein S, et al. (2005) Pre-operative thiamine deficiency in obese population undergoing laparoscopic bariatric surgery. *Surgery for Obesity and Related Diseases* Nov-Dec; 1(6): 517-22.

41. Chapman, A., Kiroff, G., Game, P., et al. (2004). Laparoscopic adjustable gastric banding in the treatment of obesity: a systematic literature review. *Surgery,* 135(3). 326-51.

42. Spaulding L. (2003) Treatment of dilated gastrojejunostomy with sclerotherapy. *Obesity Surgery* April; 13(2): 254-7; Bardaro SJ, Hong D, July L, Jan J, Patterson E. (2006) Endoscopic-sclerotherapy on dilated gastrojejunostomy as an alternative treatment for patients with weight regain. ASBS poster session.

43. http://www.asbs.org/html/story/chapter3.html

44. Hall, J., Watts, J., O'Brien, P., et al. (1990). Gastric surgery for morbid obesity. Adelaide Study. *Annals of Surgery,* 211. 419-27.

45. Perri, M., Fuller, P. (1995). Success and failure in the treatment of obesity: where do we go from here? *Med Exerc Nutr Health*, 4. 255-272; National Task Force on the Prevention and Treatment of Obesity: very low calorie diets. *(1993). Journal of the American Medical Association*, 270. 967-974; Safer, D. (1991). Diet, behavior modification and exercise. A review of obesity treatments from a long-term perspective. *South Med J*, 84(12). 1470-4; Weintraub, M., et al. (1992). Long-term weight control study IV (weeks 156-190): the second double-blind phase. *Clin Pharmacol Ther*, 51. 608-614; Powers, P., Dietel, M. ed. (1989). Conservative treatments for morbid obesity, in surgery for the morbidly obese patient. Lea & Feibiger: Philadelphia. 27-37; United States. National Institutes of Health. Clinical guidelines on the identification, evaluation, and treatment of overweight and obesity in adults: the evidence report. (1998). Bethesda, MD: US Department of Health and Human Services; Jain, A. (2004). What works for obesity? A summary of the research behind obesity interventions. BMJ Publishing Group: London, England; Pories, W., Swanson, M., MacDonald, K., et al. (1995). Who would have thought it? An operation proves to be the most effective therapy for adult onset diabetes mellitus. *Annals of Surgery*, 222(3). 339-50.

46. Pories, W., Swanson, M., MacDonald, K., et al. (1995). Who would have thought it? An operation proves to be the most effective therapy for adult onset diabetes mellitus. *Annals of Surgery*, 222(3). 339-50.

47. Lutfi R, Torquati A, Sekhar N, Richards WO. (2006) Predictors of success after laparoscopic gastric bypass: a multivariate analysis of socioeconomic factors. *Surgical Endoscopy* June; 20(6):864-7; Branson R, Potoczna N, Brunotte R. (2005) Impact of age, sex, and body mass index on outcomes at four years after gastric banding. *Obesity Surgery* Jun-July; 15(6): 834-42.

48. Pories, W., Swanson, M., MacDonald, K., et al. (1995). Who would have thought it? An operation proves to be the most effective therapy for adult onset diabetes mellitus. *Annals of Surgery*, 222(3). 339-50; Barakat, H., McLendon, V., Marks, R., Pories, W., Heath, J., Carpenter, J. (1992). Influence of morbid obesity on non-insulin-dependent diabetes mellitus on high-density lipoprotein composition and subpopulation distribution. *Metabolism*, 41(1). 37-41.

49. Ketchum ES, Morton JM. (2007) Disappointing weight loss among shift workers after laparoscopic gastric bypass surgery. May *Obesity Surgery* 17(5): 581-584.

50. *Id.*

51. *Id.*

52. *Id.*

53. *Id.*

54. *Id.*

Chapter Five – Auto Eject

1. http://www.mayoclinic.com.

2. *Mosby's Medical, Nursing & Allied Health Dictionary*, (6ᵗʰ ed.). (2002) St. Louis: Mosby.

3. http://www.healthlink.mcw.edu.

4. http://www.healthlink.mcw.edu

5. Klockhoff H, Naslund I, Jones AW. (2002) Faster absorption of ethanol and higher peak concentration in women after gastric bypass surgery. *British Journal of Clinical Pharmacology* 54:587-91.

6. Buffington, CK. (2006) Alcohol and the gastric bypass patient. *Bariatric Times* Oct; 3(8): 10.

Chapter Six — The "Build-Your-Own Cat" Kit

1. Cho S, Badel S, Golay A. (2007) Micronutrition: A global approach for obese patients. *Revue Medicale Suisse* April; 3(105): 863-7; Folope V, Coeffier M, Dechelotte P. (2007) Nutritional deficiencies associated with bariatric surgery. *Gastroenterologie Clinique et Biologique* April; 31(4): 369-77; Can your diet help you keep your hair? Hair Loss Advisor web site webcast with Peter S. Halpern, MD, New York Presbyterian Hospital, and Shari Lieberman, PhD, CNS, University of Bridgeport School of Human Nutrition. (2001) Available at: http://www.hairlossadvisor.com/hairlossadvisor/154.htm. Accessed: May 24, 2007.

2. Cho S, Badel S, Golay A. (2007) Micronutrition: A global approach for obese patients. *Revue Medicale Suisse* April; 3(105): 863-7; Jones, D. (2004) Essential Fatty Acids & Bari-EFA. Bariatrix Nutrition EFA pamphlet; Folope V, Coeffier M, Dechelotte P. (2007) Nutritional deficiencies associated with bariatric surgery. *Gastroenterologie Clinique et Biologique* April; 31(4): 369-77.

Chapter Seven — The Shadows of My Former Self

1. Merriam-Webster, A. Websters New Collegiate Dictionary. 9th Ed. Springfield, MA; Merriam-Webster Inc. 1986.

2. *Id.*

3. Song Z, Reinhardt K, Buzdon M, Liao P. (2007) Association between support group attendance and weight loss after Roux-en-Y gastric bypass. *Surgery for Obesity and Related Diseases* Mar 30 (e-pub ahead of print); Latner JD, Stunkard AJ, Wilson GT, Jackson, ML. (2006) The perceived effectiveness of continuing care and group support in the long-term self-help treatment of obesity. *Obesity (Silver Spring)* Mar; 14(3): 464-71; Elakkary E, Elhor A, Aziz F, Gazayerli MM, Silva YJ. (2006) Do support groups play a role in weight loss after laparoscopic adjustable gastric banding? *Obesity Surgery* Mar; 16(3): 331-4.

4. *Id.*

5. *Id.*

Chapter Nine — Separation Anxiety

1. Charles Horton Cooley (1864-1929). Cooley, C.H. (1902). *Human Nature and the Social Order.* New York: Scribner's; Henslen, J.M. (2005). *Sociology: A Down-to-Earth Approach.* (7th ed.). Boston: Pearson Allyn and Bacon; Best, S. (2003). *A Beginners Guide to Social Theory.* Thousand Oaks: Sage Publications.

2. *Id.*

3. Erving Goffman (1922-1982). Goffman, E. (1959). *The Presentation of Self in Everyday Life.* New York: Doubleday; Henslen, J.M. (2005). *Sociology: A Down-to-Earth Approach.* (7th ed.). Boston: Pearson Allyn and Bacon; Best, S. (2003). *A Beginners Guide to Social Theory.* Thousand Oaks: Sage Publications.

4. See Glossary for definition. Henslen, J.M. (2005). *Sociology: A Down-to-Earth Approach.* (7th ed.). Boston: Pearson Allyn and Bacon.

5. http://www.asbs.org. Medicare Expands Coverage for Lifesaving Obesity Surgery. February 21, 2006.

Chapter Ten — No Girls Allowed

1. Poulose BK, Griffin MR, Moore DE, Zhu Y, Smalley W, et al. (2005) Risk factors for post-operative mortality in bariatric surgery. *Journal of Obesity Research* July 1; 127(1): 1-7.

2. Reftopoulos Y, Gatti GG, Luketich JD, Courcoulas AP. (2005) Advanced age and sex as predictors of adverse outcomes following gastric bypass surgery. *Journal of the Society of Laparoendoscopic Surgeons* Jul-Sep; 9(3): 272-6.

3. Branson R, Potoczna, N, Brunotte R, Piec G, et al. (2005) Impact of age, sex, and body mass index on outcomes at four years after gastric banding. *Obesity Surgery* Jun-Jul; 15(6): 834-42.

4. Weller WE, Rosati C, Hannan EL. (2006) Predictors of in-hospital post-operative complications among adults undergoing bariatric procedures in New York state, 2003. *Obesity Surgery* June; 16(6): 702-8.

5. Ballantyne GH, Svahn J, Capella RF, et al. (2004) Predictors of prolonged hospital stay following open and laparoscopic bypass for morbid obesity: body mass index, length of surgery, sleep apnea, asthma, and the metabolic syndrome. *Obesity Surgery* Sept; 14(8): 1042-50.

6. Kolotkin RL, Binks M, Crosby, RD, et al. (2006) Obesity and sexual quality of life. *Obesity (Silver Spring)* Mar; 14(3): 472-9.

7. Male infertility and obesity. Reproductive Biology Associates web site. 2007. Available at: http://www.rba-online.com. Accessed: January 2007.

8. Alagna S, Cossu ML, Gallo P, et al. (2006) Biliopancreatic diversion: long-term effects on gonadal function in severely obese men. *Surgery for Obesity and Related Diseases* Mar-April; 2(2): 75-7.

9. Sallmen, M, Sandler, D., Hoppin, J, Blair A., Baird, D. (2006) Reduced fertility among overweight and obese men. *Epidemiology* Sept; 17(5): 520-3. (NIEHS study).

10. di Frega AS, Dale B, Di Matteo L, Wilding M. (2005) Secondary male factor infertility after Roux-en-Y gastric bypass for morbid obesity: case report. *Human Reproduction* April; 20(4): 997-8.

Chapter Twelve — Medication Misadventures: How to Avoid Them!

Selected Readings

1. Benet LZ, Kroetz DL, Sheiner LB. Pharmacokinetics: the dynamics of drug absorption, distribution and elimination. In: Hardman JG, Limbird LE, eds. *Goodman and Gilman's The Pharmacological Basis of Therapeutics.* 9th ed. New York: McGraw-Hill; 1996:3-27.

2. Rowland M, Tozer TN. Absorption. In: *Clinical Pharmacokinetics: Concepts and Applications.* 3rd ed. Philadelphia: Lippincott, Williams, and Wilkins; 1995: 119-36.

3. Franklin MR, Franz DN. Drug absorption, action, and disposition. In: Gennaro AR, ed. *Remington: The Science and Practice of Pharmacy.* 20th ed. Baltimore: Lippincott, Williams, and Wilkins; 2000:1098-126, 28.

4. STAT!Ref Online Electronic Medical Library. New York, NY. McGraw-Hill; 2005 - *Schwartz's Principles of Surgery;* Chapter 25: Stomach; [about 64 p.]. Available from: http://0-online.statref.com.libcat.ferris.edu.

5. Behrns KE, Smith CD, Sarr MG. Prospective evaluation of gastric acid secretion and cobalamin absorption following gastric bypass for clinically severe obesity. *Dig Dis Sci* 1994; 39: 315-320.

6. Malone M. Altered drug disposition in obesity and after bariatric surgery. *Nutr Clin Pract* 2003; 18:131-5.

7. Macgregor AM, Boggs L. Drug distribution in obesity and following bariatric surgery: a literature review. *Obes Surg* 1996; 6:17-27.

8. Miller AD, Smith KM. Medication and nutrient administration considerations after bariatric surgery. *Am J Health-Syst Pharm* 2006; 63: 1852-7.

9. McEvoy GK, editor. AHFS Drug Information 2007. Bethesda: American Society of Health-System Pharmacist; 2007.

10. Alexandrides TK, Skroubis G, Kalfarentzos F. Resolution of diabetes mellitus and metabolic syndrome following Roux-en-Y gastric bypass and a variant of biliopancreatic diversion in patients with morbid obesity. *Obes Surg* 2007 Feb; 17(2):176-84.

11. Laferrere B, Heshka S, Wang K, Khan Y, McGinty J, Teixeira J, et. al. Incretin levels and effect are markedly enhanced one month after Roux-en-Y gastric bypass surgery in obese patients with type 2 diabetes. *Diabetes Care* 2007 Apr 6; [Epub ahead of print].

12. Rostom A, Wells G, Tugwell P, Welch V, Dube C, McGowan J. The prevention of chronic NSAID induced upper gastrointestinal toxicity: a Cochrane collaboration meta-analysis of randomized controlled trials. *J Rheumatol* 2000; 27: 2203-14.

13. Lanza FL. Gastrointestinal adverse effects of bisphosphonates: etiology, incidence and prevention. *Treat Endocrinol* 2002; 1: 37-43.

Chapter Fifteen — Shrink! Shrank! Shrunk!!

1. http://www.ASBS.org. Medicare Expands Coverage for Life Saving Obesity Surgery. American Society for Bariatric Surgery. 2006. Available at: http://www.asbs.org/html/about/ncd_release.html. Accessed: May 29, 2007.

2. http://www.ASPS.org. National Plastic Surgery Statistics. American Society of Plastic Surgeons web site. 2007. Available at: http://www.plasticsurgery.org. Accessed: May 29, 2007.

3. http://www.ASAPS.org

4. *Id.*

5. http://www.ASPS.org. Statistical Brief #23: Bariatric Surgery Utilization and Outcomes in 1998 and 2004. Health Care Cost and Utilization Project, Agency for Health Care Research and Quality web site. 2007. Available at: http://www.hcup-us.ahrq.gov. Accessed: May 29, 2007; Only 15% of Bariatric Patients Follow-Up with Plastic Surgery, ASPS Reports States. American Society of Plastic Surgeons web site. 2007. Available at: http://www.plasticsurgery.org. Accessed: May 29, 2007.

Chapter Sixteen – The Final Battle: Defeat of the Clones

1. Shikora SA, Storch K, Investigational Team. (2005) Implantable gastric stimulation for the treatment of severe obesity: the American experience. *Surgery for Obesity and Related Diseases* May-June; 1(3): 334-42; Shikora SA. (2004) What are the "Yanks" doing? The US experience with the implantable gastric stimulation (IGS) for the treatment of obesity – update on the ongoing clinical trials. *Obesity Surgery* Sept; 14 Suppl 1: S40-8.

2. Hoeller E, Aigner F, Margreiter R, Weiss H. (2006) Intragastric stimulation is ineffective after failed adjustable gastric banding. *Obesity Surgery* Sept; 16(9): 1160-5.

3. Implantable System for Obesity Treatment. Enteromedics web site. 2007. Available at: http://www.enteromedics.com. Accessed: May 29, 2007.

4. Ganesh R, Rao AD, Baladas HG, Leese T. (2007) The Bioenteric Intragastric Balloon (BIB) as a treatment for obesity: poor results in Asian patients. *Singapore Medical Journal* Mar; 48(3): 227-31; Spyropoulos C, Katsakoulis E, Mead N, Vagenas K, Kalfarentzos F. (2007) Intragastric balloon for high-risk super-obese patients: a prospective analysis of efficacy. *Surgery for Obesity and Related Diseases* Jan-Feb; 3(1): 78-83 (Greece); Fernandes M, Atallah AN, Soares BG, et al. (2007) Intragastric balloon for obesity. *Cochrane Database of Systematic Reviews* Jan; 24(1): CD004931 (Brazil); Micheletto G, Perrini MN, Occhipinti V, et al. (2006) The BIB intragastric balloon. *Annali Italiani di Chirurgia* July-Aug; 77(4): 305-8 (Milan); Angrisani L, Lorenzo M, Borrelli V, et al. (2006) Is bariatric surgery necessary after intragastric balloon treatment? *Obesity Surgery* Sept; 16(9): 1135-7 (Naples); Melissas J, Mouzas J, Filis D, et al. (2006) The intragastric

balloon – smoothing the path to bariatric surgery. *Obesity Surgery* July; 16(7): 897-902 (Greece); Tosato F, Carnevale L, Monsellato I, et al. (2006) Intragastric balloon in bariatric surgery. *Il Giornale di Chirurgia* Jan-Feb; 27(1-2): 53-8 (Rome); Mui WL, So WY, Yau PY, et al. (2006) Intragastric balloon in ethnic obese Chinese: initial experience. *Obesity Surgery* Mar; 16(3): 308-13 (China); Timna M, Pomerantz I, Konikoff F. (2006) Intragastric balloon for morbid obesity. *Harefuah* Nov; 145(11): 826-30, 861 (Isreal); Nijhof HW, Steenvoorde P, Tollenaar RA. (2006) Perforation of the esophagus caused by the insertion of an intragastric balloon for the treatment of obesity. *Obesity Surgery* May; 16(5): 667-70 (The Netherlands); Allison C. (2006) Intragastric balloons: a temporary treatment for obesity. *Issues in Emerging Health Technology* Jan; (79): 1-4 (USA); Alfalah H, Philippe B, Ghazal F, et al. (2006) Intragastric balloon for preoperative weight reduction in candidates for laparoscopic gastric bypass with massive obesity. *Obesity Surgery* Feb; 16(2): 147-50 (France); Milone L, Strong V, Gagner M. (2005) Laparoscopic sleeve gastrectomy is superior to endoscopic intragastric balloon as a first stage procedure for super obese patients. *Obesity Surgery* May; 15(5): 612-17 (USA).

5. *Id.*

6. *Id.*

7. *Id.*

8. *Id.*

9. *Id.*

10. *Id.*

11. *Id.*

12. Milone L, Strong V, Gagner M. (2005) Laparoscopic sleeve gastrectomy is superior to endoscopic intragastric balloon as a first stage procedure for super obese patients. *Obesity Surgery* May; 15(5): 612-17 (USA).

13. Pryor AD, DeMaria EJ. (2007) Future treatment options for morbid obesity. *General Surgery News, Obesity Care Suppl*; June: 83-87; Malik A, Mellinger JD, Hazey JW, Dunkin BJ, MacFadyen BD Jr. (2006) Endoluminal and transluminal surgery: current status and future possibilities. *Surg Endosc* 20:1179-1192.

14. Costa B. (2007) Rimonabant: more than an anti-obesity drug? *British Journal of Pharmacology* Mar; 150(5): 535-7; Padwal RS, Majumdar SR. (2007) Drug treatments for obesity: orlistat, sibutramine, and rimonabant. *Lancet* Jan; 369(9995): 71-7; Henness S, Robinson DM, Lyseng-Williamson KA. (2006) Rimonabant. *Drugs* 66(16): 2109-19; Wiersbicki AS. (2006) Rimonabant: endocannabinoid inhibition for the metabolic syndrome. *International Journal of Clinical Practice* Dec; 60(12): 1697-706; Scheen AJ, Finer N, Hollander P, et al. (2006) Efficacy and tolerability of rimonabant in overweight or obese patients with type 2 diabetes: a randomized controlled study. *Lancet* Nov; 368(9548): 1660-72; Curioni C, Andre C. (2006) Rimonabant for overweight or obesity. *Cochrane Database of Systematic Reviews* Oct; 18(4): CD006162.

15. Wiersbicki AS. (2006) Rimonabant: endocannabinoid inhibition for the metabolic syndrome. *International Journal of Clinical Practice* Dec; 60(12): 1697-706.

16. *Id.*

17. Padwal RS, Majumdar SR. (2007) Drug treatments for obesity: orlistat, sibutramine, and rimonabant. *Lancet* Jan; 369(9995): 71-7; Wiersbicki AS. (2006) Rimonabant: endocannabinoid inhibition for the metabolic syndrome. *International Journal of Clinical Practice* Dec; 60(12): 1697-706; Curioni C, Andre C. (2006) Rimonabant for overweight or obesity. *Cochrane Database of Systematic Reviews* Oct; 18(4): CD006162.

18. Couce ME, Cottam D, Esplan J. (2006) Is ghrelin the culprit for weight loss after gastric bypass surgery: a negative answer. *Obesity Surgery* July; 16(7): 870-8; Eisenstein, J., Greenberg, A. (2003). Ghrelin: update 2003. *Nutrition Reviews,* 61(3). 101-104; Tassone, F., Broglio, F., Destefanis, S., Rovere, S., et al. (2003). Neuroendocrine and metabolic effects of acute ghrelin administration in human obesity. *Journal of Clinical Endocrinology and Metabolism,* 88(11). 5478-83; Tschop, M., Statnick, M., Suter, T., Heiman, M. (2002). GH-releasing peptide-2 increases fat mass in mice lacking NPY: indication for a crucial mediating role of hypothalamic agouti-related protein. *Endocrinology,* 143. 555-568.

19. Carlson MJ, Cummings DE. (2006) Prosepcts for an anti-ghrelin vaccine to treat obesity. *Molecular Interventions* Oct; 6(5): 249-52; Cummings, D., Weigle, D., Frayo, R., et al. (2002). Plasma ghrelin levels after diet-induced weight loss or gastric bypass surgery. *New England Journal of Medicine,* 346. 1623-1630; Eisenstein, J., Greenberg, A. (2003). Ghrelin: update 2003. *Nutrition Reviews,* 61(3). 101-104; Hanusch-Enserer, U., Cauza, E., Brabant, G., Dunky, A., et al. (2004). Plasma ghrelin in obesity before and after weight loss after laparascopical adjustable gastric banding. *Journal of Clinical Endocrinology and Metabolism,* 89(7). 3352-8.

20. Carlini VP, Gaydou RC, Schioth HB, et al. (2007) Selective serotonic reuptake inhibitor (fluoxetine) decreases the effects of ghrelin on memory retention and food intake. *Regulatory Peptides* April 5; 140(1-2): 65-73; Diano S, Farr SA, Benoit SC, et al. (2006) Ghrelin controls hippocampal spine synapse density and memory performance. *Nature Neuroscience* Mar; 9(3): 381-8; Carlini, V., Manzon, M., Varas, M., Cragnolini, A., et al. (2002). Ghrelin increases anxiety-like behavior and memory retention in rats. *Biochemical and Biophysical Research Communications,* 299(5). 739-43.

21. Dubern B, Clement K. (2007) Genetic aspects of obesity. *Presse Medicale* May 18; e-pub ahead of print; Gesta S, Bluher M, Yamamoto Y, et al. (2006) Evidence for a role of developmental genes in the origin of obesity and body fat distribution. *Proceedings of the National Academy of Science of the USA* April 25; 103(17): 667681; Perusse L, Rankinen T, Zuberi A, et al. (2005) The human obesity gene map; the 2004 update. *Obesity Research* Mar; 13(3): 381-490.

22. Adamo KB, Tesson F. (2007) Genotype-specific weight loss treatment advice: how close are we? *Applied Physiology Nutrition and Metabolism* June; 32(3): 351-366; Arner, P. (2000). Obesity – a genetic disease of adipose tissue? *British Journal of Nutrition,* 83(1). S9-16; Bouchard, C. (1993). Genes and body fat. *American Journal of Human Biology,* 5. 425-432.

Chapter Eighteen – Glossary

Mosby's Medical, Nursing & Allied Health Dictionary, (6ᵗʰ ed.). (2002). St. Louis: Mosby.

Stedman's Medical Dictionary, (26ᵗʰ ed.). (1995). Baltimore: Williams & Wilkins.

Taber's Cyclopedic Medical Dictionary, (17ᵗʰ ed.). (1993). Philadelphia: F.A. Davis Company.

NOTES

NOTES

NOTES

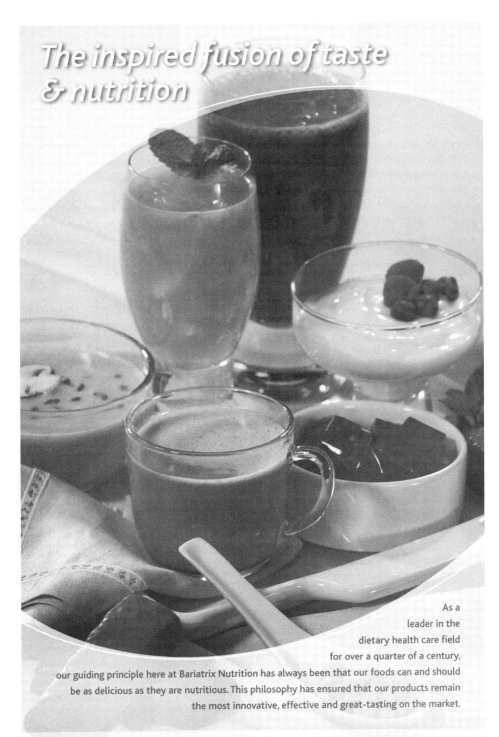

The inspired fusion of taste & nutrition

As a leader in the dietary health care field for over a quarter of a century, our guiding principle here at Bariatrix Nutrition has always been that our foods can and should be as delicious as they are nutritious. This philosophy has ensured that our products remain the most innovative, effective and great-tasting on the market.

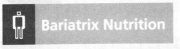

Bariatrix Nutrition

Call us or visit our web site to find out more.
40 Allen Road, South Burlington, Vermont 05403
802-862-9242 · www.bariatrix.com

There are only two ways to live your life.
One is as though nothing is a miracle.
The other is as though everything is a miracle.

ALBERT EINSTEIN